One Health: People, Animals and the Environment

One Health: People, Animals and the Environment

Editor: Elijah Evans

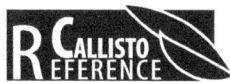

R CALLISTO
REFERENCE

www.callistoreference.com

Callisto Reference,
118-35 Queens Blvd., Suite 400,
Forest Hills, NY 11375, USA

Visit us on the World Wide Web at:
www.callistoreference.com

ISBN: 978-1-64116-811-3 (Hardback)

Cataloging-in-Publication Data

One health : people, animals and the environment / edited by Elijah Evans.
    p. cm.
Includes bibliographical references and index.
ISBN 978-1-64116-811-3
1. Zoonoses. 2. Public health. 3. Animal health. 4. Environmental health. 5. Human-animal relationships.
6. Communicable diseases in animals. 7. Communicable diseases in animals. I. Evans, Elijah.
SF740 .O54 2023
636.083 2--dc23

Table of Contents

Preface

One health (OH) is a concept which states that the health of human beings is intrinsically related to the health of animals and the environment. It involves developing and implementing policies, programs and laws in which various sectors collaborate and cooperate for improving public health outcomes. OH issues encompass environmental contamination, antimicrobial resistance, vector-borne diseases, zoonotic diseases, food security and safety, along with other health concerns that affect the environment, humans and animals. Effective prevention and management of zoonotic disease require strategies based on OH that involve experts in human health, animal health, and environmental health. The aim of these strategies is to monitor and control public health threats, and learn about the spread of diseases among people, animals, plants and the environment. The disease-centered approach to zoonoses is replaced with a system-based strategy under the concept of one health. This book is a vital tool for all researching or studying the concept of one health. Its extensive content provides the readers with a thorough understanding of the subject.

The information shared in this book is based on empirical researches made by veterans in this field of study. The elaborative information provided in this book will help the readers further their scope of knowledge leading to advancements in this field.

Finally, I would like to thank my fellow researchers who gave constructive feedback and my family members who supported me at every step of my research.

Editor

The Importance of Wildlife Disease Monitoring as Part of Global Surveillance for Zoonotic Diseases

Rupert Woods [1,2,*], Andrea Reiss [1], Keren Cox-Witton [1]◉, Tiggy Grillo [1] and Andrew Peters [3]◉

[1] Wildlife Health Australia, Mosman, NSW 2088, Australia; areiss@wildlifehealthaustralia.com.au (A.R.);
    kcox-witton@wildlifehealthaustralia.com.au (K.C.-W.); tgrillo@wildlifehealthaustralia.com.au (T.G.)
[2] World Organisation for Animal Health Working Group on Wildlife, 75017 Paris, France
[3] School of Animal and Veterinary Sciences, E. H. Graham Centre for Agricultural Innovation,
    Charles Sturt University, Boorooma St., Wagga Wagga, New South Wales 2678, Australia;
    apeters@csu.edu.au
*   Correspondence: rwoods@wildlifehealthaustralia.com.au.

Abstract: Australia has a comprehensive system of capabilities and functions to prepare, detect and respond to health security threats. Strong cooperative links and coordination mechanisms exist between the human (public health) and animal arms of the health system in Australia. Wildlife is included in this system. Recent reviews of both the animal and human health sectors have highlighted Australia's relative strengths in the detection and management of emerging zoonotic diseases. However, the risks to Australia posed by diseases with wildlife as part of their epidemiology will almost certainly become greater with changing land use and climate change and as societal attitudes bring wildlife, livestock and people into closer contact. These risks are not isolated to Australia but are global. A greater emphasis on wildlife disease surveillance to assist in the detection of emerging infectious diseases and integration of wildlife health into One Health policy will be critical in better preparing Australia and other countries in their efforts to recognize and manage the adverse impacts of zoonotic diseases on human health. Animal and human health practitioners are encouraged to consider wildlife in their day to day activities and to learn more about Australia's system and how they can become more involved by visiting www.wildlifeheathaustralia.com.au.

Keywords: Australia; emerging disease; international health regulations; Joint External Evaluation (JEE); One Health; Performance of Veterinary Services (PVS); surveillance; wildlife; zoonosis

1. Introduction

There is increasing recognition of the need to monitor as part of surveillance for emerging infectious diseases [1–4]. The majority of emerging infectious diseases are zoonoses with the predominant source shown to be wildlife [2,5]. Of specific concern is the impact and increase of wildlife-sourced zoonoses on human populations as globalisation, climate change and ecosystem alterations bring people and wildlife into closer contact. Importantly, many of the significant emerging infectious diseases in Australia have arisen in wildlife, and from within the country, rather than by overseas introductions, e.g., Hendra virus, Australian bat lyssavirus; see reviews [6,7]. For these reasons, Australia has implemented a general wildlife health surveillance system to enhance the early detection and characterization of microbial agents potentially involved with emerging diseases in free-ranging wildlife populations [6–8]. This paper briefly explains the governance for emerging zoonotic diseases and the roles played by non-human health professionals, especially those in the wildlife health sector in Australia. It concludes that though much good work has been done, there is an immediate need to improve integration of wildlife health into One Health policy as a critical step in better preparing Australia and other countries in their efforts to recognize and manage the adverse impacts of zoonotic diseases on human health.

2. Australia's Biosecurity System and Wildlife Health Systems

Australia is a federation of six states and two territories. The public and animal health (production animals, domestic animals and wildlife) systems are complex, with a number of participants across the three level of government (Australian, state or territory and local) and in different sectors (human, animal and environment) [9–11]. The nationalised, broad-ranging animal health biosecurity system and the wildlife health component have been previously described [6,12,13]. Australia's biosecurity system is complex, with activities carried out by Australian governments pre-border (offshore), border and post border (onshore) in collaboration with a large number of animal industry and other stakeholder groups, represented by a number of peak bodies. Under the Australian constitution, the Australian government is responsible for quarantine at the Australian border and also international animal health matters. State and territory governments are responsible for disease prevention, control and eradication within their boundaries. Preparedness plans and incident command structures adopted at both national and jurisdictional levels of government complement the system during emergency situations [11].

The framework ensures communication and cooperation between all levels of government and incorporates partnerships with animal industries and other stakeholders. An overarching National Animal Health Surveillance and Diagnostic Strategy Business Plan (Business Plan) guides investment in biosecurity priorities [14]. The wildlife component of the Business Plan focuses on nationally important and significant diseases of wildlife that may impact on Australia's animal industries, human health, biodiversity, trade and tourism ('wildlife diseases'). Emerging, exotic and zoonotic infectious diseases in addition to agriculturally significant diseases are emphasised.

Wildlife Health Australia (WHA) is a national body that works with Australian governments and stakeholders to improve preparedness, understanding and management of wildlife diseases. The current priority is the coordination of general surveillance and reporting of disease events in free-ranging wildlife. Over 30 surveillance partner agencies and organisations form the basis of Australia's general wildlife health surveillance system, which includes Australian, state and territory government agriculture and environment agencies, 10 zoos, eight private veterinary hospitals and seven universities around Australia. A number of targeted national programs are also in place, including a Bat Health Focus Group and the National Avian Influenza Wild Bird Surveillance Program [13]. Biosecurity, health and environment professionals are included in all of these programs, thus providing strong linkage across sectors. Recognition of the role of non-government stakeholders and the use of a partnership-type approach is a strength of the system.

A centralised, web-enabled national database of wildlife health information ('eWHIS') that is accessible across sectors by surveillance partners, both from within and outside of government, captures summary information on wildlife health and disease events submitted by surveillance partners in close to real time. About 40,000 wildlife cases are seen by WHA general surveillance partners each year [4] and one data category, 'Interesting or Unusual' wildlife cases, is designated to identify potential emerging infectious diseases. Within this category, between 200 and 300 'Interesting or Unusual' wildlife cases are reported in Australia each year.

3. Australia's Role in the Linkage and Coordination between Human and Animal Health Nationally and Internationally

Australia's capability across animal and human health has recently been evaluated by international assessors utilizing the World Health Organization's (WHO) Joint External Evaluation (JEE) against core capabilities and capacities under the International Health Regulations 2015, and the World Organisation for Animal Health's (OIE) Performance of Veterinary Services (PVS) Evaluation [9,11]. It was concluded that Australia has a comprehensive system of capabilities and functions for preparedness, detection and response to health security threats. Australia's system is strengthened through long-standing and stable cooperation links and coordination mechanisms that exist between the human and animal public health arms of the system [9]. The Australian Chief Veterinary Officer (ACVO) is Australia's delegate to the OIE (OIE Delegate). There is a need for the ACVO and Australia's state and territory Chief Veterinary Officers (CVOs) to maintain "line of sight" to the wildlife component of their animal health systems. Information provided by the wildlife surveillance system supports situation awareness and assessment of the risks posed by diseases of these animals. The ACVO coordinates Australia's OIE work and draws on other specialists in Australian Government departments and agencies, industry bodies and other sources of expertise. Strong linkage exists between the ACVO and CVOs, Australia's Chief Medical Officer and their respective departments [9]. Australia also has eight OIE Focal Points, focusing on specific animal-related topics such as wildlife, disease notification, communications and laboratories. These Focal Points support Australia's OIE Delegate and provide linkages with their counterparts in other countries through the OIE network [9].

The recent PVS evaluation also highlighted Australia's extraordinary commitment to biosecurity, serving the national interests by maintaining Australia's high animal health status. The very high level of biosecurity within Australian animal health is founded on strong partnership collaboration and formal business arrangements amongst jurisdictions and with the private sector, including primary producers, processors, suppliers of inputs and laboratories. The PVS evaluation, which also included wildlife, emphasised Australia's leadership role in the international veterinary community [11].

WHA supports the linkage and coordination between partners and across sectors by producing a regular electronic news digest that is distributed within Australia, to international members and regionally to OIE Wildlife Focal Points to share information on wildlife health and disease occurrences and issues of relevance to Australia and the region. Wildlife health surveillance data are summarised and publicly reported to the international community quarterly and yearly respectively via publications, namely Animal Health Surveillance Quarterly and Animal Health in Australia [15]. Summaries are also provided to OIE at six-monthly intervals, and WHA produces a six-month summary of Australian bat lyssavirus general surveillance data as "Bat Stats" [16]. Where possible, Australia's wildlife health data are also provided to open source databases (for example, the provision of sequence data generated by the Avian Influenza Wild Bird Surveillance Program to GenBank) and to help satisfy international reporting requirements (see [15,17]). Other relevant outputs coordinated by WHA include fact sheets and national biosecurity guidelines for wildlife health.

The processes in place for information capture, provision and reporting allow rapid and timely submission of wildlife health and disease information to the national system, assessment and notification to the relevant authorities.

4. Key Challenges and Opportunities Identified from the Australian Experience

Arguably the key challenge and opportunity emerging from Australia's experience in wildlife disease monitoring as part of surveillance for emerging infectious diseases is the difficulty in finding objective indicators of success [18]. Surveillance and response systems face considerable subjectivity if measurable outcomes, assessment and improvement of the efficacy and efficiency of wildlife disease preparedness remain lacking. Objectives for Australia's general wildlife health surveillance system are to:

- Improve Australia's ability to describe the occurrence and distribution of wildlife diseases.
- Allow early detection of unusual wildlife disease events including changes in the pattern of existing diseases and occurrence of emerging or exotic diseases.
- Provide basic data that is able to support more detailed *ad hoc* disease investigations.
- Provide data to support claims of freedom from specified diseases and answer queries from trading partners as requested.

- Identify and capture all sources of animal health information that would effectively contribute to Australia's overall understanding of its wildlife health.
- Remain highly cost effective and maximise the representativeness and coverage of the system.
- Improve and expand the capacity to collect information about feral animals, especially from non-government sources.

Seeking stakeholders' and users' input on how data and services provided by WHA improve their ability to identify and manage wildlife disease risk and preparedness is a good example of the pragmatic approach to measure success that is currently used. Effective detection and eradication of emerging infectious diseases in wildlife requires the collection of objective evidence to demonstrate the robustness of wildlife disease monitoring systems. This information, in turn, will guide adequate deployment of resources and implementation of system improvements. We are not aware of any examples of emerging infectious diseases of Australian native wildlife that have been eradicated or locally eliminated by Australian state or territory governments. A discussion of tools and tactics is beyond the scope of this opinion piece but includes options routinely deployed in production, invasive and feral animal response. Though local elimination and or proof of eradication appear to be conceptually simple measures of success, a common indicator used in human and animal health economics, economic loss averted (ELA), could also be deployed. Despite some of the challenges, the use of ELA would not only allow a greater understanding of the benefit cost of the system, but also allow comparisons to be made with other national animal and human health risk mitigation programs.

Wildlife disease surveillance faces other recognised challenges. There is incomplete knowledge of wildlife population demographics and distributions, as well as legitimate questions of surveillance sensitivity and potential biases in results. Australia uses a pragmatic approach, focusing on the development of a good general surveillance system, rapid reporting, as well as the identification and investigation of clusters of wildlife deaths or morbidity. The supporting architecture for the wildlife health surveillance system is based on Australia's livestock biosecurity framework and has historically focussed on the capture and provision of information to support trade and market access. Recognising that a general surveillance system to support one sector also supports others, a greater focus on zoonotic diseases and diseases which may impact wildlife populations and biodiversity and their inclusion in general surveillance activities would significantly strengthen the Australian system. The recent work of Craik, Palmer and Sheldrake [10] concluded that there was an immediate need to further invest in environmental biosecurity and bring it more fully into mainstream biosecurity activities in Australia. The inclusion of the environmental sector in arrangements targeting wildlife health and diseases in Australia would significantly improve the ability to detect new and emerging diseases with the potential to impact upon animal and or human health. The recent appointment of a Chief Environmental Biosecurity Officer for Australia (ACEBO) is a significant development that offers opportunities in improving the coordination and linkage between environment, health and agriculture.

More broadly, there remains significant opportunity for improvement of the position of wildlife within Australia's wider biosecurity arrangements. There are challenges, however, with maintaining a high operational functionality in Australia's complex system. The JEE concluded that despite outstanding progress in developing and implementing steps to ensure a collaborative approach between the human and animal health sectors, opportunities remain for the development of greater coordination of activities [9]. Given the risks posed by anthropogenic changes that have the potential to spark disease outbreaks in wildlife populations and the potential emergence of zoonotic diseases, each of the observations proposed by the JEE could be enhanced by the further consideration and inclusion of wildlife and environmental health:

- Development of an all-hazards health protection framework. The national framework for communicable disease control could be further developed with an increased emphasis on the risks posed by anthropogenic changes to the environment, which are linked to disease emergence in wildlife, changes in relative distribution and composition of infectious agents and species affected.

- Public and animal health workforce issues. Some specific competencies were recognized for which there is a limited workforce and future replacement may be at risk. For wildlife, this includes disease ecologists and disease and wildlife emergency response managers. Australia's PVS evaluation noted that in several jurisdictions staff levels are seen to be severely inadequate [11]. Increased investment in on-the-ground veterinary officer deployment for investigation and surveillance activities is required. Only some of Australia's environmental agencies include veterinarians and a placement within each of these agencies would also facilitate communication and linkage with counterparts in agriculture and public health agencies.

- The use of genomic data in disease surveillance, which could be better harnessed for pathogen discovery, surveillance work and elucidating the epidemiology at population interfaces, for example, at the wildlife–human and wildlife–livestock interfaces. A sequence data management and interpretation framework bridging bio-informatics and evolutionary microbiology (phylogenetics, phylogeography) is of critical importance in comprehensively holistic programs, particularly to provide an adequate ecological and evolutionary interpretation of the relationships between agents discovered in wildlife and zoonotic agents affecting human populations. All of this has the ultimate purpose of tracing the potential origins of zoonotic diseases, unveiling mechanisms as to how wildlife-associated agents may break cross species transmission barriers (host shifts) or simply quantifying and qualifying transient cross-species spillover infections. The European COMPARE project is an example of an effective approach to tackling emerging infectious diseases, ranging from risk assessment, sampling frames and surveillance, application of new generation sequencing, and data flow into databases, to the development of harmonized approaches across human, livestock and wildlife populations [19].

- Joint training and emergency animal disease response exercises across Australian Government agencies, relevant state and territory government agencies, and wildlife stakeholders, along with strategic risk assessment of current preparedness activities and arrangements for wildlife, would help to identify areas requiring improvement.

- Wildlife monitoring also presents an opportunity to assist with linkage across sectors in the areas of surveillance, preparedness and investigation. However, simpler management structures are required and the use of WHA, a public-private partnership built on One Health principles, to assist as a "trusted broker" represents a potential opportunity for the system that needs to be further developed.

- Information technology and mapping systems between Australian jurisdictions are not yet fully compatible [11]. Linkage of jurisdictional information systems to the eWHIS would remove redundancy, improve efficiency and allow analysis at a whole of country scale.

Following the completion of a JEE, the WHO recommends that countries develop a National Action Plan for Health Security (NAPHS) to address the recommendations in the JEE Mission Report. In keeping with the JEE ideology, the NAPHS is developed collaboratively across multiples sectors, with the aim of prioritising the implementation of recommendations to improve compliance with international health regulations and national health security. Specific recommendations for zoonotic diseases in Australia's NAPHS are:

- "Introduce a formal process through committee structures between human health and animal health to regularly review a joint list of priority zoonotic diseases. Consider designating zoonotic diseases of public health importance in Australia as nationally notifiable in animals.

- Establish a dedicated multisectoral national zoonosis committee or ensure reciprocal animal and human sector representation on their respective national zoonotic disease-related committees to enhance communications, bridge knowledge gaps and strengthen collaborative responses.

- Consider standardising/aligning laboratory case definitions and typing between human and animal health sectors to enhance data comparison of their surveillance systems [20]".

In addressing these recommendations, it is important for Australia that emerging infectious diseases and zoonoses of wildlife be included.

5. Conclusions

The risks to Australia posed by wildlife diseases will almost certainly become greater with anthropogenic changes such as a climate change, changes in land use, as well as societal attitudes that bring wildlife, livestock and people into closer contact [6]. The challenges of emerging infectious diseases from wildlife is, however, a global issue. A greater emphasis on wildlife disease surveillance to assist in the detection of emerging infectious diseases and integration of wildlife and environmental health into One Health policy will be critical in better preparing Australia and other countries in their efforts to recognize and manage the adverse impacts of zoonotic diseases on human health. Animal and human health professionals, including those in the community, are reminded of Australia's system of arrangements for wildlife health and are encouraged to consider wildlife health in their practices. More information on Australia's system and how they can become involved and contribute to improving the integration of wildlife health into their practice and communicate within an evolving network of partners.

Author Contributions: R.W. led the work which was co-authored by A.R., K.C.-W., T.G. and A.P.

Acknowledgments: Comments from Andrew Breed, Jenny Firman, Rachel Iglesias, Gary Lum, Mark Schipp, members of WHA's management committee and three anonymous reviewers significantly improved the manuscript.

References

1.   Kruse, H.; Kirkemo, A.M.; Handeland, K. Wildlife as source of zoonotic infections. *Emerg. Infect. Dis.* **2004**, *10*, 2067–2072. [CrossRef] [PubMed]
2.   Jones, K.E.; Patel, N.G.; Levy, M.A.; Storeygard, A.; Balk, D.; Gittleman, J.L.; Daszak, P. Global trends in emerging infectious diseases. *Nature* **2008**, *451*, 990–993. [CrossRef] [PubMed]
3.   Sleeman, J.; Brand, C.; Wright, S. Strategies for wildlife disease surveillance. In *New Directions in Conservation Medicine*; Aguirre, A., Ostfeld, R., Daszak, P., Eds.; Oxford University Press: New York, NY, USA, 2012; pp. 539–551.
4.   Cox-Witton, K.; Reiss, A.; Woods, R.; Grillo, V.; Baker, R.T.; Blyde, D.J.; Boardman, W.; Cutter, S.; Lacasse, C.; McCracken, H.; et al. Emerging infectious diseases in free-ranging wildlife–Australian zoo based wildlife hospitals contribute to national surveillance. *PLoS ONE* **2014**, *9*, e95127. [CrossRef] [PubMed]
5.   McFarlane, R.; Sleigh, A.; McMichael, T. Synanthropy of wild mammals as a determinant of emerging infectious diseases in the Asian-Australasian region. *Ecohealth* **2012**, *9*, 24–35. [CrossRef] [PubMed]
6.   Woods, R.; Grillo, T. Wildlife health in Australia. In *Medicine of Australian Mammals—CVT*; Vogelnest, L., Portas, T., Eds.; CSIRO: Sydney, Australia, 2019.
7.   Reiss, A. Emerging infectious diseases. In *Medicine of Australian Mammals—CVT*; Vogelnest, L., Portas, T., Eds.; CSIRO: Sydney, Australia, 2019.
8.   Woods, R.; Bunn, C. Wildlife health surveillance in Australia. *Microbiol. Aust.* **2005**, *26*, 56–58.
9.   World Health Organization. *Joint External Evaluation of IHR Core Capacities of Australia: Mission Report, 24 November–1 December 2017*; World Health Organization: Geneva, Switzerland, 2018.
10. Craik, W.; Palmer, D.; Sheldrake, R. *Priorities for Australia's Biosecurity System: An Independent Review of the Capacity of the National Biosecurity System and Its Underpinning Intergovernmental Agreement*; Department of Agriculture and Water Resources: Canberra, Australia, 2017.
11. Schneider, H.; Batho, H.; Stermshorn, B.; Thiermann, A. *PVS Evaluation Report, Australia*; World Organisation for Animal Health: Paris, France, November, 2015.
12. Animal Health Australia. *Animal Health in Australia 2016*; Animal Health Australia: Canberra, Australia, 2017.

13. Wildlife Health Australia. National Wildlife Health Information System. Available online: https://www. wildlifehealthaustralia.com.au/ProgramsProjects/eWHISWildlifeHealthInformationSystem.aspx (accessed on 22 November 2018).

14. Department of Agriculture and Water Resources. *National Animal Health Surveillance and Diagnostics Business Plan 2016–2019*; Department of Agriculture and Water Resources: Canberra, Australia, 2016.

15. Animal Health Australia. *Animal Health in Australia 2017*; Animal Health Australia: Canberra, Australia, 2018.

16. WHA Bat Health Focus Group. *ABLV Bat Stats*; WHA Bat Health Focus Group: Sydney, Australia, 2018.

17. Grillo, T.; Arzey, K.E.; Hansbro, P.M.; Hurt, A.C.; Warner, S.; Bergfeld, J.; Burgess, G.W.; Cookson, B.; Dickason, C.J.; Ferenczi, M.; et al. Avian influenza in Australia: A summary of 5 years of wild bird surveillance. *Aust. Vet. J.* **2015**, *93*, 387–393. [CrossRef] [PubMed]

18. Nguyen, N.T.; Duff, J.P.; Gavier-Widén, D.; Grillo, T.; He, H.; Lee, H.; Ratanakorn, P.; Rijks, J.M.; Ryser-Degiorgis, M.-P.; Sleeman, J.M. *Report of the Workshop on Evidence-Based Design of National Wildlife Health Programs*; US Department of the Interior US Geological Survey: Reston, VA, USA, 2017.

19. Compare. About Compare. Available online: https://www.compare-europe.eu/about (accessed on 19 December 2018).

20. Department of Health. *Australia's National Action Plan for Health Security 2019–2023*; Department of Health: Canberra, Australia, 2018.

2

Identification of Residues in Lassa Virus Glycoprotein Subunit 2 that are Critical for Protein Function

Katherine A. Willard [1,†]📷, **Jacob T. Alston** [1,†], **Marissa Acciani** [1] and **Melinda A. Brindley** [2,*]📷

[1] Department of Infectious Diseases, College of Veterinary Medicine, University of Georgia, Athens, GA 30602, USA; kwillard@uga.edu (K.A.W.); jacob.t.alston@gmail.com (J.T.A.); marissa.acciani@uga.edu (M.A.)

[2] Department of Infectious Diseases, Department of Population Health, Center for Vaccines and Immunology, College of Veterinary Medicine, University of Georgia, Athens, GA 30602, USA

* Correspondence: mbrindle@uga.edu.

† These authors contributed equally to this work.

Abstract: Lassa virus (LASV) is an Old World arenavirus, endemic to West Africa, capable of causing hemorrhagic fever. Currently, there are no approved vaccines or effective antivirals for LASV. However, thorough understanding of the LASV glycoprotein and entry into host cells could accelerate therapeutic design. LASV entry is a two-step process involving the viral glycoprotein (GP). First, the GP subunit 1 (GP1) binds to the cell surface receptor and the viral particle is engulfed into an endosome. Next, the drop in pH triggers GP rearrangements, which ultimately leads to the GP subunit 2 (GP2) forming a six-helix-bundle (6HB). The process of GP2 forming 6HB fuses the lysosomal membrane with the LASV envelope, allowing the LASV genome to enter the host cell. The aim of this study was to identify residues in GP2 that are crucial for LASV entry. To achieve this, we performed alanine scanning mutagenesis on GP2 residues. We tested these mutant GPs for efficient GP1-GP2 cleavage, cell-to-cell membrane fusion, and transduction into cells expressing α-dystroglycan and secondary LASV receptors. In total, we identified seven GP2 mutants that were cleaved efficiently but were unable to effectively transduce cells: GP-L280A, GP-L285A/I286A, GP-I323A, GP-L394A, GP-I403A, GP-L415A, and GP-R422A. Therefore, the data suggest these residues are critical for GP2 function in LASV entry.

Keywords: Lassa virus; arenavirus; viral glycoprotein; viral entry; viral fusion; fusion protein

1. Introduction

Mammalian arenaviruses are divided into two subgroups based on geographic distribution: Old World and New World [1]. Both subgroups contain human pathogens capable of causing severe hemorrhagic fever with high morbidity and mortality. Lassa virus (LASV), the pathogen that causes Lassa fever, is an Old World arenavirus endemic to West Africa. Each year, LASV infects several hundred-thousand people resulting in nearly 5000 deaths [2,3]. The 2018 outbreak in Nigeria was more extensive and had a higher case fatality rate (CFR) than normally recorded (CFR of confirmed cases was approximately 25% as of July 2018) [4], which exemplifies the need to develop LASV antivirals and vaccines. Human infections predominantly occur through zoonotic spread from the rodent host *Mastomys natalensis*, and potentially *Hylomyscus pamfi* and *Mastomys erythroleucus* [5,6]. Transmission can occur through direct contact with infected rodent hosts or exposure to rodent excreta/blood. In addition, person-to-person spread can occur through contact with infectious bodily fluids, putting healthcare workers at higher risk [7,8]. Due to the lack of vaccines and effective therapeutics, LASV is categorized as a class A pathogen [9].

The arenavirus particle consists of a host cell-derived lipid envelope encasing a bi-segmented RNA genome in an ambisense orientation. The envelope contains mature trimeric viral glycoprotein

(GP) spikes that are responsible for attachment and entry into the host cell. The glycoprotein precursor (GPC) is produced as a type I membrane protein and is processed twice by host cell peptidases. First, a cellular peptidase in the endoplasmic reticulum (ER) cleaves the stable signal peptide (SSP) subunit from the precursor. Second, subtilisin kexin isozyme-1/site-1 protease (SKI-1/S1P) in the cis-Golgi cleaves GP1 from GP2 [10–12]. The arenavirus signal peptide is not degraded; instead, it becomes part of the trimeric glycoprotein complex serving as a chaperone assisting with protein processing, trafficking, and pH sensing [13–16]. The GP1 and GP2 subunits mediate receptor interactions and membrane fusion, respectively [17–21].

To enter the host cell, enveloped viruses must mediate fusion between the viral envelope and cellular membrane. The arenavirus glycoprotein contains two heptad repeat (HR) domains and an amino-terminal fusion peptide (N-FP) [22], characteristic of class I fusion proteins [19,20], and similar to those of retroviruses, filoviruses, paramyxoviruses, and influenza [17]. Unlike typical class I fusion proteins, the arenavirus GP2 also contains an internal fusion loop (I-FP), which helps mediate fusion [23,24]. Under low-pH, the arenavirus glycoprotein undergoes major conformational changes prior to initiating viral fusion [25]. Interaction between GP1 and lysosomal associated membrane protein 1 (LAMP1) dissociates GP1 from the trimer, activating the GP2 fusion protein [26,27]. During GP2 rearrangement, the fusion peptide/loop inserts into the host membrane. Once multiple GP2 subunits are triggered, the glycoproteins collapse into an energetically favorable conformation known as a six-helix bundle (6HB) [19]. Full collapse of the glycoprotein complex forms a fusion pore, which enables genome release into the cytoplasm [28].

The pre-fusion LASV GP and post-fusion GP2 of lymphocytic choriomeningitis virus (LCMV), a closely related Old World arenavirus, have been crystalized [19,29]. These two structures illustrate the major GP2 conformational changes that occur during fusion. Previous studies on arenavirus GP2 subunits have characterized both the C-terminal domain, required for interactions with SSP, and hydrophobic amino acids within the fusion peptide and fusion loop [23,30]. However, there has not been an extensive characterization of the GP2 subunit as a whole. Therefore, we produced a panel of GP mutants using either insertional or alanine-scanning mutagenesis and functionally characterized them to identify conserved residues that are critical for the fusion process. We identified several residues, that when changed to alanine, did not affect protein processing but inhibited GP2-mediated-fusion, suggesting these residues may be important for GP2 structural rearrangement or lipid interactions.

2. Results

To identify critical residues in LASV GP2, we produced a panel of mutants. This panel included four hemagglutinin (HA) constructs in which the HA epitope tag was inserted at specific locations within GP2. It also included twenty-nine constructs in which conserved charged amino acids were changed to alanine; in two of these constructs, tandem charged residues were mutated together. Finally, we made twenty-six constructs in which hydrophobic amino acids were changed to alanine, which again included two constructs with tandem hydrophobic residues mutated in a single construct.

2.1. Insertional Mutagenesis

The prefusion structure of LASV GP1-GP2 is compact, with the GP2 alpha helices stacked under the GP1 subunit [29]. Although the likelihood of inserting a peptide tag without disturbing the structure and function was low, we added HA peptides at two locations in the ectodomain. The first was inserted after position 303, which we predicted would fill the center core of the structure. The second was inserted after position 375, which added an HA peptide at the tip of the T-loop, close to the membrane in a surface exposed region (Figure 1A). We also added HA peptides to the cytoplasmic tail. One HA peptide was added at the C-terminus (residue 491), a position that is known to tolerate FLAG tag additions. An HA tag was also engineered after residue 487, to maintain the charged residues at the C-terminus. To characterize these HA mutants, we first assessed whether they were efficiently expressed on the cell surface and cleaved by SKI-1/S1P, releasing GP2. Only GP$_{FLAG}$-491-HA was processed at levels comparable to parental GP$_{FLAG}$ (Figure 1B,D). All of the remaining HA mutants had low (<50%) GP2 production levels compared to parental GP$_{FLAG}$ (Table 1). Incubating cells expressing LASV GP with a low-pH buffer mimics the lysosomal low-pH environment and triggers GP fusion, resulting in robust syncytia formation [31]. Fusion efficiency is determined by comparing the extent of syncytia formation caused by the mutant GP to parental GP. Production of parental GP$_{FLAG}$ protein induced extensive fusion that resulted in large syncytia after low-pH treatment. GP$_{FLAG}$-491-HA was the only HA construct that induced fusion similarly to parental GP$_{FLAG}$ (Figure 1C,D) as expected based on the surface levels. Taken together, these results suggest that the addition of the HA tag at these locations prevents efficient GP production and processing.

Figure 1. Functional analysis of LASV GP2 HA mutants. (**a**) Schematic of LASV GPC and amino acid sequence of GP2. The signal peptidase cleaves the SSP (red arrow) whereas SKI/S1P cleaves GP1-GP2 (yellow arrow). The known GP2 domains have been color coded, N-terminal fusion peptide (red); internal fusion loop (orange); heptad repeat 1 (blue); the T-loop (magenta); heptad repeat 2 (green); and the transmembrane domain is in italics (grey). The HA tags were inserted before the amino acids labeled with a ^, * denote charged, and # hydrophobic amino acids examined with alanine scanning. (**b**) Representative image of surface biotinylation to assess LASV glycoprotein processing to form GP2. GP1GP2 is the uncleaved glycoprotein precursor. LASV GP$_{FLAG}$ was detected with an anti-FLAG antibody, M2, against the C-terminal GP2 3x FLAG tag. (**c**) Representative images of HA mutants in the cell-to-cell fusion assay. GP$_{FLAG}$ is the parental LASV glycoprotein and mock represents cells transfected with only GFP (no glycoprotein). (**d**) LASV GP2 HA mutant cleavage and fusion efficiencies compared to parental GP$_{FLAG}$. Error bars represent the standard error of the mean (SEM) from at least three independent trials.

Table 1. Summary of Fusion and GP cleavage of HA mutants.

Mutant	GP2 Protein Expression [1]	Cleavage Efficiency [1]	Fusion Activity [1]
303-HA	14.3 ± 3.5	62.8 ± 6.1	6 ± 2.6
375-HA	1.1 ± 0.1	25.4 ± 5.6	0 ± 3.6
487-HA	1.6 ± 0.4	50.2 ± 9.1	0 ± 3.2
491-HA	55.0 ± 16.1	98.5 ± 3.5	76.3 ± 7.1

[1] All values are displayed as percentage of GP_{FLAG} control $\pm$ SEM.

2.2. Characterization of Charged Constructs

In order to define individual residues important for GP2 refolding, we made more subtle mutations with alanine scanning mutagenesis. Since charged amino acids are important for protein organization and function [32], we began by mutating 29 highly conserved charged amino acid residues throughout the fusion-active subunit of LASV. We expressed the 29 constructs in Vero cells and monitored the levels of GP present on the cell surface to determine the production and cleavage efficiencies of the constructs (Figure 2A). All mutant glycoproteins except for GP-E308A and GP-H467A/R468A were cleaved producing GP2. GP-H467A/R468A did not produce detectable GP1GP2 or GP2, suggesting this mutation prevents proper protein folding and induced degradation. In contrast, GP-E308A produced a bright GP1GP2 band, which was not cleaved into GP2, indicating that GP1GP2 was produced and trafficked to the surface, but was not cleaved by SKI/S1P (Figure 2A, Table 2).

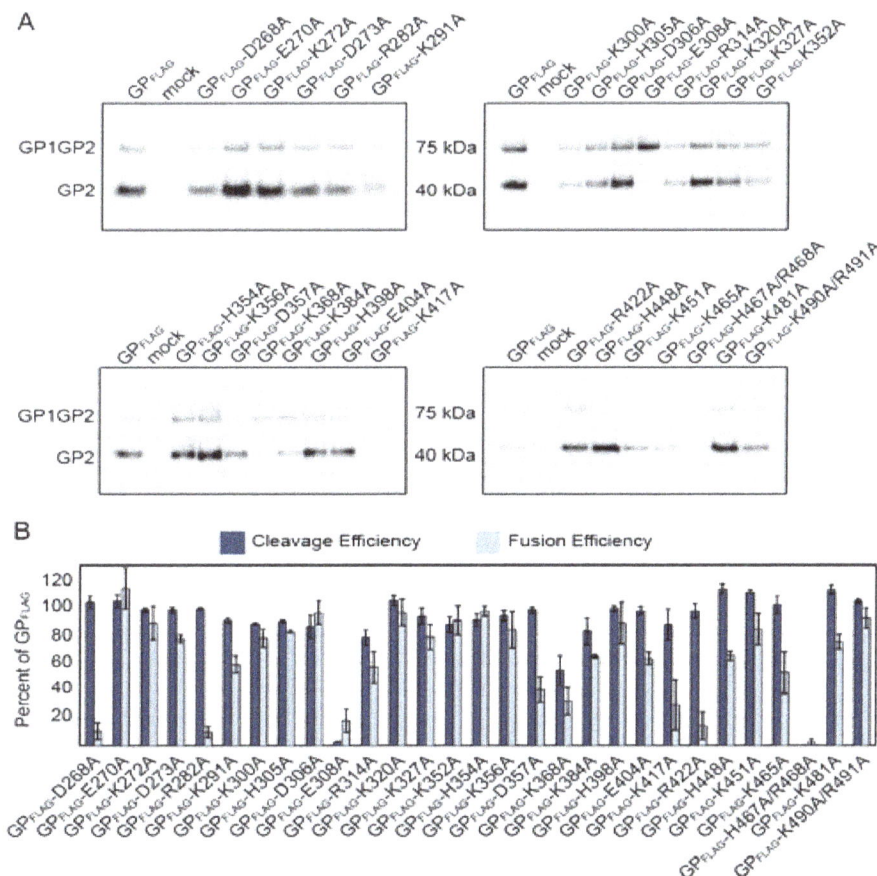

Figure 2. Functional analysis of charged residues in GP2. (**a**) Cell surface proteins were cross-linked to biotin and purified with streptavidin beads. Purified proteins were separated on SDS-PAGE and probed with an anti-FLAG antibody to detect GP, representative immunoblots are shown. (**b**) LASV GP2 mutant cleavage and fusion efficiencies compared to parental GP_{FLAG}. Error bars represent the SEM from at least three independent trials.

Table 2. Summary of GP2 Expression, GP Cleavage, Cell-to-cell Fusion, and Transduction Data.

Mutant [1]	Mutant Type [2]	GP2 Protein Expression [3]	Cleavage Efficiency [3]	Fusion Activity [3]	Transduction Efficiency [3]	
					HAP1	HAP1-ΔDAG
F262A	H	198.3 ± 62.5	108.8 ± 3.1	88.9 ± 6.4	87.2 ± 5.2	94.7 ± 9.3
L266A	H	56.2 ± 6.7	96.3 ± 3.2	81.1 ± 8.4	71.5 ± 8.5	67.7 ± 11.4
D268A	*C*	*118.6 ± 46.2*	*103.4 ± 4.2*	*10.8 ± 5.0*	*94.1 ± 1.8*	*86.0 ± 5.5*
E270A	C	187.4 ± 41	104.1 ± 4.2	113.3 ±14.8	80.7 ± 6.7	71.1 ± 8.9
K272A	C	136.2 ± 17.3	97.7 ± 1.5	88.5 ± 11.8	88.5 ± 6.5	87.6 ± 13.2
D273A	C	101.4 ± 12.8	97.7 ± 2	77.1 ± 2.7	91.5 ± 4.2	76.2 ± 15.6
L280A	*H*	*45 ± 12.2*	*90.7 ± 4.7*	*12.1 ± 7.9*	*6.1 ± 3.3*	*7.6 ± 7.1*
R282A	*C*	*80.7 ± 11.2*	*98.6 ± 0.7*	*10.1 ± 3.6*	*74.2 ± 5*	*53.5 ± 9.6*
L285A/I286A	*H*	*63.7 ± 13.5*	*98.9 ± 4.7*	*18.4 ± 5.4*	*4.2 ± 2.6*	*0.5 ± 0.5*
K291A	C	43.4 ± 15.3	90.2 ± 1.8	58.5 ± 16.2	88.5 ± 6	92.8 ± 6.8
K300A	C	49 ± 16.5	88.1 ± 0.6	77.6 ± 6.5	100.8 ± 4.9	86.4 ± 10.6
H305A	C	95.8 ± 34.7	89.6 ± 0.7	82.2 ± 1.2	53.8 ± 8.8	43.2 ± 3.9
D306A	C	98.5 ± 31.1	85.8 ± 8.3	96 ± 8.1	67.8 ± 9.6	73.2 ± 8.9
E308A	C	0 ± 0	3.0 ± 1.0	18.2 ± 8.3		
F309A	H	0 ± 0	0 ± 0	6.2 ± 2.1		
L313A	H	63.9 ± 10	97.6 ± 1.4	50.8 ± 9.3	49.5 ± 12.8	41.5 ± 8.8
R314A	C	35.7 ± 11.8	78.1 ± 5.4	56.8 ± 11.2		
K320A	C	118.6 ± 27.3	104.4 ± 3.5	96 ± 9.1	90.4 ± 3.4	75.3 ± 21
I323A	*H*	*116.4 ± 26.2*	*95.6 ± 3.5*	*20 ± 7.3*	*0.5 ± 0.3*	*0 ± 0*
L326A	H	57.3 ± 13.3	68.6 ± 8.1	84.1 ± 4.6	82.6 ± 6	73.6 ± 9.4
K327A	C	69.8 ± 12.8	93.4 ± 5.6	78.3 ± 9	95.0 ± 5.5	83.1 ± 8.7
I334A	H	18.8 ± 6.6	65 ± 8.8	84.7 ± 10		
I337A	H	12.2 ± 4.9	34.2 ± 11.5	46.5 ± 9.6		
L344A/I345A	H	0 ± 0	0 ± 0	14.7 ± 4.8		
L349A	H	54.7 ± 15.1	89.3 ± 5.8	99.1 ± 2.2	64.4 ± 12.2	76.9 ± 4.6
K352A	C	32.1 ± 8.2	87.3 ± 5.3	90.3 ± 10.7	56.5 ± 9.5	68.5 ± 9.5
H354A	C	79.9 ± 26	90.8 ± 4.3	96.9 ± 3.5	89.7 ± 4.9	92.2 ± 8.7
L355A	H	14.8 ± 4.1	53.9 ± 8.7	25.2 ± 4.9		
K356A	C	85.7 ± 37.1	93.6 ± 3.6	83.5 ± 13.3	36.8 ± 4.0	29.4 ± 5.5
D357A	C	39.4 ± 13.3	97.6 ± 2.2	40.6 ± 9.1		
I358A	H	68.2 ± 11.7	99 ± 2.3	96.3 ± 3.7	75.1 ± 8.5	66.7 ± 9.9
I361A	H	117.5 ± 28.8	106 ± 2.1	98.1 ± 3.1	21.3 ± 11	24.1 ± 7.2
K368A	C	13.6 ± 2.8	54.3 ± 10.7	32.5 ± 9.6		
L372A	H	0 ± 0	0 ± 0	17.3 ± 7.8		
L382A	H	25.6 ± 8.9	66.8 ± 6.5	72.9 ± 10.5		
K384A	C	24.2 ± 3.3	82.3 ± 9.2	64.6 ± 1.4	70.1 ± 3.3	55.1 ± 9.4
L387A	H	71.4 ± 16.4	97.4 ± 3.9	94.8 ± 10.8	43.3 ± 11.7	37.6 ± 5.9
L394A	*H*	*45.7 ± 4.9*	*93.8 ± 5.3*	*12.8 ± 6.7*	*2 ± 1*	*0 ± 0*
H398A	C	165 ± 93.7	98.7 ± 1.8	88.3 ± 14.8	90.5 ± 2.0	79.3 ± 5.6
I403A	*H*	*57.8 ± 13.7*	*94.9 ± 6.7*	*12.3 ± 8.2*	*12.4 ± 1.4*	*13.8 ± 5.4*
E404A	C	43.5 ± 19.8	97 ± 3	63.1 ± 4.3	96.3 ± 3.3	93.9 ± 2.9
I411A	H	63.7 ± 20.1	92.7 ± 6.4	38.1 ± 11.9		
L415A	*H*	*34.1 ± 10.7*	*81.3 ± 7.5*	*14.6 ± 7.8*	*0.3 ± 0.2*	*0 ± 0*
K417A	C	22.1 ± 12.4	87.3 ± 11	29.5 ± 18		
R422A	*C*	*286.2 ± 138.8*	*97 ± 5.5*	*14.6 ± 10.1*	*23.4 ± 4.1*	*19.2 ± 6.2*
H448A	C	560.5 ± 235.9	113 ± 3.7	64.9 ± 3.1	8.9 ± 5.6	9.8 ± 5.5
L449A	H	41.6 ± 16.9	82.2 ± 5	86.2 ± 8	89.3 ± 4.3	88.2 ± 7.4
K451A	C	225.4 ± 48.5	110.9 ± 1.6	84.1 ± 11.2	94.4 ± 4.9	81.3 ± 8.8
I452A	H	40.1 ± 13.5	90.8 ± 5.9	79.5 ± 10.1		
I458A	H	95.7 ± 26.7	103 ± 3.1	88.9 ± 5.2	90.9 ± 4.2	97.9 ± 5.0
K465A	C	91.6 ± 28.9	101.4 ± 6	52.7 ± 14.8	3.8 ± 1.3	11.3 ± 2.1
H467A/R468A	C	0 ± 0	0 ± 0	2.4 ± 2.4		
L469A	H	19.2 ± 3.1	81.7 ± 7.2	40.6 ± 5.9		
K481A	C	393.2 ± 200.5	112.3 ± 3.3	74.9 ± 5.2	94.9 ± 6.7	83.8 ± 11.5
K490A/R491A	C	223.7 ± 64.1	103.6 ± 1.2	91.8 ± 7.1	102.8 ± 5.1	86.8 ± 9.3

[1] Mutations that impaired GP2 function (>80% cleavage efficiency and <20% fusion activity) are bold and italicized.
[2] Table 1 abbreviations. H: Hydrophobic; C: Charged. [3] All values are displayed as a percentage of GP control ± SEM.

To determine if the charged constructs produced functional GP, we assessed the fusion activity using the cell-to-cell based fusion assay. The majority of the mutant GPs produced syncytia at levels similar to parental GP (Figure 2B), suggesting the alanine substitutions at those positions did not impede interaction with the target membrane or low-pH induced protein conformational changes. Of the constructs that were efficiently processed into GP2, only three (GP-D268A, GP-R282A, and GP-R422A) reduced fusion (<20%) compared to parental LASV GP. D268 was adjacent to the N-terminal fusion peptide and R282 was within the internal fusion-loop, suggesting these charged residues were important for GP2 to effectively anchor into the target membrane. R422 was located between HR2 and the transmembrane domain, but was not resolved in either the pre-fusion or post-fusion structures. Alanine substitution at R422 retained GP1-GP2 processing and surface expression, but the decrease in cell-to-cell fusion suggests the arginine was important for the fusion process.

2.3. Characterization of Hydrophobic Residues

Hydrophobic residues within viral class I fusion proteins are involved in protein folding and are critical for the viral fusion peptides/loops to effectively insert into the target membrane [33]. Previous studies identified hydrophobic residues within the fusion domains and C-terminus of the LASV GP2 subunit that are required for fusion [23]. We built upon this work and characterized 26 mutations throughout the GP2 subunit to identify conserved, hydrophobic residues involved in GP structure and function. Once again, we analyzed cell surface expression and cleavage of the glycoprotein constructs by purifying proteins found on the surface of transfected cells. The majority of the mutated GP proteins were cleaved, but three constructs (GP-F309A, GP-L344A/I345A, and GP-L372A) did not produce detectable GP2 (Figure 3A, Table 2). GP-L344A/I345A and GP-L372A produced the GP1GP2 protein precursor indicating the mutation prevents recognition by SKI/S1P. GP-F309A was not detected in the surface material, indicating that the mutation is deleterious to GP precursor production or trafficking (Figure 3A).

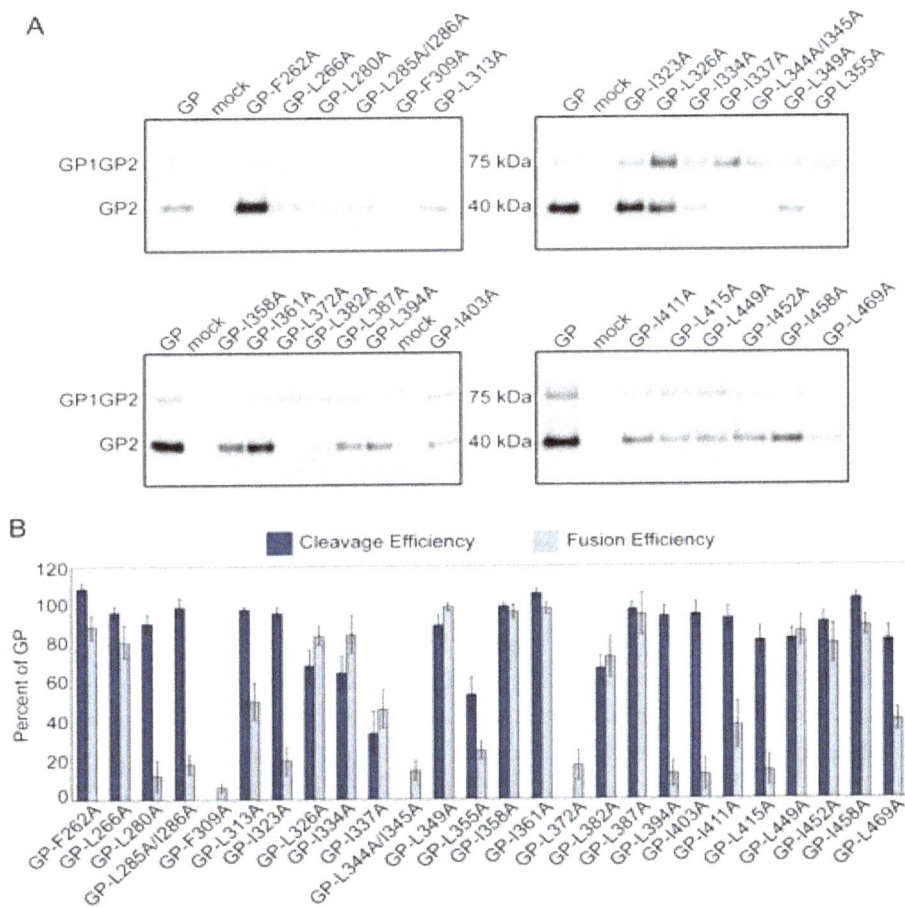

Figure 3. Functional analysis of conserved hydrophobic GP2 mutations. (**a**) Cell surface proteins were cross-linked to biotin and purified with streptavidin beads. Purified proteins were separated on SDS-PAGE and probed with anti-GP2 antibody (22.5D) representative immunoblots are shown. (**b**) LASV GP2 mutant cleavage and fusion efficiencies compared to parental GP. Error bars represent the SEM from at least three independent trials.

The cell-to-cell fusion assay results suggested many of the hydrophobic mutations reduced or eliminated syncytia formation. In total, there were six hydrophobic constructs, GP-L280A, GP-L285A/I286A, GP-I323A, GP-L394A, GP-I403A, and GP-L415A, that were efficiently cleaved (>80%) but fused <20% compared to parental LASV GP (Figure 3B). Constructs GP-L280A and GP-L285A/I286A reduced the hydrophobicity of the internal fusion loop, potentially preventing adequate insertion in the target membrane. I323 in HR1 and I403 and L415 in HR2 may have decreased efficient 6HB formation. L394 is a hydrophobic residue just outside of HR2 and may also inhibit 6HB formation.

2.4. Transduction Efficiencies of Charged and Hydrophobic Mutants

Our cell-to-cell fusion assay examines GP2's ability to undergo the low-pH induced conformational changes needed for fusion, but in an artificial system [34]. Lassa virus-to-cell fusion occurs in the lysosome, which contains different cellular proteins and lipids [35,36]. Therefore, to test whether the GP2 mutations affect viral entry, we pseudotyped our GP constructs onto vesicular stomatitis virus (VSV) particles lacking their native glycoprotein. VSV-LASV GP particles require LASV receptors for entry and trafficking to an endo-lysosomal compartment for efficient GP triggering. We used HAP1 and HAP1-ΔDAG haploid cell lines in our transduction assays to examine different entry mechanisms. Both cell lines have been extensively characterized for LASV entry [18,37]. HAP1 cells express the primary LASV receptor, α-dystroglycan (α-DG), and LASV entry occurs most efficiently when this receptor is present. HAP1-ΔDAG cells lack α-DG but contain secondary receptors that enable LASV entry through less efficient routes [18,31].

The LASV glycoprotein precursor must be cleaved into GP1 and GP2 to induce fusion. Therefore, we examined transduction efficiency for two sets of constructs: parental-like (constructs that produced over 80% cleaved GP2 and over 50% fusion efficiency compared to parental GP) and fusion-defective (constructs that produced over 80% cleaved GP2 but had less than 20% fusion efficiency compared to parental GP). We hypothesized that the parental-like mutants should be able to effectively transduce these cells whereas the fusion-defective mutants would have comparatively low transduction efficiencies. Because GP2 is not directly involved in receptor interactions, we expected few differences in the transduction efficiencies between HAP1 and HAP1-ΔDAG cell lines.

We examined the transduction efficiencies of 20 charged (Figure 4A, Table 2) and 10 hydrophobic parental-like constructs (Figure 4B, Table 2). The majority of the charged mutant constructs transduced cells relative to the level of GP produced in the cells. However, three constructs, GP-H305A, GP-K356A, and GP-K465A produced near wild-type levels of cleaved GP, but transduced poorly, suggesting these residues may be important in particle incorporation or fusion activity in the lysosome. Surprisingly the GP-H448A construct was unable to transduce either HAP cell line despite high cell surface production. The majority of hydrophobic constructs also transduced cells at rates similar to the levels of cleaved GP (Figure 4B). Only GP-I361A, a residue adjacent to HR-N, was cleaved and fused at parental GP levels but inefficiently transduced cells. As expected, construct transduction efficiencies did not significantly differ between cell lines, confirming that the GP2 mutations are not altering receptor interactions.

While we expected poorly-fusing mutant GPs to demonstrate equally reduced transduction, two mutant GPs, GP-D268A and GP-R282A, transduced cells efficiently (>80% and >50% respectively) (Figure 4C, Table 2). Both of these charged residues are part of the fusion peptide region; D268 is adjacent to the N-FP and R282 is within the fusion loop. The lipid and protein content of the plasma membrane and lysosomal membrane are distinct [36]. Thus, the removal of the charged residue may have altered the low-pH induced conformation of the fusion peptide, preventing proper insertion at the plasma membrane, but retaining activity in the lysosomal membrane.

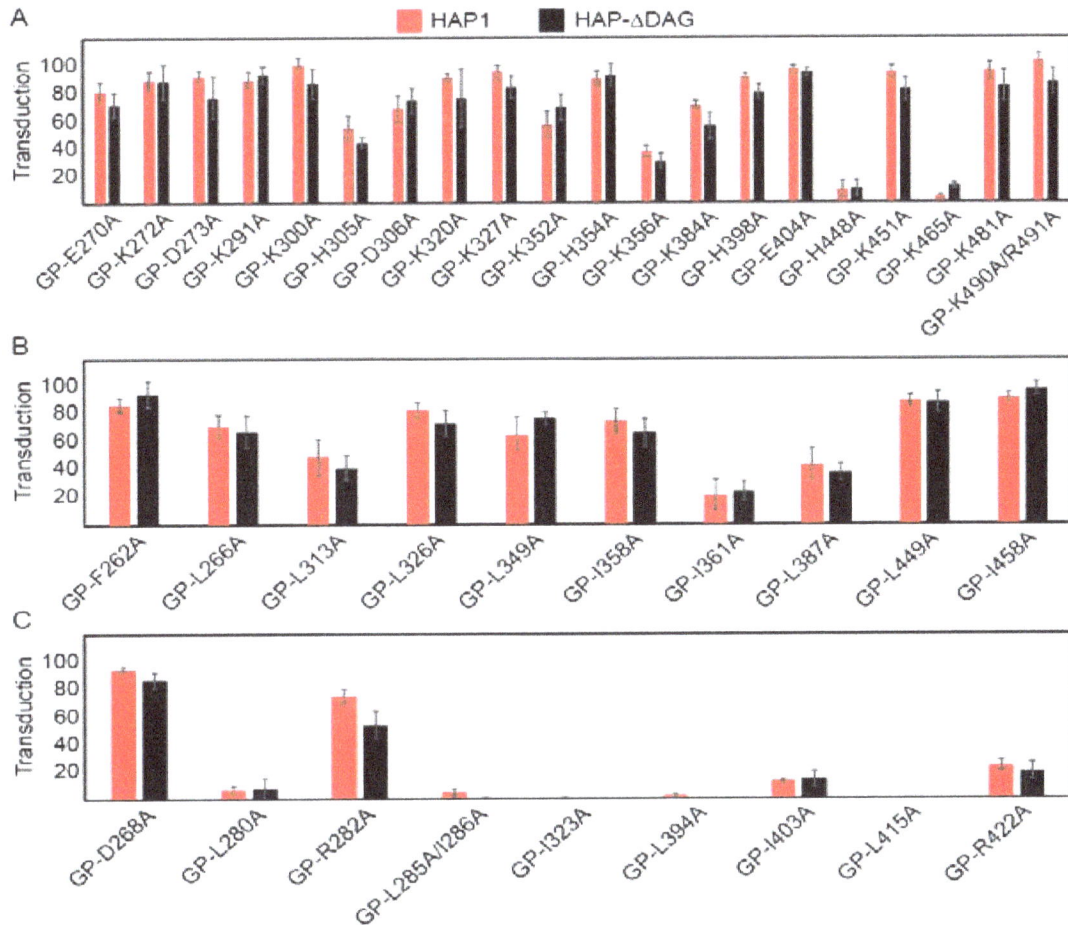

Figure 4. Transduction efficiencies of parental-like charged (**a**), parental-like hydrophobic (**b**), and fusion-defective (**c**) GP2 mutants. HAP1 and HAP1-ΔDAG1 cells were transduced with VSVΔG-LASV GP constructs encoding GFP. Transduction was quantified using flow cytometry by gating for GFP-positive cells. Transduction efficiency for each construct was normalized to parental LASV GP particle transduction for each cell line. All data are based on the average and standard error of the mean of at least three replicate experiments.

3. Discussion

In this study, we produced and characterized a library of 59 LASV GP2 mutants to identify residues involved in GP2 function. We identified 14 residues (E308, F309, I334, I337, L344/I345, L355, K368, L372, L382, K417, H467/R468, and L469) that are critical for GP folding, trafficking, or SKI/S1P recognition, evidenced by the lack of GP2 present in cell surface material. Twenty-one charged or hydrophobic residues could be changed to alanine without significantly altering protein production, localization or function, suggesting that GP2 can tolerate mutations at those locations. In total, nine constructs were efficiently cleaved (at least 80% of parental GP), yet failed to produce syncytia at levels similar to parental GP. Many of these residues, including D268, L280, R282, and L285/I286, are part of the fusion peptide domain. Both L280 and L285-I286 within I-FP impaired both cell-to-cell and virus-to-cell fusion, suggesting these hydrophobic residues may be critical for I-FP insertion, as expected (Figure 5). Surprisingly, GP-D268A and GP-R282A mutant proteins failed to induce cell-to-cell fusion, but were efficient in virus-to-cell fusion when incorporated onto VSV particles. These data suggest the charged residues are required for mediating fusion at the plasma membrane that is predominantly saturated lipids and sterols, but are less important when fusing in the lysosomal membrane, which contains low levels of cholesterol [36,38]. Similar lipid-dependent fusion occurs with other viruses; efficient insertion of the Dengue fusion peptide requires specific lipids within the late endosomes and fails to mediate low-pH fusion at the plasma membrane [39].

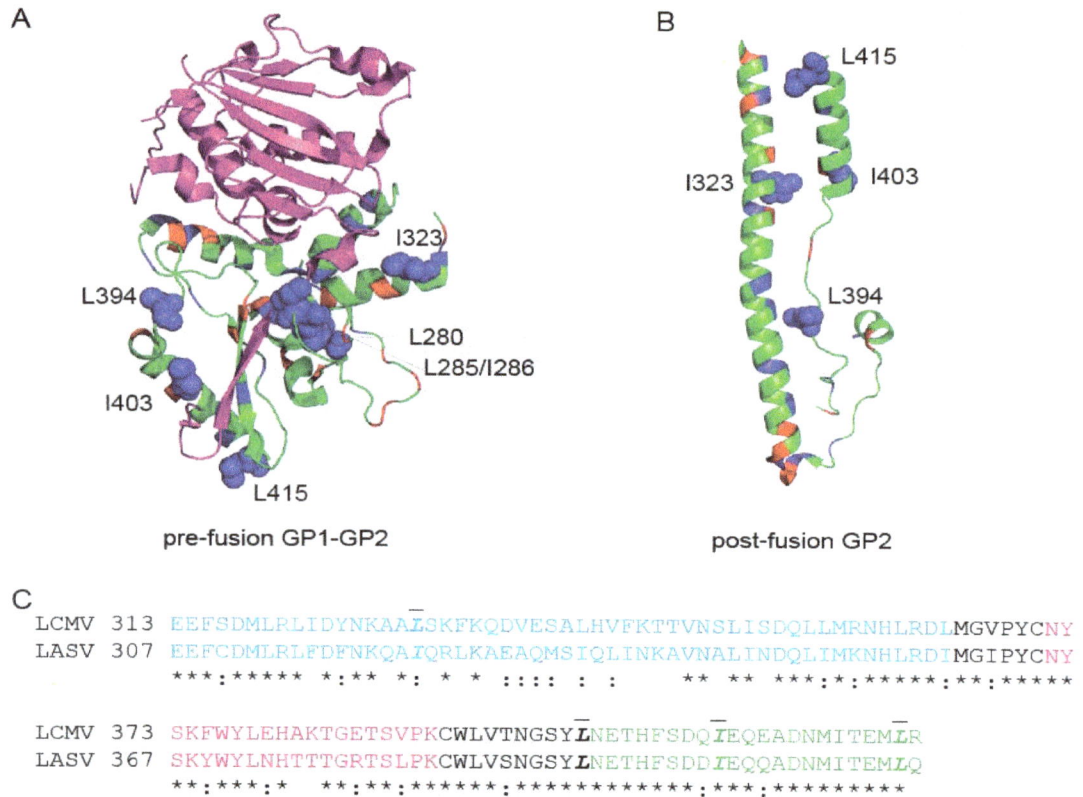

Figure 5. Mapping the fusion-defective charged and hydrophobic mutations on pre-fusion LASV GP2 and post-fusion LCMV homology model. (**a**) The LASV GP1-GP2 monomeric pre-fusion crystal structure (PDB 5vk2) [29] The GP1 subunit is shown in purple and the GP2 subunit is shown in green. The residues targeted in this study are highlighted, charged residues (red) and hydrophobic (blue). Residues found to be critical for GP2 fusion activity are shown in spheres (L280, L285/I286, I323, L394, I403, and L415) (**b**) The LCMV (an Old World arenavirus closely-related to LASV) GP2 post-fusion crystal structure (PDB 3mko) [19]. Homologous residues are highlighted as in part (a). (**c**) Amino acid alignment of LCMV GP2 region crystallized with corresponding region of LASV GP2. Identical residues are indicated with a (*), whereas conservative replacements are indicated by (:). Residues labeled in the structure are in bold-italics and contain a dash above the residues. All structures were rendered with PyMol.

While many of the residues that impacted fusion localized to the fusion peptide, five residues were part of other GP2 domains (Figure 5). I323 is part of the HR1 domain, I403 and L415 are in the HR2 domain, and L394 is the amino acid preceding HR2 (Figure 5). These residues may be critical for 6HB formation [19]. Residue R422 falls right next to the membrane but was not resolved in either crystal structure. Removal of the charged residue may impact the final 6HB structure and inhibit fusion.

Of the seven constructs that produced cleaved GP2 but failed to transduce cells (GP-L280A, GP-L285A/I286A, GP-I323A, GP-L394A, GP-I403A, GP-L415A, and GP-R422A), six were hydrophobic residues. While all of the constructs retained high cleavage efficiencies, several (GP-L280A, GP-L285A/I286A, GP-L394A, GP-I403A, and GP-L415A) produced decreased levels of GP on the surface, which may contribute to the decreased transduction.

Three of our hydrophobic constructs, GP-F262A, GP-L266A, and GP-L280A were previously characterized [23]. Klewitz et al. found GP-F262A and GP-L266A produced very little protein on the surface and had no fusion activity [23]. However, our cleavage data suggests that both GP-F262A and GP-L266A are surface-expressed near or above parental GP levels and induced both cell-to-cell and virus-to-cell fusion (Figure 3A). These phenotypic differences may be due to a difference in our transfection protocols, harvesting cells at 36 h versus 24 h, which allows more time for GP to traffic to the cell surface. We both found GP-L280A produced cleaved GP2, albeit at a decreased level, but was unable to induce fusion. Therefore, while the hydrophobic nature of the N-FP and I-FP is important, some individual residues can be made less hydrophobic while preserving functionality. Both data sets agree that the internal fusion peptide region is important for protein function.

Taken together, these data demonstrate that both conserved hydrophobic and charged residues throughout GP2 are required for optimal protein function. Specifically, the data highlighted specific residues near or within the I-FP, HR1, and HR2 domains that play critical roles in fusion.

4. Materials and Methods

Cell Lines and Transfections

Vero cells stably expressing human SLAM were maintained in Dulbecco−s modified Eagle−s medium (DMEM) with 5% (v/v) fetal bovine serum (FBS) and incubated at 37 °C and 5% CO_2 [40]. HAP1 and HAP1-ΔDAG1 cells (Horizon Discovery, Cambridge, UK) were maintained in Iscove's media supplemented with 10% (v/v) FBS and incubated at 37 °C and 5% CO_2. All transfections were performed with GeneJuice (Millipore, Burlington, MA) according to the manufacturer's instructions.

Expression Vectors and Mutagenesis

The LASV GPC protein coding sequence was codon optimized for mammalian expression and cloned into a pcDNA3.1 intron vector. A CMV promoter initiated gene expression, and we included a β-globin intron in the 5′ untranslated region (UTR) to increase protein production [31]. We added a carboxy-terminal 3xFLAG tag to the GP2 cytoplasmic tail to biochemically detect HA and charged constructs. HA insertions and point mutations were created with QuikChange mutagenesis and PfuTurbo-HS polymerase (Agilent, Santa Clara, CA). We verified the presence of each mutation with DNA sequence analysis, and a complete sequence information is available upon request.

Surface Biotinylation

Vero cells were transfected (as described above) with plasmid DNA encoding the indicated LASV GPC construct. Thirty-six hours following transfection, cells were washed with cold PBS and incubated with 0.5 mg/mL sulfosuccinimidyl-2-(biotinamido) ethyl-1,3-dithiopropionate (ThermoFisher, Waltham, MA) for 30 min on ice to tag cell surface proteins with biotin [41]. The reaction was quenched with Tris-HCl, and cells were lysed in M2 lysis buffer (50 mM Tris, pH 7.4, 150 mM NaCl, 1 mM EDTA, 1% Triton X-100) at 4°C, then centrifuged (20,000× g, 15 min, 4°C). The clarified lysate was rotated with streptavidin sepharose beads (GE Healthcare, Chicago, IL) for 60 min. Following incubation, the streptavidin sepharose beads were washed in buffer 1 (100 mM Tris, 500 mM lithium chloride, 0.1% Triton X-100) and then in buffer 2 (20 mM HEPES (pH 7.2), 2 mM EGTA, 10 mM magnesium chloride, 0.1% Triton X-100). The samples were then incubated in urea buffer (200 mM Tris, pH 6.8, 8 M urea, 5% sodium dodecyl sulfate (SDS), 0.1 mM EDTA, 0.03% bromophenol blue, 1.5% dithiothreitol) for 30 min at 55°C and analyzed using an immunoblot.

Antibodies and Immunoblots

After surface biotinylation, samples were separated by gel electrophoresis on 4-20% Nu-PAGE gels (ThermoFisher, Waltham, MA) and transferred to polyvinylidene difluoride (PVDF) membranes (GE Healthcare). HA and charged GP constructs were detected with an antibody against the Flag epitope tag (M2; Sigma, Burlington, MA) and a mouse IgG horseradish peroxidase (HRP)-conjugated secondary antibody (Jackson ImmunoResearch, West, Grove, PA). Hydrophobic constructs were detected with an antibody against LASV GP2 (22.5D), kindly provided by Dr. James Robinson (Tulane University), and a human IgG HRP-conjugated secondary antibody (Jackson). Immunoblots were visualized with SuperSignal West Dura Extended Duration Substrate (ThermoFisher, Waltham, MA) and a ChemiDoc digital imaging system (Bio-Rad, Hercules, CA). Immunoblots were quantified using ImageLab software (Bio-Rad, Hercules, CA).

Cell-to-Cell Fusion Assay

Vero cells were co-transfected with LASV GP mutants and pmaxGFP (4:1 ratio). Forty hours following transfection, media was removed and replaced with PBS (pH 4) and incubated (37 °C and 5% CO_2) for 30 min to allow glycoprotein triggering. The PBS was replaced with warm DMEM and cells were incubated for an additional 3 h to enable membrane rearrangement and syncytia formation. Four representative pictures of the fusion were taken using Zoe microscope (Bio-Rad) (20× magnification) and unfused cells were counted. Fusion efficiency was quantified using the following equation:

$$Fusion = \frac{(unfused\ cells\ in\ GFP\ transfected - unfused\ cells\ in\ mutant\ transfected)}{(unfused\ cells\ in\ GFP\ transfected - unfused\ cells\ in\ parental\ GPC\ transfected)} \times 100$$

Each mutant was assessed for fusion in at least three independent experiments.

VSV Pseudoparticle Production and Transductions

GP constructs lacking the C-terminal 3xFlag tag were used to make vesicular stomatitis virus (VSV) pseudotyped particles. Vero cells were transfected with LASV GP DNA. Thirty-six hours following transfection the cells were transduced with VSVΔG-GFP particles pseudotyped with VSV-G (MOI 1) for one hour (courtesy of Dr. Michael Whitt; KeraFAST, Boston, MA) [42]. The particle-containing media was then replaced with fresh DMEM. VSVΔG-GFP particles displaying the LASV GP were collected 8 h following the transduction. These particles were applied onto HAP1 and HAP1-ΔDAG1 cells. A larger volume of particles (4 times as much) was used to transduce HAP1-ΔDAG1 cells to overcome the decreased transduction efficiency when cells are missing the primary α-DG receptor [18]. The number of GFP positive cells was enumerated in a flow cytometer. Results are displayed as the percent of GFP positive cells present in a population of 10,000 live cell events compared to parental GP transduction.

Author Contributions: Conceptualization, M.A.B.; Methodology, M.A.B.; Validation, K.A.W., J.T.A., and M.A.B.; Formal Analysis, K.A.W., J.T.A., and M.A.B.; Investigation, K.A.W., J.T.A., M.A., and M.A.B.; Resources, M.A.B.; Data Curation, K.A.W., J.T.A., and M.A.B.; Writing-Original Draft Preparation, K.A.W. and J.T.A.; Writing—Review and Editing, K.A.W. and M.A.B.; Visualization, K.A.W. and J.T.A.; Supervision, M.A.B.; Project Administration, M.A.B.; Funding Acquisition, M.A.B.

Acknowledgments: We thank the CVM Cytometry Core Facility for technical assistance, members of the Brindley lab for helpful comments on the manuscript, and Dr. James Robinson at Tulane University for providing antibodies against LASV GP.

References

1.   Maes, P.; Alkhovsky, S.V.; Bao, Y.; Beer, M.; Birkhead, M.; Briese, T.; Buchmeier, M.J.; Calisher, C.H.; Charrel, R.N.; Choi, I.R.; et al. Taxonomy of the family Arenaviridae and the order Bunyavirales: Update 2018. *Arch. Virol.* **2018**, *163*, 2295–2310. [CrossRef] [PubMed]

2.   Ogbu, O.; Ajuluchukwu, E.; Uneke, C.J. Lassa fever in West African sub-region: An overview. *J. Vector Borne Dis.* **2007**, *44*, 1–11. [PubMed]

3.   Fichet-Calvet, E.; Rogers, D.J. Risk maps of Lassa fever in West Africa. *PLoS Negl. Trop. Dis.* **2009**, *3*, e388. [CrossRef] [PubMed]

4.   Lassa Fever—Nigeria. Available online: http://www.who.int/csr/don/20 april-2018-lassa-fever-nigeria/en/ (accessed on 2 July 2018).

5.   Olayemi, A.; Cadar, D.; Magassouba, N.; Obadare, A.; Kourouma, F.; Oyeyiola, A.; Fasogbon, S.; Igbokwe, J.; Rieger, T.; Bockholt, S.; et al. New Hosts of The Lassa Virus. *Sci. Rep.* **2016**, *6*, 25280. [CrossRef] [PubMed]

6. Monath, T.P.; Newhouse, V.F.; Kemp, G.E.; Setzer, H.W.; Cacciapuoti, A. Lassa virus isolation from Mastomys natalensis rodents during an epidemic in Sierra Leone. *Science* **1974**, *185*, 263–265. [CrossRef] [PubMed]

7. Ajayi, N.A.; Ukwaja, K.N.; Ifebunandu, N.A.; Nnabu, R.; Onwe, F.I.; Asogun, D.A. Lassa fever—Full recovery without ribavarin treatment: A case report. *Afr. Health Sci.* **2014**, *14*, 1074–1077. [CrossRef]

8. Prescott, J.B.; Marzi, A.; Safronetz, D.; Robertson, S.J.; Feldmann, H.; Best, S.M. Immunobiology of Ebola and Lassa virus infections. *Nat. Rev. Immunol.* **2017**, *17*, 195–207. [CrossRef]

9. Yun, N.E.; Walker, D.H. Pathogenesis of Lassa fever. *Viruses* **2012**, *4*, 2031–2048. [CrossRef]

10. Burri, D.J.; Pasqual, G.; Rochat, C.; Seidah, N.G.; Pasquato, A.; Kunz, S. Molecular characterization of the processing of arenavirus envelope glycoprotein precursors by subtilisin kexin isozyme-1/site-1 protease. *J. Virol.* **2012**, *86*, 4935–4946. [CrossRef]

11. Kunz, S.; Edelmann, K.H.; de la Torre, J.C.; Gorney, R.; Oldstone, M.B. Mechanisms for lymphocytic choriomeningitis virus glycoprotein cleavage, transport, and incorporation into virions. *Virology* **2003**, *314*, 168–178. [CrossRef]

12. Lenz, O.; ter Meulen, J.; Klenk, H.D.; Seidah, N.G.; Garten, W. The Lassa virus glycoprotein precursor GP-C is proteolytically processed by subtilase SKI-1/S1P. *Proc. Natl. Acad. Sci. USA* **2001**, *98*, 12701–12705. [CrossRef] [PubMed]

13. Bederka, L.H.; Bonhomme, C.J.; Ling, E.L.; Buchmeier, M.J. Arenavirus stable signal peptide is the keystone subunit for glycoprotein complex organization. *MBio* **2014**, *5*, e02063. [CrossRef] [PubMed]

14. Eichler, R.; Lenz, O.; Strecker, T.; Eickmann, M.; Klenk, H.D.; Garten, W. Identification of Lassa virus glycoprotein signal peptide as a trans-acting maturation factor. *EMBO Rep.* **2003**, *4*, 1084–1088. [CrossRef] [PubMed]

15. Eichler, R.; Lenz, O.; Strecker, T.; Garten, W. Signal peptide of Lassa virus glycoprotein GP-C exhibits an unusual length. *FEBS Lett.* **2003**, *538*, 203–206. [CrossRef]

16. Messina, E.L.; York, J.; Nunberg, J.H. Dissection of the role of the stable signal peptide of the arenavirus envelope glycoprotein in membrane fusion. *J. Virol.* **2012**, *86*, 6138–6145. [CrossRef] [PubMed]

17. Hastie, K.M.; Igonet, S.; Sullivan, B.M.; Legrand, P.; Zandonatti, M.A.; Robinson, J.E.; Garry, R.F.; Rey, F.A.; Oldstone, M.B.; Saphire, E.O. Crystal structure of the prefusion surface glycoprotein of the prototypic arenavirus LCMV. *Nat. Struct. Mol. Biol.* **2016**. [CrossRef] [PubMed]

18. Jae, L.T.; Raaben, M.; Herbert, A.S.; Kuehne, A.I.; Wirchnianski, A.S.; Soh, T.K.; Stubbs, S.H.; Janssen, H.; Damme, M.; Saftig, P.; et al. Virus entry. Lassa virus entry requires a trigger-induced receptor switch. *Science* **2014**, *344*, 1506–1510. [CrossRef] [PubMed]

19. Igonet, S.; Vaney, M.-C.; Vonrhein, C.; Bricogne, G.; Stura, E.A.; Hengartner, H.; Eschli, B.; Rey, F.A. X-ray structure of the arenavirus glycoprotein GP2 in its postfusion hairpin conformation. *Proc. Natl. Acad. Sci. USA* **2011**, *108*, 19967–19972. [CrossRef] [PubMed]

20. Eschli, B.; Quirin, K.; Wepf, A.; Weber, J.; Zinkernagel, R.; Hengartner, H. Identification of an N-terminal trimeric coiled-coil core within arenavirus glycoprotein 2 permits assignment to class I viral fusion proteins. *J. Virol.* **2006**, *80*, 5897–5907. [CrossRef] [PubMed]

21. Cao, W.; Henry, M.D.; Borrow, P.; Yamada, H.; Elder, J.H.; Ravkov, E.V.; Nichol, S.T.; Compans, R.W.; Campbell, K.P.; Oldstone, M.B. Identification of alpha-dystroglycan as a receptor for lymphocytic choriomeningitis virus and Lassa fever virus. *Science* **1998**, *282*, 2079–2081. [CrossRef]

22. Glushakova, S.E.; Lukashevich, I.S.; Baratova, L.A. Prediction of arenavirus fusion peptides on the basis of computer analysis of envelope protein sequences. *FEBS Lett.* **1990**, *269*, 145–147. [CrossRef]

23. Klewitz, C.; Klenk, H.D.; ter Meulen, J. Amino acids from both N-terminal hydrophobic regions of the Lassa virus envelope glycoprotein GP-2 are critical for pH-dependent membrane fusion and infectivity. *J. Gen. Virol.* **2007**, *88*, 2320–2328. [CrossRef] [PubMed]

24. Glushakova, S.E.; Omelyanenko, V.G.; Lukashevitch, I.S.; Bogdanov, A.A., Jr.; Moshnikova, A.B.; Kozytch, A.T.; Torchilin, V.P. The fusion of artificial lipid membranes induced by the synthetic arenavirus −fusion peptide−. *Biochim. Biophys. Acta* **1992**, *1110*, 202–208. [CrossRef]

25. Li, S.; Sun, Z.; Pryce, R.; Parsy, M.L.; Fehling, S.K.; Schlie, K.; Siebert, C.A.; Garten, W.; Bowden, T.A.; Strecker, T.; et al. Acidic pH-Induced Conformations and LAMP1 Binding of the Lassa Virus Glycoprotein Spike. *PLoS Pathog.* **2016**, *12*, e1005418. [CrossRef] [PubMed]

26. Cohen-Dvashi, H.; Israeli, H.; Shani, O.; Katz, A.; Diskin, R. The role of LAMP1 binding and pH sensing by the spike complex of Lassa virus. *J. Virol.* **2016**. [CrossRef] [PubMed]

27. Hulseberg, C.E.; Feneant, L.; Szymanska, K.M.; White, J.M. Lamp1 Increases the Efficiency of Lassa Virus Infection by Promoting Fusion in Less Acidic Endosomal Compartments. *MBio* **2018**, 9. [CrossRef] [PubMed]

28. White, J.M.; Delos, S.E.; Brecher, M.; Schornberg, K. Structures and mechanisms of viral membrane fusion proteins: Multiple variations on a common theme. *Crit. Rev. Biochem. Mol. Biol.* **2008**, *43*, 189–219. [CrossRef] [PubMed]

29. Hastie, K.M.; Zandonatti, M.A.; Kleinfelter, L.M.; Heinrich, M.L.; Rowland, M.M.; Chandran, K.; Branco, L.M.; Robinson, J.E.; Garry, R.F.; Saphire, E.O. Structural basis for antibody-mediated neutralization of Lassa virus. *Science* **2017**, *356*, 923–928. [CrossRef]

30. York, J.; Nunberg, J.H. A novel zinc-binding domain is essential for formation of the functional Junin virus envelope glycoprotein complex. *J. Virol.* **2007**, *81*, 13385–13391. [CrossRef]

31. Acciani, M.; Alston, J.T.; Zhao, G.; Reynolds, H.; Ali, A.M.; Xu, B.; Brindley, M.A. Mutational Analysis of Lassa Virus Glycoprotein Highlights Regions Required for Alpha-Dystroglycan Utilization. *J. Virol.* **2017**, *91*. [CrossRef]

32. Aftabuddin, M.; Kundu, S. Hydrophobic, hydrophilic, and charged amino acid networks within protein. *Biophys. J.* **2007**, *93*, 225–231. [CrossRef] [PubMed]

33. Apellaniz, B.; Huarte, N.; Largo, E.; Nieva, J.L. The three lives of viral fusion peptides. *Chem. Phys. Lipids* **2014**, *181*, 40–55. [CrossRef] [PubMed]

34. Mindell, J.A. Lysosomal acidification mechanisms. *Annu. Rev. Physiol.* **2012**, *74*, 69–86. [CrossRef] [PubMed]

35. Van Meer, G. Transport and sorting of membrane lipids. *Curr. Opin. Cell Biol.* **1993**, *5*, 661–673. [CrossRef]

36. Holthuis, J.C.; Menon, A.K. Lipid landscapes and pipelines in membrane homeostasis. *Nature* **2014**, *510*, 48–57. [CrossRef] [PubMed]

37. Jae, L.T.; Raaben, M.; Riemersma, M.; van Beusekom, E.; Blomen, V.A.; Velds, A.; Kerkhoven, R.M.; Carette, J.E.; Topaloglu, H.; Meinecke, P.; et al. Deciphering the glycosylome of dystroglycanopathies using haploid screens for lassa virus entry. *Science* **2013**, *340*, 479–483. [CrossRef] [PubMed]

38. Schoer, J.K.; Gallegos, A.M.; McIntosh, A.L.; Starodub, O.; Kier, A.B.; Billheimer, J.T.; Schroeder, F. Lysosomal membrane cholesterol dynamics. *Biochemistry* **2000**, *39*, 7662–7677. [CrossRef]

39. Zaitseva, E.; Yang, S.T.; Melikov, K.; Pourmal, S.; Chernomordik, L.V. Dengue virus ensures its fusion in late endosomes using compartment-specific lipids. *PLoS Pathog.* **2010**, *6*, e1001131. [CrossRef]

40. Ono, N.; Tatsuo, H.; Hidaka, Y.; Aoki, T.; Minagawa, H.; Yanagi, Y. Measles viruses on throat swabs from measles patients use signaling lymphocytic activation molecule (CDw150) but not CD46 as a cellular receptor. *J. Virol.* **2001**, *75*, 4399–4401. [CrossRef]

41. Brindley, M.A.; Plattet, P.; Plemper, R.K. Efficient replication of a paramyxovirus independent of full zippering of the fusion protein six-helix bundle domain. *Proc. Natl. Acad. Sci. USA* **2014**, *111*, E3795–E3804. [CrossRef]

42. Whitt, M.A. Generation of VSV pseudotypes using recombinant DeltaG-VSV for studies on virus entry, identification of entry inhibitors, and immune responses to vaccines. *J. Virol. Methods* **2010**, *169*, 365–374. [CrossRef] [PubMed]

3

Japanese Encephalitis Virus in Australia: From Known Known to Known Unknown

Andrew F. van den Hurk [1,*] , Alyssa T. Pyke [1] , John S. Mackenzie [2] , Sonja Hall-Mendelin [1] and Scott A. Ritchie [3]

[1]   Public Health Virology, Forensic and Scientific Services, Department of Health, Queensland Government, PO Box 594, Archerfield, QLD 4108, Australia; Alyssa.Pyke@health.qld.gov.au (A.T.P.); Sonja.Hall-Mendelin@health.qld.gov.au (S.H.-M.)

[2]   Faculty of Medical Sciences, Curtin University, and Division of Microbiology and Infectious Diseases, PathWest, Locked Bag2009, Nedlands, WA 6909, Australia; J.Mackenzie@curtin.edu.au

[3]   College of Public Health, Medical and Veterinary Sciences, and Australian Institute of Tropical Health and Medicine, James Cook University, PO Box 6811, Cairns, QLD 4870, Australia; scott.ritchie@jcu.edu.au

*   Correspondence: andrew.vandenhurk@health.qld.gov.au.

Abstract: Japanese encephalitis virus (JEV) is a major cause of neurological disease in Asia. It is a zoonotic flavivirus transmitted between water birds and/or pigs by *Culex* mosquitoes; humans are dead-end hosts. In 1995, JEV emerged for the first time in northern Australia causing an unprecedented outbreak in the Torres Strait. In this article, we revisit the history of JEV in Australia and describe investigations of JEV transmission cycles in the Australian context. Public health responses to the incipient outbreak included vaccination and sentinel pig surveillance programs. Virus isolation and vector competence experiments incriminated *Culex annulirostris* as the likely regional vector. The role this species plays in transmission cycles depends on the availability of domestic pigs as a blood source. Experimental evidence suggests that native animals are relatively poor amplifying hosts of JEV. The persistence and predominantly annual virus activity between 1995 and 2005 suggested that JEV had become endemic in the Torres Strait. However, active surveillance was discontinued at the end of 2005, so the status of JEV in northern Australia is unknown. Novel mosquito-based surveillance systems provide a means to investigate whether JEV still occurs in the Torres Strait or is no longer a risk to Australia.

Keywords: Japanese encephalitis virus; zoonosis; mosquito; transmission; Australia

1. Introduction

Japanese encephalitis virus (JEV) is a single-strand, positive-sense RNA virus of the genus *Flavivirus*, family *Flaviviridae*. The virus is responsible for approximately 68,000 clinical cases annually and is the leading cause of encephalitis in a number of countries in Southeast Asia, the Indian sub-continent and the Indonesian archipelago [1]. Predominantly asymptomatic, less than 1% of human infections result in clinical disease which can range broadly in severity from a mild febrile illness to acute meningomyeloencephalitis. Of symptomatic cases, 20–30% are fatal, and among the survivors, approximately 30–50% will have ongoing neurological sequelae.

Prevalent in tropical and subtropical parts of Asia and the Pacific rim [2], JEV exists in a zoonotic transmission cycle between ardeid wading birds, such as herons and egrets, and *Culex* mosquitoes, particularly, *Culex tritaeniorhynchus* and *Cx. vishnui* which utilize rice fields for larval development [3]. Domestic pigs are important amplifying hosts, due to rates of infection of 90–100%, development of viremia levels sufficient to infect mosquitoes and constant annual turnover leading to a continual supply of immunologically naïve pigs as susceptible hosts. Recent experiments have demonstrated that JEV can be transmitted directly between pigs via oronasal secretions further enhancing the status of pigs as amplifying hosts [4]. Although the epidemiological significance of this finding needs to be definitively established, it suggests that virus transmission can potentially occur in the absence of suitable mosquito vectors. Humans and horses can develop fatal disease, but they are considered dead end hosts of JEV because they do not produce adequate viral levels required to infect mosquitoes. Thus, JEV is considered an important zoonotic pathogen and a concerted One Health approach is required for sustained disease suppression [5].

In Australia, JEV is mostly viewed as an issue for travelers to endemic regions and occasional overseas acquired cases are reported [6–8]. However, in 1995, JEV was first recognized in natural transmission cycles in northern Australia when a widespread outbreak occurred on the islands of the Torres Strait, the body of water that separates Cape York Peninsula and the New Guinea landmass (Figure 1). Three human cases, two of which were fatal, occurred on the island of Badu. This event was unprecedented, as Murray Valley encephalitis virus (MVEV) and West Nile virus Kunjin subtype (WNV_{KUN}) were considered the only encephalitogenic flaviviruses southeast of Wallacea, the region that separates the Asian and Australasian zoogeographical regions. In the current paper, we revisit the epidemiology of JEV in the Australasian region and summarize research conducted to elucidate the factors that led to its emergence and apparent disappearance.

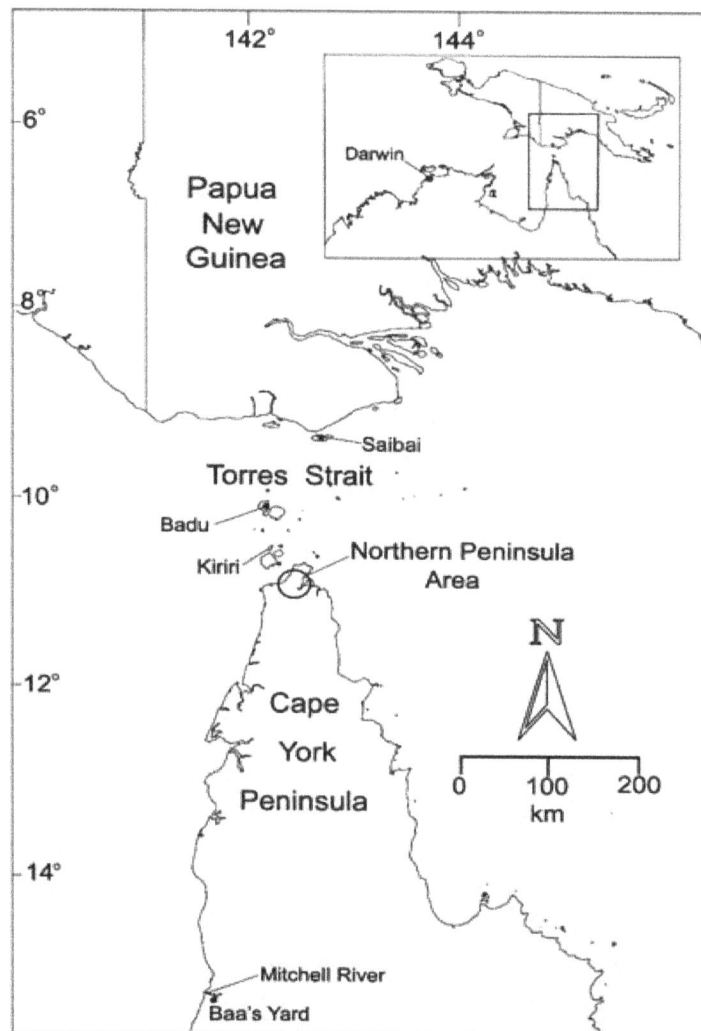

Figure 1. Map of Northern Australia and southern Papua New Guinea showing locations mentioned in the text. The Northern Peninsula Area includes the communities of Bamaga, Injinoo, New Mapoon, Seisia, and Umagico.

2. The Emergence of JEV in Northern Australia

In March 1995, Public Health authorities were notified of three cases of encephalitis on Badu in the Torres Strait [9]. Given previous MVEV activity in northern Australia, it was initially suspected that this virus was the etiological agent. However, virus isolation from serum samples from two asymptomatic residents of the island and mosquitoes yielded JEV isolates. Several other residents and domestic pigs were also found to be JEV seropositive by enzyme linked immunosorbent assay (ELISA) and hemagglutination inhibition (HAI) assay. Whilst it is known that flavivirus cross-reactivity can obscure serological findings and complicate result interpretation, a proportion of these serum samples also demonstrated specific neutralizing antibodies at notably higher titers to JEV than to MVEV or WNV$_{KUN}$, providing further definitive evidence that JEV had caused the outbreak [9]. Virus genotyping revealed that the Badu 1995 human and mosquito isolates clustered within genotype II [9]. *Culex annulirostris* was the only mosquito that yielded JEV at a carriage rate of 2.97 per 1000 mosquitoes, indicating that this was the potential mosquito vector [10]. Subsequent, broader serosurveys of humans and pigs revealed that the outbreak was widespread across the Torres Strait, although Badu appeared to have conditions conducive to epizootic JEV transmission. This included an immunologically naïve human population and a large immunologically naïve domestic pig population, with numerous pigpens located close to houses. There were also widespread productive larval habitats of *Cx. annulirostris*, created by poorly maintained drains, damaged septic systems, and groundwater sites which had become nutrient rich due to feces from horses that had been introduced to the island in the year preceding the outbreak [11]. Emergency vector control strategies included treatment of larval sites with the insect growth regulator, *s*-methoprene, and thermal fogging of adults with the pyrethroid, bioresmethrin.

Following this incipient outbreak, several strategies were employed to limit JEV transmission, both on Badu and on other islands. A vaccination program using the formalin inactivated mouse brain-derived vaccine (Biken Institute, Japan) commenced in December 1995 and by March 1996, 93% of residents of the outer islands who commenced the schedule had received at least 2 doses [12]. To detect further JEV activity, a sentinel pig program was established on 4 islands of the Torres Strait, as well as proximal to mainland Australian communities on the tip of Cape York Peninsula [13]. To reduce the availability of larval habitats, maintenance and drainage works were initiated on Badu, although the swampy ground present over much of the island limited the impact of this strategy on adult mosquito populations [11]. In 1996 and 1997, JEV activity, as evidenced by seroconversions of sentinel pigs, appeared restricted to the northernmost island of Saibai.

The unexpected emergence of JEV in the Australasian region prompted investigations of the origins of the virus and potential mechanisms of introduction. Between 1996 and 1998, almost 400,000 mosquitoes were processed from the Western Province of Papua New Guinea (PNG) yielding 3 isolates [14]. Furthermore, there was evidence of human infection in PNG, as demonstrated by JEV-specific antibodies in sera collected as far back as 1989 [15] and by clinical cases of encephalitis (J Oakley and S. Flew, unpublished data cited by [14]. Thus, it appeared that the New Guinea landmass was the source of the incursions. Furthermore, backtrack simulations by Ritchie and Rochester [16] suggested that wind-borne mosquitoes carried by low pressure systems from New Guinea could have been the mechanism of virus introduction.

In 1998, widespread JEV activity again occurred in the Torres Strait and, for the first time, on the Australian mainland [17]. There were two clinical human cases recognized serologically during this outbreak, with the first being in an unvaccinated child on Badu and the second being a fisherman at the mouth of the Mitchell River on western Cape York Peninsula. Sentinel pigs on many outer islands seroconverted to the virus, whilst seroconversion of pigs on Kiriri Island signaled the first evidence of transmission occurring on the inner Torres Strait islands. On the mainland, sentinel pigs on the Northern Peninsula Area (NPA) and at Baa's Yard near the Mitchell River, seroconverted to JEV, and the virus was isolated from 3 pigs at Seisia on the NPA. Collections on Badu yielded 42 isolates of JEV from 31,898 mosquitoes, with all but one coming from *Cx. sitiens* subgroup mosquitoes (primarily *Cx.*

annulirostris); the other isolate was from *Aedes vigilax* [18]. In contrast, no JEV was detected in 35,235 mosquitoes processed from the Australian mainland [19]. Nucleotide sequence analysis and molecular genotyping of mosquito and pig 1998 isolates revealed that they also belonged to genotype II. A high nucleotide identity was also demonstrated between the sequences of the 1998 and 1995 Torres Strait viruses, and to the Australian mainland and PNG sequences, highly suggesting that the origin of JEV incursions into Northern Australia may have been PNG [17,18]. Following the 1998 outbreak, and with a view to reducing contact and transmission between pigs, mosquitoes, and humans, domestic pigs were relocated from proximal to houses to communal pig pens >2 km away from the community.

The magnitude of the 1998 outbreak of JEV in the Torres Strait and Cape York Peninsula was unprecedented in both spatial scale and intensity. JEV activity was recorded from southern PNG, across most of the Torres Strait and south to western Cape York Peninsula [14,17], suggesting a unique and extreme event. The outbreak appeared to represent the convergence of high populations of *Culex* mosquitoes and widespread JEV transmission in southern PNG, coupled with a strong tropical cyclone in the Gulf of Carpentaria that may have transported JEV infected mosquitoes from PNG into the Torres Strait and deep into Cape York Peninsula. Late 1997 to early 1998 featured a strong *El-Nino* event that caused severe drought in the Western Province of PNG [20]. Normally flooded wetlands may have been reduced to stagnant pools of highly organic water favorable for the production of *Cx. sitiens* subgroup mosquitoes. Indeed, mosquito collections in February 1998 in Western Province were very high, with many traps catching over 10,000 mosquitoes per night [16], from which JEV was isolated [14]. This event was also coupled with the occurrence of Tropical Cyclone Sid in the western Gulf of Carpentaria in late December 1997. The large wind field of this category 2 cyclone was potentially sufficient to transport mosquitoes from southern New Guinea to west central Cape York Peninsula, where JEV activity occurred at the mouth of the Mitchell River [16]. The coincidental occurrence of two extreme events, drought induced JEV transmission in southern PNG and a cyclone in the Gulf of Carpentaria that could transport the mosquitoes from New Guinea landmass deep into the Cape York Peninsula, make a repeat of this event unlikely.

After no recognized activity in 1999, JEV reappeared in the Torres Strait in 2000. Although virus was not isolated from 7652 *Cx. annulirostris* collected from Badu, a single JEV isolate was obtained from 84 *Cx. gelidus* mosquitoes [21]. Collections from Saibai Island also yielded an isolate, albeit from *Cx. sitiens* subgroup mosquitoes [22]. JEV isolates were also obtained from the acute sera of three pigs on Badu. Interestingly, molecular genotyping of the two mosquito and pig sera 2000 isolates demonstrated they belonged to genotype I and did not cluster with the previous Australian 1995 and 1998 genotype II viruses. Importantly, this demonstrated the introduction of a new JEV genotype into Australia and highlighted the continued risk and vulnerability of the region to further JEV incursions [22,23].

Between 2001 and 2005, sentinel pigs and/or deployment of a newly developed remote mosquito trapping system were effective in detection of JEV on Badu Island every year [24]. In 2004, the virus was again detected on mainland Australia, when pigs located on the NPA seroconverted to JEV and a single isolate was obtained from a pool of *Cx. sitiens* subgroup mosquitoes collected from the Bamaga rubbish dump [25]. This was the first time that JEV had been isolated from mosquitoes collected from the Australian mainland. Molecular phylogenetic analysis revealed that the virus clustered with a 2004 Badu pig isolate, and 2000 mosquito and pig sequences in genotype I. As no further evidence of genotype II in the region had been demonstrated since 1998, these findings suggested this genotype may have been subsequently replaced by genotype I.

The sentinel pig program and remote mosquito trapping trials were discontinued in the Torres Strait at the end of the 2005, whilst the sentinel pigs were removed from the NPA in 2011. However, given the continual risk of re-emergence, in 2012, mosquito-based surveillance was re-deployed, albeit using a different system (refer to Section 3.3) in the NPA by the Northern Australia Quarantine Service. Despite multiple detections of MVEV and WNV$_{KUN}$ in the NPA traps which were most notable in 2015 [26], there has been no evidence of recent JEV activity (T. Kerlin and K. Rickart, unpublished data). Traps were also run on Badu, but only during the 2012–2013 wet season. No JEV was detected during this period of deployment. Thus, the status of JEV in the Torres Strait since 2005 is unknown.

3. Elucidating the Ecology of JEV Transmission Cycles in Australia

3.1. Vertebrate Host Studies

Numerous vertebrate species have been investigated as amplifying hosts of JEV in endemic regions, although ardeid birds and pigs are considered the most important [2]. When JEV appeared in northern Australia, it was feared that the large populations of feral pigs and wading birds on the mainland would provide an abundance of amplifying hosts to allow the virus to become established in natural transmission cycles. An unknown quantity and continuing concern is the role that other vertebrates, particularly native species, could play in these transmission cycles. Unfortunately, laboratory based vertebrate studies are very complex, requiring high level biocontainment, which restricts them to a limited number of laboratories in Australia. Thus, there has only been limited experimentation on the course of JEV infection in Australian vertebrates. In experiments conducted well before JEV emerged in Australia, the Nankeen Night Heron, *Nycticorax caledonicus*, was shown to produce viremia levels that could potentially infect recipient mosquitoes [27]. Later, the response of marsupials to JEV infection was investigated at the Australian Animal Health Laboratories (AAHL). It was shown that eastern grey kangaroos, agile wallabies and tammar wallabies either did not develop detectable viremia or were only capable of producing viremia levels below the threshold required to infect questing mosquitoes (PW Daniels, D Middleton, D Boyle, K Newberry, D Williams, R Lunt, unpublished data cited by Mackenzie et al. [28]). In contrast, possums produced a higher viremia when compared to the macropods tested. The only other native species examined as a potential amplifying host in laboratory-based experiments was the black flying fox, *Pteropus alecto* [29]. Only 1 of 15 flying foxes produced a detectable viremia which was sufficient to infect recipient mosquitoes. Interestingly, 3 other flying foxes were able to infect recipient mosquitoes, even though they did not produce a viremia that was detectable using a highly sensitive real-time reverse transcriptase PCR. Despite exhibiting low infection rates following experimental exposure, flying foxes could still play a role in the ecology of JEV in Northern Australia, as they roost in camps containing 1000s of individuals, are prevalent on a number of islands of the Torres Strait and are known to migrate from the New Guinea landmass.

The importance of pigs as amplifying hosts of JEV and the existence of large, abundant feral populations across Northern Australia prompted pig infection studies with a regional context. Of particular interest, was whether prior exposure to endemic MVEV or WNV$_{KUN}$ viruses affected pig susceptibility to JEV infection and how this may impact on their immune responses. In experiments performed at AAHL, JEV was readily detected in pigs following primary JEV infection, but not in pigs previously infected with MVEV or WNV$_{KUN}$ that were later challenged with JEV [30]. Coupled with suppressed JEV viremia levels, elevation of existing cross-reactive JEV neutralizing antibodies were further demonstrated in these pigs. Notably, these findings suggest that prior exposure to MVEV or WNV$_{KUN}$ may elicit protective immunity against JEV in pigs. Together with the suppression of viremia levels, this indicates that pre-immune pigs may not be effective amplifying hosts and therefore are unlikely to play a major role in JEV transmission.

3.2. Incrimination of Mosquito Vectors

In the majority of regions where JEV is known to circulate, *Cx. tritaeniorhynchus* and *Cx. vishnui* are the key mosquito vectors, however, these species, do not occur in Northern Australia. Based on its role as the primary vector of MVEV and WNV$_{KUN}$ [31], it was suspected that an alternate species, *Cx. annulirostris*, was the primary vector during the original Torres Strait 1995 outbreak. This hypothesis was further supported by the fact that this was the only species from which JEV isolates were recovered during this initial outbreak and to date, has been the species yielding the most isolates obtained in Northern Australia. Subsequent laboratory-based vector competence experiments using genotype II JEV isolated from Badu Island in 1998 confirmed the status of *Cx. annulirostris* as the likely primary vector in Australia [32]. Interestingly, Hemmerter et al. [33] demonstrated that *Cx. annulirostris* contains at least 5 mitochondrial cytochrome oxidase I lineages, with some having a wide distribution in the Australasian regions, whilst others appeared more restricted geographically. It was revealed that three of these lineages occurred in southern PNG, the Torres Strait and Cape York Peninsula. The authors hypothesized that these lineages may vary in their vector competence for JEV, thus potentially explaining the southern limits of the virus on the Australian mainland. Phenotypic evidence to corroborate this hypothesis was provided by Johnson et al. [34] who showed that the dominant mainland Australian lineage of *Cx. annulirostris* was a relatively poor laboratory vector of the genotype I JEV.

Studies of other species which yielded isolates demonstrated that *Cx. gelidus* was a highly efficient laboratory vector [34] whereas *Ae. vigilax* had a comparatively low transmission rate [32]. Although other species, such as *Cx. sitiens* and *Cx. quinquefasciatus* were efficient laboratory vectors [32] and have been implicated as secondary vectors in SE Asia, their status as vectors in Northern Australia remains largely unknown. Finally, electrophoretic analysis of collections of *Cx. annulirostris* that yielded JEV revealed that the closely related and morphologically similar *Cx. palpalis* was present, sometimes at high levels [35]. Thus, this species could also be considered a potential JEV vector. Similar to the situation in endemic locations, the evidence from virus detection in field collected mosquitoes and vector competence experiments incriminates members of the genus *Culex* as the primary vectors of JEV in Northern Australia.

3.3. The Influence of Mosquito Host Feeding Patterns on JEV Transmission in Northern Australia

The propensity for the mosquito to feed on the vertebrate host is critical to its role as a virus vector. Analysis of host feeding patterns of *Cx. annulirostris* from numerous locations in northern Australia revealed that, for the most part, pigs and birds accounted for only a small percentage of positive blood meals [36,37]. Instead, most of the blood meals obtained by *Cx. annulirostris* originated from marsupials, particularly the Agile Wallaby, *Macropus agilis* [37,38]. As mentioned previously, experiments conducted at AAHL had previously shown that Agile wallabies produced only low-level viremia. Thus, predilection for *Cx. annulirostris* to feed on wallabies may have dampened transmission, particularly on the mainland, by diverting host seeking mosquitoes away from pigs. Interestingly, there are no wallabies on Badu, so this possible dampening effect would not have impacted transmission dynamics on the island.

The only locations where significant feeding on pigs was recorded in northern Australia was from locations adjacent to domestic pigs or where feral pigs congregated, such as rubbish dumps. In endemic areas in Southeast Asia, intense JEV transmission is usually driven by pig feeding rates >30%. Thus, it was not surprising when analysis of *Cx. annulirostris* host feeding patterns during periods of recognized JEV transmission also revealed relatively high porcine feeding rates, as high as 80% [36,37]. The proportion of *Cx. annulirostris* feeding on pigs was significantly reduced when the domestic pigs were relocated from the Badu community to a communal piggery some 2.5 km away [21]. However, this did not appear to eliminate virus transmission close to human habitation, as infected mosquitoes were subsequently collected within the community [39], although it may have diminished the potential for transmission. It was suggested that domestic pigs needed to be moved further away to be out of the flight range of *Cx. annulirostris*, which can be as much as 12 km [40].

3.4. Development of Mosquito-Based JEV Surveillance Systems

Undoubtedly, the sentinel pig surveillance program played a considerable role in providing evidence of JEV activity and, in some cases, seroconversion in herds preceded human cases [17]. However, the use of sentinel pigs for detection of viral activity has several limitations affecting their continued deployment, particularly in remote areas [24]. Firstly, the fact that pigs are a key amplifying host of the virus is an obvious risk which may exacerbate and contribute to ongoing transmission. Secondly, sentinel animal programs can be highly expensive to establish and maintain, impacting on local resources and resulting in a major financial burden to biosecurity and public health authorities. Efficient running and effectiveness of sentinel animal programs may also be affected by labor-intensive bleeding and collection procedures which can lead to occupational health and safety issues and, if delayed, can greatly affect downstream result interpretation and disease management strategies. The inherent difficulty in distinguishing JEV from MVEV and WNV_{KUN} infections in serological assays due to cross-reacting antibodies may also obscure accurate laboratory interpretations and require further testing by highly specialized reference laboratories [30].

A surveillance system involving detection of viral RNA in mosquitoes collected in continuously run mosquito traps has been developed as an alternative to using sentinel pigs. The original iterations of this mosquito-based system involved processing all mosquitoes collected in solar or propane-powered traps [24]. However, these traps had the capacity to collect >150,000 mosquitoes in a week, so diagnostic capacity was overwhelmed. To circumvent the need to process hundreds of pools, a system was developed that takes advantage of the sugar feeding behavior of mosquitoes [41]. In this system, mosquitoes are collected in CO_2-baited traps, where they can feed on honey-soaked nucleic acid preservation cards, which are submitted for detection of viral RNA [42]. A number of modifications have been made to the trapping system, resulting in the current trap design, the sentinel mosquito arbovirus capture kit (SMACK) which does not require electricity and maximizes survivability of collected mosquitoes, thus increasing the likelihood of multiple feedings on the cards [26,43].

The sugar-based arbovirus system has been trialled in several locations around Australia and has detected a number of arboviruses, including MVEV and WNV_{KUN}, the alphaviruses, Ross River and Barmah Forest viruses, and the bunyavirus Gan Gan [26,42,44,45]. Detection of WNV_{KUN} in traps deployed near Darwin, Northern Territory, without concurrent detection in sentinel chickens demonstrated that the system is potentially more sensitive than sentinel animals in some instances [45]. Furthermore, if enough viral RNA is expectorated on the cards, it can provide a template for nucleotide gene sequencing in phylogenetic studies. The sugar-based arbovirus system using SMACK traps is now deployed operationally at 12 remote locations in Queensland, including communities in the NPA. Although JEV has not been detected in cards removed from field-deployed traps, results from laboratory-based studies showed that this virus could readily be detected in saliva expectorated by sugar-feeding mosquitoes [41]. This indicates that the sugar-based system has direct utility for JEV surveillance.

In the current sugar-based arbovirus system, the small amounts of virus expectorated on the nucleic acid preservation cards means that some samples deemed positive are at the limit of detection in molecular assays [45]. To increase the sensitivity of the sugar-based surveillance system for arbovirus detection, investigations are currently underway into the utility of mosquito excreta as an alternative sample type to saliva [46]. Early results have demonstrated that both WNV_{KUN} and dengue viruses can be detected in excreta at a higher rate than it is detected in the saliva, and possibly represents the greater volume of liquid excreted by mosquitoes (1.5 µL) compared with the volume of saliva expectorated (4.7 nL) [46,47].

4. Conclusions

To date, the detection of JEV in mosquitoes collected in a mosquito trap on Badu in March 2005 signified the final time that virus activity was unequivocally detected in Northern Australia. Overall, the virus was detected in 10 out of 11 years between 1995 and 2005 indicating that JEV had either become established in enzootic cycles in the Torres Strait or was re-introduced during the period almost annually when conditions were suitable.

Despite the status of the JEV in the Torres Strait being largely unknown, the ongoing vaccination program has likely limited the number of human cases. The vaccines currently utilized in the Torres Strait are the live attenuated, recombinant vaccine (IMOJEV) and the inactivated, African green monkey kidney (Vero) cell culture-derived vaccine (JEspect) [48]. Vaccination is recommended for residents of the outer islands and non-residents who spend a cumulative total of 30 days in the Torres Strait during the wet season (December to May) and, as such, is offered as part of an immunization program in risk areas.

The lack of evidence of JEV activity on Badu since 2005 likely represents limited surveillance rather than natural disappearance of the virus from the region. Human infection with JEV resulting in clinical disease is rigorously investigated and is defined as clinical evidence of non-encephalitic and encephalitic disease coupled with definitive laboratory testing [49]. However, the majority of JEV infections are asymptomatic and the only human virus isolates obtained from the initial 1995 outbreak were from two asymptomatic patients and these were only recovered after wider, retrospective sampling and surveillance of Torres Strait island residents was performed. Thus, some other form of active surveillance could potentially provide evidence as to whether the virus is still circulating in the Torres Strait.

When JEV first emerged in northern Australia it was initially feared that the virus would proliferate in mosquito–pig–bird cycles and become established on the mainland [50] similar to events involving establishment of WNV in bird-mosquito cycles in the United States [51]. Despite these predictions, viral activity appears to have remained restricted to the Torres Strait, with the occasional incursion onto Cape York Peninsula. There is no evidence to suggest that the virus has become established on the mainland, let alone reaching endemic status in any other areas of the country. Several ecological reasons for this apparent lack of establishment have been proposed and include: (a) competition between the endemic flaviviruses, MVEV and WNV_{KUN}, with JEV for susceptible vertebrate hosts; (b) host feeding patterns of *Cx. annulirostris* whereby they feed on hosts other than pigs, that cannot amplify JEV; and (c) different lineages of *Cx. annulirostris* which vary in their vector competence for the different genotypes of JEV [3]. Alternatively, the lack of detection on the mainland could represent the limited geographical area covered by the current sugar-based surveillance program. Whilst a vaccination program is in place for Torres Strait island residents, immunologically naïve populations exist on the mainland. Thus, it would be prudent to continue the current JEV surveillance program on Cape York Peninsula, and consider expanding its geographical scope with increased sensitivity to provide future early warning and enhanced public health prevention of disease.

The investigations presented in the current paper are, in effect, examples of One Health in action. Indeed, a One Health approach has been successfully used to understand JEV transmission and to provide tools to combat epidemics [5], and it has been suggested that the employment of One Health strategies, particularly those concerned with improving coordination and collaboration across different disciplines and jurisdictions, are essential to planning and initiating interventions to mitigate risk and in improving prevention and control of mosquito-borne arboviruses [52].

Author Contributions: Conceptualization, A.F.v.d.H., A.T.P., J.S.M., S.H.-M. and S.A.R.; Writing—Original Draft Preparation, A.F.v.d.H.; Writing—Review & Editing, A.F.v.d.H., A.T.P., J.S.M., S.H.-M. and S.A.R.

Acknowledgments: The authors wish to thank Tim Kerlin, Keith Rickart and Jamie McMahon for information on recent JEV surveillance in Northern Australia. They also thank Frederick Moore for comments on the manuscript.

References

1.   Campbell, G.L.; Hills, S.L.; Fischer, M.; Jacobson, J.A.; Hoke, C.H.; Hombach, J.M.; Marfin, A.A.; Solomon, T.; Tsai, T.F.; Tsu, V.D.; et al. Estimated global incidence of Japanese encephalitis: A systematic review. *Bull. World Health Organ.* **2011**, *89*, 766–774. [CrossRef]

2.   Mackenzie, J.S.; Williams, D.T.; Smith, D.W. Japanese encephalitis virus: The geographic distribution, incidence, and spread of a virus with a propensity to emerge in new areas. *Perspect. Med. Virol.* **2006**, *16*, 201–268. [CrossRef]

3. Van den Hurk, A.F.; Ritchie, S.A.; Mackenzie, J.S. Ecology and geographical expansion of Japanese encephalitis virus. *Ann. Rev. Entomol.* **2009**, *54*, 17–35. [CrossRef] [PubMed]

4. Ricklin, M.E.; García-Nicolás, O.; Brechbühl, D.; Python, S.; Zumkehr, B.; Nougairede, A.; Charrel, R.N.; Posthaus, H.; Oevermann, A.; Summerfield, A. Vector-free transmission and persistence of Japanese encephalitis virus in pigs. *Nat. Commun.* **2016**, *7*, 10832. [CrossRef] [PubMed]

5. Impoinvil, D.E.; Baylis, M.; Solomon, T. Japanese encephalitis: On the One Health agenda. *Curr. Top. Microbiol. Immunol.* **2013**, *365*, 205–247. [CrossRef]

6. Fleming, K. Japanese encephalitis in an Australian soldier returned from Vietnam. *Med. J. Aust.* **1975**, *2*, 19–23. [PubMed]

7. Hanson, J.P.; Taylor, C.T.; Richards, A.R.; Smith, I.L.; Boutlis, C.S. Japanese encephalitis acquired near Port Moresby: Implications for residents and travellers to Papua New Guinea. *Med. J. Aust.* **2004**, *181*, 282.

8. Macdonald, W.B.G.; Tink, A.R.; Ouvrier, R.A.; Menser, M.A.; de Silva, L.M.; Naim, H.; Hawkes, R.A. Japanese encephalitis after a two-week holiday in Bali. *Med. J. Aust.* **1989**, *150*, 334–339.

9. Hanna, J.N.; Ritchie, S.A.; Phillips, D.A.; Shield, J.; Bailey, M.C.; Mackenzie, J.S.; Poidinger, M.; McCall, B.J.; Mills, P.J. An outbreak of Japanese encephalitis in the Torres Strait, Australia, 1995. *Med. J. Aust.* **1996**, *165*, 256–260.

10. Ritchie, S.A.; Phillips, D.; Broom, A.; Mackenzie, J.; Poidinger, M.; van den Hurk, A. Isolation of Japanese encephalitis virus from *Culex annulirostris* in Australia. *Am. J. Trop. Med. Hyg.* **1997**, *56*, 80–84. [CrossRef]

11. Ritchie, S.A.; van den Hurk, A.F.; Shield, J. The 1995 Japanese encephalitis outbreak: Why Badu? *Arbovirus Res. Aust.* **1997**, *7*, 224–227.

12. Hanna, J.; Barnett, D.; Ewald, D. Vaccination against Japanese encephalitis in the Torres Strait. *Comm. Dis. Intell.* **1996**, *19*, 447.

13. Shield, J.; Hanna, J.; Phillips, D. Reappearance of the Japanese encephalitis virus in the Torres Strait, 1996. *Comm. Dis. Intell.* **1996**, *20*, 191.

14. Johansen, C.A.; van den Hurk, A.F.; Ritchie, S.A.; Zborowski, P.; Paru, R.; Bockari, M.J.; Drew, A.C.; Khromykh, T.I.; Mackenzie, J.S. Isolation of Japanese encephalitis virus from mosquitoes (Diptera: Culicidae) collected in the Western Province of Papua New Guinea, 1997–1998. *Am. J. Trop. Med. Hyg.* **2000**, *62*, 631–638. [CrossRef] [PubMed]

15. Johansen, C.; Ritchie, S.; Hurk, A.v.d.; Bockarie, M.; Hanna, J.; Phillips, D.; Melrose, W.; Poidinger, M.; Scherret, J.; Hall, R.; et al. The Search for Japanese encephalitis virus in the Western Province of Papua New Guinea, 1996. *Arbovirus Res. Aust.* **1997**, *7*, 131–136.

16. Ritchie, S.A.; Rochester, W. Wind-blown mosquitoes and introduction of Japanese encephalitis into Australia. *Emerg. Infect. Dis.* **2001**, *7*, 900–903. [CrossRef]

17. Hanna, J.N.; Ritchie, S.A.; Phillips, D.A.; Lee, J.M.; Hills, S.; van den Hurk, A.F.; Pyke, A.; Johansen, C.A.; Mackenzie, J.S. Japanese encephalitis in north Queensland, Australia, 1998. *Med. J. Aust.* **1999**, *170*, 533–536. [CrossRef]

18. Johansen, C.A.; van den Hurk, A.F.; Pyke, A.T.; Zborowski, P.; Phillips, D.A.; Mackenzie, J.S.; Ritchie, J.S. Entomological Investigations of an outbreak of Japanese encephalaitis virus in the Torres Strait, Australia, in 1998. *J. Med. Entomol.* **2001**, *38*, 581–588. [CrossRef]

19. Van den Hurk, A.F.; Johansen, C.A.; Zborowski, P.; Phillips, D.A.; Pyke, A.T.; Mackenzie, J.S.; Ritchie, S.A. Flaviviruses isolated from mosquitoes collected during the first outbreak of Japanese encephalitis virus on Cape York Peninsula, Australia. *Am. J. Trop. Med. Hyg.* **2001**, *64*, 125–130. [CrossRef]

20. Barr, J. Drought Assessment: The 1997-98 El Nino Drought in Papua New Guinea and the Solomon Islands. *Aust. J. Emerg. Manag.* **1999**, *14*, 31–37.

21. Van den Hurk, A.F.; Nisbet, D.J.; Johansen, C.A.; Foley, P.N.; Ritchie, S.A.; Mackenzie, J.S. Japanese encephalitis on Badu Island, Australia: The first isolation of Japanese encephalitis virus from *Culex gelidus* in the Australasian region and the role of mosquito host-feeding patterns in virus transmission cycles. *Trans. Royal. Soc. Trop. Med. Hyg.* **2001**, *95*, 595–600. [CrossRef]

22. Johansen, C.A.; Nisbet, D.J.; Foley, P.N.; van den Hurk, A.F.; Hall, R.A.; Mackenzie, J.S.; Ritchie, S.A. Flavivirus isolations from mosquitoes collected from Saibai Island in the Torres Strait, Australia, during an incursion of Japanese encephalitis virus. *Med. Vet. Entomol.* **2004**, *18*, 281–287. [CrossRef]

23. Pyke, A.T.; Williams, D.T.; Nisbet, D.J.; van den Hurk, A.F.; Taylor, C.T.; Johansen, C.A.; Macdonald, J.; Hall, R.A.; Simmons, R.J.; Mason, R.J.V.; et al. The appearance of a second genotype of Japanese encephalitis virus in the Australasian region. *Am. J. Trop. Med. Hyg.* **2001**, *65*, 747–753. [CrossRef] [PubMed]

24. Ritchie, S.A.; van den Hurk, A.F.; Zborowski, P.; Kerlin, T.J.; Banks, D.; Walker, J.A.; Lee, J.M.; Montgomery, B.L.; Smith, G.A.; Pyke, A.T.; et al. Operational trials of remote mosquito trap systems for Japanese encephalitis virus surveillance in the Torres Strait, Australia. *Vector Borne Zoonotic Dis.* **2007**, *7*, 497–506. [CrossRef] [PubMed]

25. Van den Hurk, A.F.; Montgomery, B.L.; Northill, J.A.; Smith, I.L.; Zborowski, P.; Ritchie, S.A.; Mackenzie, J.S.; Smith, G.A. The first isolation of Japanese encephalitis virus from mosquitoes collected from mainland Australia. *Am. J. Trop. Med. Hyg.* **2006**, *75*, 21–25. [CrossRef]

26. Johnson, B.J.; Kerlin, T.; Hall-Mendelin, S.; van den Hurk, A.F.; Cortis, G.; Doggett, S.L.; Toi, C.; Fall, K.; McMahon, J.L.; Townsend, M.; et al. Development and field evaluation of the sentinel mosquito arbovirus capture kit (SMACK). *Parasit. Vectors* **2015**, *8*, 509. [CrossRef]

27. Boyle, D.B.; Dickerman, R.W.; Marshall, I.D. Primary viraemia responses of herons to experimental infection with Murray Valley encephalitis, Kunjin and Japanese encephalitis viruses. *Aust. J. Exp. Biol. Med. Sci.* **1983**, *61*, 655–664. [CrossRef]

28. Mackenzie, J.S.; Johansen, C.A.; Ritchie, S.A.; van den Hurk, A.F.; Hall, R.A. The emergence and spread of Japanese encephalitis virus in Australasia. *Curr. Top. Microbiol. Immunol.* **2002**, *267*, 49–73. [CrossRef]

29. Van den Hurk, A.F.; Smith, C.S.; Field, H.E.; Smith, I.L.; Northill, J.A.; Taylor, C.T.; Jansen, C.C.; Smith, G.A.; Mackenzie, J.S. Transmission of Japanese encephalitis virus from the black flying fox, *Pteropus alecto*, to *Culex annulirostris* mosquitoes, despite the absence of detectable viremia. *Am. J. Trop. Med. Hyg.* **2009**, *81*, 457–462. [CrossRef]

30. Williams, D.T.; Daniels, P.W.; Lunt, R.A.; Wang, L.-F.; Newberry, K.M.; Mackenzie, J.S. Experimental infections of pigs with Japanese encephalitis virus and closely related Australian flaviviruses. *Am. J. Trop. Med. Hyg.* **2001**, *65*, 379–387. [CrossRef]

31. Van den Hurk, A.F.; Jansen, C.C. Arboviruses of Oceania. In *Neglected Tropical Diseases—Oceania*; Loukas, A., Ed.; Springer Nature: Basel, Switzerland, 2016; pp. 193–235. [CrossRef]

32. Van den Hurk, A.F.; Nisbet, D.J.; Hall, R.A.; Kay, B.H.; Mackenzie, J.S.; Ritchie, S.A. Vector competence of Australian mosquitoes (Diptera: Culicidae) for Japanese encephalitis virus. *J. Med. Entomol.* **2003**, *40*, 82–90. [CrossRef] [PubMed]

33. Hemmerter, S.; Slapeta, J.; van den Hurk, A.F.; Cooper, R.D.; Whelan, P.I.; Russell, R.C.; Johansen, C.A.; Beebe, N.W. A curious coincidence: Mosquito biodiversity and the limits of the Japanese encephalitis virus in Australasia. *BMC Evol. Biol.* **2007**, *7*, 100. [CrossRef] [PubMed]

34. Johnson, P.H.; Hall-Mendelin, S.; Whelan, P.I.; Frances, S.P.; Jansen, C.C.; Mackenzie, D.O.; Northill, J.A.; van den Hurk, A.F. Vector competence of Australian *Culex gelidus* Theobald (Diptera: Culicidae) for endemic and exotic arboviruses. *Aust. J. Entomol.* **2009**, *48*, 234–240. [CrossRef]

35. Chapman, H.F.; Kay, B.H.; Ritchie, S.A.; van den Hurk, A.F.; Hughes, J.M. Definition of species in the *Culex sitiens* subgroup (Diptera: Culicidae) from Papua New Guinea and Australia. *J. Med. Entomol.* **2000**, *37*, 736–742. [CrossRef] [PubMed]

36. Hall-Mendelin, S.; Jansen, C.C.; Cheah, W.Y.; Montgomery, B.L.; Hall, R.A.; Ritchie, S.A.; van den Hurk, A.F. *Culex annulirostris* (Diptera: Culicidae) host feeding patterns and Japanese encephalitis virus ecology in northern Australia. *J. Med. Entomol.* **2012**, *49*, 371–377. [CrossRef] [PubMed]

37. Van den Hurk, A.F.; Johansen, C.A.; Zborowski, P.; Paru, R.; Foley, P.N.; Beebe, N.W.; Mackenzie, J.S.; Ritchie, S.A. Mosquito host-feeding patterns and implications for Japanese encephalitis virus transmission in northern Australia and Papua New Guinea. *Med. Vet. Entomol.* **2003**, *17*, 403–411. [CrossRef]

38. Van den Hurk, A.F.; Smith, I.L.; Smith, G.A. Development and evaluation of real-time polymerase chain reaction assays to identify mosquito (Diptera: Culicidae) blood meals originating from native Australian mammals. *J. Med. Entomol.* **2007**, *44*, 85–92. [CrossRef]

39. Van den Hurk, A.F.; Ritchie, S.A.; Johansen, C.A.; Mackenzie, J.S.; Smith, G.A. Domestic pigs and Japanese encephalitis virus infection, Australia. *Emerg. Infect. Dis.* **2008**, *14*, 1736–1738. [CrossRef]

40. Bryan, J.H.; O'Donnell, M.S.; Berry, G.; Carvan, T. Dispersal of adult female *Culex annulirostris* in Griffith, New South Wales, Australia: A further study. *J. Am. Mosq. Control. Assoc.* **1992**, *8*, 398–403.

41. Van den Hurk, A.F.; Johnson, P.H.; Hall-Mendelin, S.; Northill, J.A.; Simmons, R.J.; Jansen, C.C.; Frances, S.P.; Smith, G.A.; Ritchie, S.A. Expectoration of flaviviruses during sugar feeding by mosquitoes (Diptera: Culicidae). *J. Med. Entomol.* **2007**, *44*, 845–850. [CrossRef]

42. Hall-Mendelin, S.; Ritchie, S.A.; Johansen, C.A.; Zborowski, P.; Cortis, G.; Dandridge, S.; Hall, R.A.; van den Hurk, A.F. Exploiting mosquito sugar feeding to detect mosquito-borne pathogens. *Proc. Natl. Acad. Sci. USA* **2010**, *107*, 11255–11259. [CrossRef] [PubMed]

43. Ritchie, S.A.; Cortis, G.; Paton, C.; Townsend, M.; Shroyer, D.; Zborowski, P.; Hall-Mendelin, S.; van den Hurk, A.F. A simple non-powered passive trap for the collection of mosquitoes for arbovirus surveillance. *J. Med. Entomol.* **2013**, *50*, 185–194. [CrossRef] [PubMed]

44. Huang, B.; Firth, C.; Watterson, D.; Allcock, R.; Colmant, A.M.; Hobson-Peters, J.; Kirkland, P.; Hewitson, G.; McMahon, J.; Hall-Mendelin, S.; et al. Genetic characterization of archived Bunyaviruses and their potential for emergence in Australia. *Emerg. Infect. Dis.* **2016**, *22*, 833–840. [CrossRef] [PubMed]

45. Van den Hurk, A.F.; Hall-Mendelin, S.; Townsend, M.; Kurucz, N.; Edwards, J.; Ehlers, G.; Rodwell, C.; Moore, F.A.; McMahon, J.L.; Northill, J.A.; et al. Applications of a sugar-based surveillance system to track arboviruses in wild mosquito populations. *Vector Borne Zoonotic Dis.* **2014**, *14*, 66–73. [CrossRef] [PubMed]

46. Ramirez, A.L.; Hall-Mendelin, S.; Doggett, S.L.; Hewitson, G.R.; McMahon, J.L.; Ritchie, S.A.; van den Hurk, A.F. Mosquito excreta: A sample type with many potential applications for the investigation of Ross River virus and West Nile virus ecology. *PLoS Negl. Trop. Dis.* **2018**, *12*, e0006771. [CrossRef] [PubMed]

47. Fontaine, A.; Jiolle, D.; Moltini-Conclois, I.; Lequime, S.; Lambrechts, L. Excretion of dengue virus RNA by *Aedes aegypti* allows non-destructive monitoring of viral dissemination in individual mosquitoes. *Sci. Rep.* **2016**, *6*, 24885. [CrossRef]

48. Australian Technical Advisory Group on Immunisation. *Australian Immunisation Handbook*; Australian Government Department of Health: Canberra, Australia, 2018. Available online: https://immunisationhandbook.health.gov.au/ (accessed on 18 February 2019).

49. Australian Government Department of Health. Japanese Encephalitis Virus Infection Case Definition—V1.1. Available online: http://www.health.gov.au/internet/main/publishing.nsf/Content/cda-surveil-nndss-casedefs-cd_je.htm (accessed on 18 February 2019).

50. Mackenzie, J.S.; Broom, A.K.; Hall, R.A.; Johansen, C.A.; Lindsay, M.D.; Phillips, D.A.; Ritchie, S.A.; Russell, R.C.; Smith, D.W. Arboviruses in the Australian region, 1990 to 1998. *Comm. Dis. Intell.* **1998**, *22*, 93–100.

51. Mackenzie, J.S.; Gubler, D.J.; Petersen, L.R. Emerging flaviviruses: The spread and resurgence of Japanese encephalitis, West Nile and dengue viruses. *Nature Med.* **2004**, *10*, S98–S109. [CrossRef]

52. Mackenzie, J.S.; Lindsay, M.D.A.; Smith, D.W.; Imrie, A. The ecology and epidemiology of Ross River and Murray Valley encephalitis viruses in Western Australia: Examples of One Health in action. *Trans. R. Soc. Trop. Med. Hyg.* **2017**, *111*, 248–254. [CrossRef]

Policy and Science for Global Health Security: Shaping the Course of International Health

Kavita M. Berger [1,*], James L. N. Wood [2], Bonnie Jenkins [3,4], Jennifer Olsen [5], Stephen S. Morse [6], Louise Gresham [7], J. Jeffrey Root [8], Margaret Rush [1], David Pigott [9,10], Taylor Winkleman [11], Melinda Moore [12,†], Thomas R. Gillespie [13,14], Jennifer B. Nuzzo [15], Barbara A. Han [16], Patricia Olinger [17], William B. Karesh [18], James N. Mills [13], Joseph F. Annelli [19], Jamie Barnabei [20], Daniel Lucey [21] and David T. S. Hayman [22,*]

[1] Gryphon Scientific, LLC, 6930 Carroll Avenue, Suite 810, Takoma Park, MD 20912, USA; margaret@gryphonscientific.com

[2] Disease Dynamics Unit, Department of Veterinary Medicine, University of Cambridge, Madingley Road, Cambridge CB3 0ES, UK; jlnw2@cam.ac.uk

[3] Brookings Institution, 1775 Massachusetts Avenue NW, Washington, DC 20036, USA; bonniedjenkins@gmail.com

[4] Women of Color Advancing Peace, Security and Conflict Transformation, 3695 Ketchum Court, Woodbridge, VA 22193, USA

[5] Rosalynn Carter Institute for Caregiving, Georgia Southwestern State University, 800 GSW State University Drive, Americus, GA 31709, USA; jenolsen.drph@gmail.com

[6] Department of Epidemiology, Mailman School of Public Health, Columbia University, 722 West 168th St., New York, NY 10032, USA; ssm20@cumc.columbia.edu

[7] Ending Pandemics and San Diego State University, San Diego, CA 92182, USA; lgresham@sdsu.edu

[8] U.S. Department of Agriculture, National Wildlife Research Center, Fort Collins, CO 80521, USA; Jeff.Root@aphis.usda.gov

[9] Institute for Health Metrics and Evaluation, Department of Health Metrics Sciences, University of Washington, 2301 Fifth Avenue, Suite 600, Seattle, WA 98121, USA; pigottdm@uw.edu

[10] Wellcome Centre for Human Genetics, Nuffield Department of Medicine, University of Oxford, Roosevelt Drive, Oxford OX3 7BN, UK

[11] Next Generation Global Health Security Network, Washington, DC 20001, USA; t.winkleman.dvm@gmail.com

[12] RAND Corporation, 1200 South Hayes St., Arlington, VA 22202, USA

[13] Population Biology, Ecology, and Evolution Program, Emory University, Atlanta, GA 30322, USA; thomas.gillespie@emory.edu (T.R.G.); wildlifedisease@gmail.com (J.N.M.)

[14] Department of Environmental Health, Rollins School of Public Health, 1518 Clifton Road, Atlanta, GA 30322, USA

[15] Center for Health Security, Johns Hopkins University School of Public Health, Pratt Street, Baltimore, MD 21202, USA; jnuzzo1@jhu.edu

[16] Cary Institute of Ecosystem Studies, Box AB Millbrook, NY 12545, USA; hanb@caryinstitute.org

[17] Environmental, Health and Safety Office (EHSO), Emory University, 1762 Clifton Rd., Suite 1200, Atlanta, GA 30322, USA; patty.olinger@emory.edu

[18] EcoHealth Alliance, 460 West 34th Street, New York, NY 10001, USA; karesh@ecohealthalliance.org

[19] Practical One Health Solutions, LLC, New Market, MD 21774, USA; pohsolutions@gmail.com

[20] Plum Island Animal Disease Center, Department of Homeland Security, Greenport, NY 11944, USA; jbarnabei87@gmail.com

[21] Department of Medicine Infectious Disease, Georgetown University, 600 New Jersey Avenue, NW Washington, DC 20001, USA; daniel.lucey8@gmail.com

[22] EpiLab, Infectious Disease Research Centre, School of Veterinary Science, Massey University, Private Bag, 11 222, Palmerston North 4442, New Zealand

* Correspondence: kberger@gryphonscientific.com (K.M.B.); d.t.s.hayman@massey.ac.nz (D.T.S.H.);

† Deceased, 17 January 2019.

Abstract: The global burden of infectious diseases and the increased attention to natural, accidental, and deliberate biological threats has resulted in significant investment in infectious disease research. Translating the results of these studies to inform prevention, detection, and response efforts often can be challenging, especially if prior relationships and communications have not been established with decision-makers. Whatever scientific information is shared with decision-makers before, during, and after public health emergencies is highly dependent on the individuals or organizations who are communicating with policy-makers. This article briefly describes the landscape of stakeholders involved in information-sharing before and during emergencies. We identify critical gaps in translation of scientific expertise and results, and biosafety and biosecurity measures to public health policy and practice with a focus on One Health and zoonotic diseases. Finally, we conclude by exploring ways of improving communication and funding, both of which help to address the identified gaps. By leveraging existing scientific information (from both the natural and social sciences) in the public health decision-making process, large-scale outbreaks may be averted even in low-income countries.

Keywords: One Health; zoonoses; Ebola virus; emerging infectious diseases

1. Introduction

For decades, researchers have been studying infectious diseases affecting people, domestic and wild animals, and plants. Researchers have characterized emerging infectious diseases from viruses such as Human Immunodeficiency Virus (HIV) [1] and Severe Acute Respiratory Syndrome (SARS) coronavirus (CoV) [2,3], and bacteria such as *Escherichia coli* O104:H4 in Germany and France [4,5]. Approximately 75% of emerging pathogens have their origins in non-human reservoir hosts and are classic examples of zoonoses [6]. Furthermore, antimicrobial resistance among zoonotic diseases has become a significant health security challenge [7–9]. Combined with vaccine research and development (R&D) and immunization campaigns, scientific studies have contributed to the prevention or reduction of disease transmission globally [10–12]. Existing scientific knowledge and experience could be built upon to prevent or mitigate future outbreaks. However, under pressure to respond quickly to emerging outbreaks, decision-makers struggle to identify effective and relevant medical and non-medical public health response measures because they may not have available information about the causative agents, assessments of potential health and/or economic effects, effective biosafety and infection control measures, information about societally appropriate control measures, and ready risk communication measures for their constituents. Three primary types of gaps (data and models, safety and security, and cultural awareness) limit the translation of research findings in the decision-making process before, during, and after emergencies.

The 2014–2016 West-African Ebola virus disease (EVD) outbreak reinforced the concept that a major pathogen outbreak in one country can affect other countries throughout the region and world, and highlighted the aforementioned gaps in leveraging existing knowledge and practices to facilitate outbreak response [13,14]. This outbreak demonstrated that urban settings, socio-cultural traditions, and local migration affect outbreak dynamics. These lessons, along with the development and use of an experimental Ebola virus vaccine, contributed to very different responses in the 2018 outbreaks in the Democratic Republic of Congo (DRC) [15]. However, conflict and an unsafe public health response environment in the DRC towards the end of 2018 and into 2019 have led to a significant increase of known cases to over 1000 [16]. As long as the security situation ensues, the number of cases will continue to increase and the ability of researchers to collect information about circulating strains will be hampered.

In addition, advancing genomic sequencing capabilities are used to generate increasing amounts of data about bacteria, viruses, and other microorganisms in different locations. For example, the

U.S. government has supported sequencing and modelling studies to identify different strains of pathogens in nature and evaluate their potential to initiate or drive outbreaks of local and international concern. The Canadian government, World Health Organization, U.S. government, non-governmental organizations (e.g., ProMED-mail), private companies, and research groups have leveraged data analytics platforms to analyze these and other available data and attempt to identify potential outbreaks before they become significant public health problems [17–20]. These platforms integrate epidemiological or syndromic data from a variety of sources, both official (e.g., Ministry of Health reports) and unofficial (e.g., media reports) sources, to help identify potential outbreaks as early as possible. The utility of these and related efforts relies on access to data, the sharing of which is governed by different international and national-level policies, and on awareness among policy-makers that scientific information, however uncertain, can inform initial and ongoing assessments of infectious disease risk and response [21,22]. These platforms do not appear to incorporate systematically the results from environmental scanning, modeling, and other related research fields. These platforms vary by the purpose, their intended stakeholders, the data they integrate, their analytic capabilities and methodologies, their accuracy, and other factors, all of which have different utility to public health decision-makers [23–25].

Although these results often are published in academic literature, decision-makers may not be aware that the studies exist, may not have access to the publication or the information contained therein, may not know how best to integrate the information into their decision-making processes, and/or may prefer to rely on scientific studies conducted by government, rather than non-governmental, researchers. Therefore, the existence of research, biosurveillance platforms, and official reporting mechanisms for infectious disease events does not necessarily indicate that these activities intersect and inform each other.

As observed after the launch of the 2014 Global Health Security Agenda (GHSA) and associated action packages, much of the scientific information accessed by human and animal health officials and public health decision-makers was, and continues to be, generated by local and/or central diagnostic laboratories [26–28]. Continuing to address gaps in these capabilities can lead to significant advances in disease prevention, such as a recent response to Nipah virus in India [29]. However, different sectors (specifically, academic, industry, and non-profit organizations) comprise the science and technology communities that develop and provide the tools necessary for detection, characterization, and analysis of infectious disease events. The results of this basic and applied research are published in scientific articles and discussed at scientific conferences, and genetic sequences and other similar information are deposited in databases, many of which exist for various model systems (e.g., plants and animals) and microbes. The scientists who conduct these studies become experts in their fields, often having the skills to help understand the significance of unusual outbreaks with known pathogens and to characterize new pathogens that resemble the ones they study. For example, in 2003, researchers on three continents who studied known respiratory pathogens were able to identify the first member of the coronavirus family causing widespread pneumonia in humans, the SARS-CoV [2,3,30–33]. In addition, researchers who study insects contribute to the scientific knowledge about how mosquitoes and ticks transmit pathogens such as Zika virus and *Borrelia burgdorferi* (the causative agent of Lyme disease), respectively. However, the expertise of the independent researchers (i.e., researchers who are not embedded within public or veterinary health agencies) and the data they produce often are not included in the decision-making process for outbreak response, unless prior relationships exist between the researchers and the public health decision-makers and practitioners.

The disconnect between research investment in human and animal health decision-making about infectious disease outbreaks and translation of data and expertise generated from research in the decision-making process may limit some early detection and response activities needed to prevent and control infectious disease outbreaks. This article describes the current state of scientific input in the public health decision-making process and highlights the different types of organizations involved in communicating scientific information before and during outbreaks. Based on the identified gaps, we consider approaches for promoting communication and trust-building between scientists (both governmental and non-governmental scientists) and policy-makers to ensure that existing data and knowledge can be brought to bear when preparing for, assessing, and responding to infectious disease incidents. Among these approaches, promoting objective, open communication among policy-makers and researchers (from the natural and social sciences) before, during, and after public health emergencies are critical for achieving the goals of the GHSA and related initiatives focused on reducing natural, accidental, and deliberate biological risks, frequently through the lens of One Heath.

2. Science Informing Global Health Security Decision Making

Information Pathways and Decision-Making in Crises

The flow of scientific information into the global health security decision-making process relies on several key factors, including: (a) networks of experts who are familiar to decision-makers and trusted experts in their respective fields; (b) information that is accessible to organizations and individuals involved in public health response; (c) decision-makers' ability to understand and evaluate scientific information; and (d) the use of scientific information by individual(s) responsible for assessing the public health situation and operational decisions. In this paper, we distinguish between scientific information (i.e., data) collected during an outbreak, and information generated by clinical or fundamental research prior to an outbreak and published in publicly-available literature, regardless of whether it is open access or available for a fee. In addition, we group together organizations involved in data generation, whether through research or epidemiological studies, which includes academic, industrial, non-profit, human and animal diagnostic, and government laboratories. We distinguish these scientists from public health decision-makers and practitioners, who play roles in policy-making and/or health response operations. All of these stakeholders are critical to the effective translation of data to public health emergency prevention, detection, and response.

Under non-emergency conditions, scientific and technical information usually is provided to policy and decision-makers of all levels (e.g., health and agricultural agencies, political leaders, and lawmakers) through a variety of means, including white papers, briefings, informal communication, published papers, and scientific conferences [34,35]. However, the flow of scientific information during emergencies is different, often reflecting the immediacy of the situation. The GHSA and International Health Regulations (IHR) provide a defined process, through guidance, for the generation and reporting of public health emergencies of potential international concern. No clear process exists for compiling and evaluating previously published scientific data to inform public health decision-making. Without trusted networks of experts and organizations that communicate scientific information to policy-makers objectively, interest groups which provide information selectively, may be the prevailing voice [36,37]. This situation may result in policy-makers developing trusted relationships with individuals and organizations with biases, which may limit objective and thorough examination of the human, animal, agricultural, or environmental health problem(s). At the same time, many researchers, though not all, do not engage with policy-makers because they do not believe they play a role in policy or decision-making and/or believe that decision-makers may not be willing to listen to their insights. This lack of engagement can limit the quality and objectivity of information being conveyed to decision-makers.

Limitations in effective translation of scientific information under emergency and non-emergency conditions determine its use in decision-making. For example, if information is perceived as partial (i.e., incomplete and/or highly uncertain) or people communicating the information are perceived as biased, decision-makers may question the utility of the data or disregard it completely. Similarly, data inconsistent with beliefs, traditions, or political agendas may be disregarded and/or discredited to maintain cultural and social realities. For example, a number of parents choose to not vaccinate their children for unsubstantiated reasons, including a disbelief in the necessity of the vaccines, perception that vaccines cause infections rather than prevent them, and belief that vaccines may cause autism [38]. Conversely, more complete data sets, more objective communication of the data, and clearer descriptions of the uncertainty of the data and analytic results may engender greater confidence in the information contributing to the decision-making process, especially if communicated effectively and appropriately for the audience.

In emergency situations, when timing and dynamics change, confidence in scientific information and advice is extremely important. Decision-makers frequently do not have time to identify and familiarize themselves with existing scientific information. Consequently, gaps in knowledge may develop, leading to uncertainty about the utility of scientific data. Similarly, uncertainty in known data also may lead decision-makers to question the utility of the scientific data. In addition, the process for sharing information with decision-makers may be cumbersome, inefficient, or nonexistent, all hampering scientifically-informed decision making. Although these limitations exist in non-emergency situations, they are exacerbated in emergencies. Therefore, during emergencies, decision-makers rely more on established relationships with experts for sourcing scientific information, which may include relevant knowledge and expertise (e.g., 2003 SARS-CoV outbreak) or only public health data, ignoring other sources (e.g., 2014–2016 West Africa EVD outbreak).

3. Key Gaps and Impediments to Science-Driven Decision Making

3.1. Data and Models

Incorporating social, natural, computational, and mathematical science analyses, including collection and characterization of specimens [39], into public health decision-making processes may help prevent future outbreaks of infectious diseases [40]. Full integration of information is difficult to achieve because of a lack of cross-pollination of disciplines and sectors [41]. Under-resourced individuals and organizations (including diagnostic and research laboratories, particularly in low-resource countries) may not have the capacity to conduct needed scientific assessments and communicate results to key audiences, which significantly limits the sharing and use of scientific information by researchers, health officials, and decision-makers. In addition, to evaluate the potential risk of emerging outbreaks, researchers and decision-makers must interpret new scientific findings from multidisciplinary studies and modeling data, which may vary in uncertainty based on the availability and veracity of the input data [42]. The relative lack of inter-disciplinary research and data analysis [43,44] in research of public health relevance contributes to these challenges of data interpretation and risk assessment.

Scientific methodologies, such as ecological niche modeling and spatial regression analyses, could contribute to better situational awareness in public health crises [45–48]. Combining these analyses with existing case studies may improve outbreak prediction and prevention (e.g., recent assessments of mosquito vectors for Zika virus in the United States) [49]. These and other types of modeling approaches [50,51] help to identify the information needs for which little data exist by leveraging results from other studies and revealing key knowledge gaps that, if filled, could improve accuracy and reduce the uncertainty of computational models [42,44,52,53]. As data are generated and analytic capabilities improve, uncertainty associated with modeling and data analysis decreases. Therefore, investments in cross-disciplinary research on ecology, wildlife and domestic animals, human health, behavioral sciences, implementation science, and cultural anthropology are essential for understanding how humans interact with their environments and how these interactions facilitate the emergence of previously unknown, wildlife-derived pathogens in the human population [54–58]. Similar trends can be observed with integration of social and biomedical sciences research, where research on behavioral change can inform compliance with medical interventions [59–61]. Communicating these and other data clearly and concisely to public health decision-makers is important for translating research investments to public health practice [62].

3.2. Safety and Security

From a risk management and infection control perspective, data on the capability of nations to respond to emerging or re-emerging infectious disease events are incomplete and the local traditions that inform control measures generally are not integrated into formal public health responses [63–69]. However, these data play a key role in implementing measures that meet the objectives of the 2005 IHR, OIE (World Organization for Animal Health) Standards, and the GHSA objectives and Action Packages (https://ghsagenda.org/). In 2016, a Commission on a Global Health Risk Framework for the Future highlighted the neglected dimension of security in global health [70]. Still, the ability to protect scientists, healthcare providers, the community, and the environment from exposure to pathogens that could harm public health and safety often is overlooked. However, this situation may change through efforts such as the GHSA 2024 Framework [71].

Critical to successful outbreak prevention and management is recognizing the need to identify, test, and employ biosafety and biosecurity measures that are sustainable and adoptable in local conditions, account for local infrastructure, laws, and social structure, and prevent accidental and deliberate release of studied pathogens. Outbreak investigations for Ebola virus, Middle East Respiratory Syndrome coronavirus (MERS-CoV), and SARS-CoV demonstrated the need for locally effective biosafety measures that protect healthcare workers, diagnostic laboratory workers, and animal health workers from exposure to the outbreak viruses, and biosecurity measures that prevent access to pathogens by malicious actors. Applied research may identify measures that enhance current risk management efforts, such as laboratory and clinical biosafety, biosecurity, and biorisk management.

3.3. Cultural Awareness

Social science research can provide a better understanding of local culture and traditions, which strongly influence pathogen transmission and acceptance of medical and public health interventions [43]. During the 2014–2016 West African EVD outbreak, a lack of cultural awareness about local end-of-life traditions led to ineffective or unintentionally dangerous public health interactions and undocumented infections [72–74]. Eventually, the public health community began identifying approaches to communicate the risk of virus transmission from touching infected bodies, mitigate transmission events through culturally acceptable means, and reduce fear of death through appropriately chosen infection control methods (e.g., use of white, instead of black, body bags in West Africa [75]). Early engagement with communities and social scientists who study the culture, tradition, and linguistics of people from affected areas would help inform communication by decision-makers, mitigation strategies used by public health responders, and trust-building with the local population. Furthermore, leveraging the knowledge gained from these social science disciplines could enhance efforts to build trust among affected individuals rather than allow the persistence of distrust between local communities and foreign health workers [76,77]. Similar approaches should be used towards domestic and wild animal research, with animal and conservation ethics and local cultural and traditions considered.

Research involving bioethics and social equity helps scientists incorporate ethical principles in the design and conduct studies involving human participants affected by public health emergencies [78]. Such studies are critically important for research examining the effectiveness of candidate vaccines and medicines, understanding pathogen transmission and infection in natural settings, and testing non-pharmaceutical interventions for disease prevention and mitigation. Although such studies have been conducted for years, the U.S. National Academies of Science, Engineering, and Medicine highlighted research needs for preparedness and response to public health emergencies and associated bioethical considerations [79]. This focus on the bioethics of disaster research has prompted non-governmental and governmental organizations alike to evaluate challenges and identify solutions to promote ethical practices in research during public health emergencies. Building on this and other social science research can promote the development and implementation of clinical and public health research that takes into account the culture, society, and benefits to and needs of research participants.

4. Potential Solutions

The purpose of much of infectious disease research is to identify pharmaceutical and non-pharmaceutical approaches for preventing, detecting and monitoring, and responding to public health outbreaks of national, regional, and international concern. Data that could inform prevention, detection, and response activities are generated by several different types of studies, including mathematical modeling, epidemiological studies, environmental scanning, life-sciences studies (e.g., microbial genomics), and cultural anthropology. By integrating known, published data in these fields, considering key knowledge gaps and existing areas of uncertainty, scientists can assist public health responders and decision-makers in understanding initial cases and feasible infection control measures. However, the results of these investments have limited utility if they are not being conveyed to policy-makers before the occurrence of and during an emergency. Without this information, human and animal health officials and health care professionals are left to diagnose emerging outbreaks using sub-optimal approaches and driving response efforts that might be unnecessarily ineffective and promulgating distrust in health response efforts.

Three approaches for addressing these gaps are communication, funding, and translation efforts. Although not explicitly described in this paper, international and national policies on data access and decisions made for political or national security purposes present additional challenges to fully informed decision-making. Some of the solutions described in this section may help reduce, but not eliminate, these challenges, highlighting the realities inherent in global governance of public health preparedness and response. Nevertheless, the proposed solutions could improve communication between researchers and decision-makers and enhance translation of research investments to inform public health practice before, during, and after emergencies.

4.1. Communication

Communication strategies that include better articulation and dissemination of existing scientific knowledge and modeling approaches (including their use, gaps, and limitations), their relevance to public health emergencies, and the inherent uncertainties in scientific assessment greatly would enhance high-level public health decision-making before, during, and after emergencies [34]. Better awareness about the types of public health decisions, associated information needs, operational constraints, time pressures of decision-makers, and limitations of current scientific knowledge would enable researchers to communicate scientific information more effectively. Understanding what is required of data and how data are best communicated in public health emergencies would provide researchers with the necessary operational context in which decision-makers must evaluate and base their decisions. With greater appreciation for the limitations of and information needs during the decision-making process, researchers can identify, integrate and distill data of greatest relevance to the specific emergency.

Effective communication can be achieved through active interaction or written documents, and fostered in a variety of venues, including scientific conferences, science and society workshops, and governmental meetings. Although some of these efforts currently are used, their effectiveness can be improved by tailoring communication to the audience. Interactions cultivated among stakeholders before emergencies could promote the development of trusted relationships between decision-makers and scientists, which can serve as the foundation for reach-back during public health emergencies. In addition, interactions through networks, such as the GHSA and associated groups, could promote open lines of communication between governmental health security officials and scientists, facilitating information-sharing and enabling greater understanding of key questions with which decision-makers struggle [35]. These interactions are most effective if they are in place before crises occur and maintained after an emergency ends, which can lead to greater trust and familiarity between policy-makers and researchers and more opportunities for information-sharing in non-emergency situations. Throughout, promoting diversity of scientific expertise and experiences within these communications networks is critical for ensuring that policy-makers receive unbiased, objective information upon which to base their decisions.

4.2. Funding and Open Access

Research investments can enhance detection, characterization, assessment, and response to infectious diseases. However, several challenges exist with the current approaches: (1) limited funding is available for basic research for a majority of infectious diseases, particularly neglected tropical diseases and wildlife-associated, epizootic (animal only) diseases; (2) limited funding opportunities exist for multi-disciplinary, multi-sectoral research and education; (3) limited support is provided for social science research that is relevant to prevention and mitigation of infectious disease outbreaks; (4) research funding continuously changes for many infectious diseases, limiting the sustainability of individual efforts (e.g., the 2018 U.S. President's proposed budget included funding cuts for efforts to prevent and respond to EVD outbreaks even as the 2018 outbreak in the DRC emerged [80,81]); (5) lack of communication from scientists to non-technical audiences, including policy-makers; and (6) lack of evaluation metrics for assessing the effectiveness of scientific input into the public health process.

To counter these challenges, government agencies, intergovernmental organizations, private funders, and philanthropic organizations should develop forward-looking, longer-term initiatives that support basic and applied research in a variety of natural and social sciences, and in efforts promoting integration and translation of scientific data to public health emergency prevention, detection, and response. Although not routinely done, proactive and stable funding for these and other scientific inquiries provides opportunities to increase the knowledge-base from which decision-makers can draw when considering appropriate infection control actions, a suggestion supported by several scientific organizations. For example, longer-term studies, such as those on New World hantaviruses, have produced a great deal of information relevant to public health [82], including changing infection prevalence with species richness [83], the preponderance of infected males [84], and the role of climatic changes in causing fluctuations in rodent reservoir populations and their links to localized, sporadic disease outbreaks. Although these studies were initiated as part of a reactive response to an acute outbreak—in this case, hantavirus pulmonary syndrome—in 1993–1994, the information produced addresses key knowledge gaps that can inform future outbreaks. Similarly, research supported during and after EVD outbreaks has generated data on wildlife reservoir hosts and people's perceptions of health and healthcare practices, both of which could inform future outbreak assessments and response efforts. In addition, funders should establish a process through which the results and assessments can be communicated to public health decision-makers, leveraging the recent movement towards open access publication requirements. As a positive example, the Bill and Melinda Gates Foundation and The Wellcome Trust require all grantees to make their results publicly available, enabling access to various stakeholders, including decision-makers [85–87]. However, access to information does not ensure their use by decision-makers. In addition, new data protection laws may counteract these open access policies of funders and journals [88].

Specific approaches for promoting greater translation of research include scientific staff support for decision-makers, fellowship opportunities, cross-disciplinary cooperation, and strategic funding mechanisms (e.g., contracts and cooperative agreements). Scientists and funders should identify and support the integration and translation of science from multiple sectors, fields, and disciplines to identify key information gaps for global health security and provide the scientific foundation for assessing infectious disease risks. Funding support for training and fellowships can promote explicit scientific input into decision-making and encourage open sharing of data with other researchers and health officials. Researchers and research institutions should aim to shift the culture of data sharing by promoting the open sharing of data with public health practitioners as an academic product on par with publications, decreasing the potential for politicization or biased use of data [70]. Data sharing has been raised with H5N1 influenza A virus, Ebola virus, and Zika virus [89], and informed by efforts to promote equitable benefit of results from the sharing of data and samples from emerging outbreaks [90,91]. In 2014, the U.S. government passed the DATA (Data Transparency and Accountability) Act, which requires that data from federally-funded efforts be made open and available. The U.S. government's DATA.gov website (https://www.data.gov/) is the platform that was developed to store and provide access to the datasets. In addition, agencies such as U.S. Geological Survey now have an 'eternal data' archive called Science Base (https://www.sciencebase.gov/catalog/). Despite these efforts, national policies restricting data access and sharing to foreign entities present new challenges to equitable and reciprocal data sharing, especially as biological research increasingly relies on data science approaches [92].

Approaches for improving communication between researchers and policy-makers, the funding landscape, and open access policies could help promote research that addresses key knowledge gaps in health security policy and practice, and translate funded research to global health decision-making.

4.3. Translation of Data

Looking forward, the 2024 Framework of the Global Health Security Agenda stresses communication, political and financial advocacy, and engagement of a more diverse set of stakeholders [71]. In part, these efforts intend to increase national-level investment and support for addressing shortcomings in human and animal health capabilities that currently limit effective prevention, detection, and response to public health emergencies of international concern. However, the new structure developed to progress towards these GHSA efforts could be enhanced further by including the research community as a critical stakeholder and focusing attention on data sharing among the research, public health, veterinary health, agriculture, and environmental health communities. Active engagement of the scientific arms of research and diagnostic entities (regardless of their sector, whether academic, industry, or government laboratories) with local and national public and veterinary health entities could enable better translation of scientific information to address public health needs. Recent calls for integrating veterinary and human health research to improve One Health efforts, including policy development and implementation, have been published [93,94]. Training on and implementation of data translation, improved strategies for communicating data and their associated limitations and/or statistical significance, and active participation of the scientific community in public health decision-making processes could reveal opportunities for leveraging data in an informative and timely manner.

5. Conclusions

The global burden of infectious diseases and the increased attention to natural, accidental, and deliberate biological threats has resulted in scientific and financial investment in infectious disease research. However, the results of these studies often are not translated to prevention, detection, and response efforts. Furthermore, the needs, receptivity, and stakeholders involved in sharing scientific data before and during emergencies differ, which can lead to barriers towards research translation to human and animal health practice. Overcoming these barriers is necessary to prevent and mitigate emerging and re-emerging infectious diseases, including the recent epidemics caused by Zika virus in the Americas, Yellow fever virus (YFV) in Angola and the DRC, and Ebola virus in the DRC. The public health burden caused by influenza virus has led to the creation of WHO collaborating centers through which data on naturally circulating strains and results from basic and applied research are shared, informing influenza surveillance efforts. In addition, scientific data associated with the Zika virus disease outbreak has been placed in the public domain to facilitate prevention and control of the outbreak. However, these data sharing efforts are inconsistent across outbreaks, as demonstrated by the lack of similar data sharing practice in the YFV outbreak in Africa [95]. Furthermore, sharing of data is not the same as effective communication of the data.

Despite the increased investment for infectious disease research, significant knowledge gaps remain in host–pathogen interactions, urbanization and climactic influences on pathogen transmission, pathogen evolution, interactions between wild and domestic animals and humans, existence of unknown but naturally occurring pathogens, and other areas of interest. These knowledge gaps introduce uncertainty about what can be concluded from available data, which in turn can raise doubt in the utility of research results and validity of science-based conclusions during decision-making, especially in emergency situations. Advanced engagement and communication between researchers and policy-makers could help identify critical knowledge gaps that could reduce uncertainty levels and promote better trust between scientists and decision-makers. Encouraging and training scientists to recognize and translate research findings to public health decision-makers enhances these efforts. Effective communication and long-term funding are important for providing decision-makers with a clear understanding of what is known and what needs to be determined to improve prevention, detection, and response efforts of current and future outbreaks.

Author Contributions: Conceptualization, all authors; Writing—Original Draft preparation, K.M.B. and D.T.S.H.; Writing—Review and Editing, all authors.

Acknowledgments: The driver for this paper and its broad authorship was a workshop held in June 2015, titled "Joint RAPIDD-GHSA Workshop: Policy Implications of Detecting Hemorrhagic Fever Viruses in Wildlife and Domestic Animals". The workshop was held under the auspices of the National Institutes of Health and Department of Homeland Security-funded Research and Policy for Infectious Disease Dynamics (RAPIDD) program and in coordination with the U.S. Department of State. We thank Audrey Thevenon (National Academy of Sciences, Engineering, and Medicine), Rocco Casagrande (Gryphon Scientific), Christopher Hofmann (U.S. Department of State), Ellis McKenzie (National Institutes of Health, sadly deceased), and Bryan Grenfell (Princeton University) for their support.

References

1. Barré-Sinoussi, F.; Chermann, J.-C.; Rey, F.; Nugeyre, M.T.; Chamaret, S.; Gruest, J.; Dauguet, C.; Axler-Blin, C.; Vézinet-Brun, F.; Rouzioux, C. Isolation of a T-lymphotropic retrovirus from a patient at risk for acquired immune deficiency syndrome (AIDS). *Science* **1983**, *220*, 868–871. [CrossRef]
2. Rota, P.A.; Oberste, M.S.; Monroe, S.S.; Nix, W.A.; Campagnoli, R.; Icenogle, J.P.; Peñaranda, S.; Bankamp, B.; Maher, K.; Chen, M.-H.; et al. Characterization of a novel coronavirus associated with severe acute respiratory syndrome. *Science* **2003**, *300*, 1394–1399. [CrossRef] [PubMed]
3. Peiris, J.S.M.; Lai, S.T.; Poon, L.L.M.; Guan, Y.; Yam, L.Y.C.; Lim, W.; Nicholls, J.; Yee, W.K.S.; Yan, W.W.; Cheung, M.T.; et al. Coronavirus as a possible cause of severe acute respiratory syndrome. *Lancet* **2003**, *361*, 1319–1325. [CrossRef]
4. Rohde, H.; Qin, J.; Cui, Y.; Li, D.; Loman, N.J.; Hentschke, M.; Chen, W.; Pu, F.; Peng, Y.; Li, J.; et al. Open-source genomic analysis of shiga-toxin–producing *E. coli* O104:H4. *N. Engl. J. Med.* **2011**, *365*, 718–724. [CrossRef]
5. Frank, C.; Faber, M.; Askar, M.; Bernard, H.; Fruth, A.; Gilsdorf, A.; Höhle, M.; Karch, H.; Krause, G.; Prager, R. Large and ongoing outbreak of haemolytic uraemic syndrome. *Euro Surveill.* **2011**, *16*, 19878. [PubMed]
6. Taylor, L.H.; Latham, S.M.; Woolhouse, M.E. Risk factors for human disease emergence. *Philos. Trans. R. Soc. Lond. Ser. B Biol. Sci.* **2001**, *356*, 983–989. [CrossRef]
7. World Health Organization. Antimicrobial Resistance. Available online: https://www.who.int/en/news-room/fact-sheets/detail/antimicrobial-resistance (accessed on 31 March 2019).
8. Asokan, G.V.; Kasimanickam, R.K. Emerging infectious diseases, antimicrobial resistance and millennium development goals: Resolving the challenges through one health. *Cen. Asian J. Glob. Health* **2013**, *2*, 76. [CrossRef]

9. European Centre for Disease Prevention and Control. Zoonoses: Antimicrobial Resistance Shows no Signs of Slowing Down. Available online: https://ecdc.europa.eu/en/news-events/zoonoses-antimicrobial-resistance-shows-no-signs-slowing-down (accessed on 31 March 2019).
10. Greenwood, B. The contribution of vaccination to global health: Past, present and future. *Philos. Trans. R. Soc. Lond. B Biol. Sci.* **2014**, *369*, 20130433. [CrossRef]
11. Francis, D.P. Success and failures: Worldwide vaccine development and application. *Biologicals* **2010**, *38*, 523–528. [CrossRef]
12. Greenwood, B.; Salisbury, D.; Hill, A.V.S. Vaccines and global health. *Philos. Trans. R. Soc. Lond. B Biol. Sci.* **2011**, *366*, 2733–2742. [CrossRef] [PubMed]
13. Heymann, D.L.; Chen, L.; Takemi, K.; Fidler, D.P. Global health security: The wider lessons from the West African Ebola virus disease epidemic. *Lancet* **2015**, *385*, 1884–1901. [CrossRef]
14. Backer, J.A.; Wallinga, J. Spatiotemporal analysis of the 2014 Ebola epidemic in West Africa. *PLoS Comput. Biol.* **2016**, *12*, e1005210. [CrossRef]
15. World Health Organization. Ebola Vaccine Provides Protection and Hope for High-Risk Communities in the Democratic Republic of the Congo. Available online: http://www.who.int/news-room/feature-stories/detail/ebola-vaccine-provides-protection-and-hope-for-high-risk-communities-in-the-democratic-republic-of-the-congo (accessed on 14 August 2018).
16. Centers for Disease Control and Prevention. Ebola Outbreak in Eastern Democratic Republic of Congo tops 1000 cases. Available online: https://www.cdc.gov/media/releases/2019/s0322-ebola-congo.html (accessed on 31 March 2019).
17. Pellerin, C. DTRA Scientists Develop Cloud-Based Biosurveillance Ecosystem. Available online: https://dod.defense.gov/News/Article/Article/681832/dtra-scientists-develop-cloud-based-biosurveillance-ecosystem/ (accessed on 17 March 2019).
18. Public Health Agency of Canada. About GPHIN. Available online: https://gphin.canada.ca/cepr/aboutgphin-rmispenbref.jsp?language=en_CA (accessed on 14 August 2018).
19. World Health Organization. Global Outbreak Alert and Response Network (GOARN). Available online: http://www.who.int/ihr/alert_and_response/outbreak-network/en/ (accessed on 14 August 2018).
20. ProMED. International Society for Infectious Diseases. Available online: http://www.promedmail.org/ (accessed on 14 February 2019).
21. Holmes, E.C.; Rambaut, A.; Andersen, K.G. Pandemics: spend on surveillance, not prediction. *Nature* **2018**, *558*, 180–182. [CrossRef]
22. Rivers, C.; Scarpino, S. Modelling the trajectory of disease outbreaks works. *Nature* **2018**, *559*, 477. [CrossRef]
23. Milinovich, G.J.; Soares Magalhaes, R.J.; Hu, W. Role of big data in the early detection of Ebola and other emerging infectious disease. *Lancet Glob. Health* **2015**, *3*, PE20–PE21. [CrossRef]
24. Lazer, D.; Kennedy, R.; King, G.; Vespignani, A. The parable of google flu: Traps in big data analysis. *Science* **2014**, *343*, 1203–1205. [CrossRef]
25. Dion, M.; AbdelMalik, P.; Mawudeku, A. Big data and the global public health intelligence network (GPHIN). *Can. Commun. Dis. Rep.* **2015**, *41*, 209–214. [CrossRef]
26. Kennedy, E.D.; Morgan, J.; Knight, N.W. Global health security implementation: Expanding the evidence base. *Health Security* **2018**. [CrossRef]
27. Edelson, M.; Lee, L.M.; Herten-Crabb, A.; Heymann, D.L.; Harper, D.R. Strengthening global public health surveillance through data and benefit sharing. *Emerg. Infect. Dis.* **2018**, *24*, 1324–1330. [CrossRef]
28. Rodier, G.; Greenspan, A.L.; Hughes, J.M.; Haymann, D.L. Global public health security. *Emerg. Infect. Dis.* **2007**, *13*, 1447–1452. [CrossRef]
29. Sadanadan, R.; Arunkumar, G.; Laserson, K.F.; Heretik, K.H.; Singh, S.; Mourya, D.T.; Gangakhedkar, R.R.; Gupta, N.; Sharma, R.; Dhuria, M. Towards global health security: Response to the May 2018 Nipah virus outbreak linked to pteropus bats in Kerala, India. *BMJ Glob. Health* **2018**, *3*, e001086. [CrossRef]
30. Fouchier, R.A.M.; Kuiken, T.; Schutten, M.; van Amerongen, G.; van Doornum, G.J.J.; van den Hoogen, B.G.; Peiris, M.; Lim, W.; Stöhr, K.; Osterhaus, A.D.M.E. Koch's postulates fulfilled for SARS virus. *Nature* **2003**, *423*, 240. [CrossRef]
31. Drosten, C.; Günther, S.; Preiser, W.; Van Der Werf, S.; Brodt, H.-R.; Becker, S.; Rabenau, H.; Panning, M.; Kolesnikova, L.; Fouchier, R.A. Identification of a novel coronavirus in patients with severe acute respiratory syndrome. *N. Eng. J. Med.* **2003**, *348*, 1967–1976. [CrossRef]

32. Falsey, A.R.; Walsh, E.E. Novel coronavirus and severe acute respiratory syndrome. *Lancet* **2003**, *361*, 1312–1313. [CrossRef]

33. Ksiazek, T.G.; Erdman, D.; Goldsmith, C.S.; Zaki, S.R.; Peret, T.; Emery, S.; Tong, S.; Urbani, C.; Comer, J.A.; Lim, W. A novel coronavirus associated with severe acute respiratory syndrome. *N. Eng. J. Med.* **2003**, *348*, 1953–1966. [CrossRef]

34. Whitty, C.J. What makes an academic paper useful for health policy? *BMC Med.* **2015**, *13*, 1. [CrossRef]

35. Cook, C.N.; Mascia, M.B.; Schwartz, M.W.; Possingham, H.P.; Fuller, R.A. Achieving conservation science that bridges the knowledge–action boundary. *Conserv. Biol.* **2013**, *27*, 669–678. [CrossRef]

36. Contandriopoulos, D.; Brousselle, A.; Brenton, M.; Larouche, C.; Champagne, G.; Rivard, G. Policy-making: polarization and interest group influence: Damien Contradriopoulos. *Eur. J. Public Health* **2017**, *27* (Suppl. 3). [CrossRef]

37. Kushel, M.; Bindman, A.B. Healthcare lobbying: Time to make patients the special interest. *Am. J. Med.* **2004**, *116*, 496–497. [CrossRef]

38. World Health Organization. Global Vaccine Safety. Available online: https://www.who.int/vaccine_safety/initiative/detection/immunization_misconceptions/en/ (accessed on 8 February 2018).

39. DiEuliis, D.; Johnson, K.R.; Morse, S.S.; Schindel, D.E. Opinion: Specimen collections should have a much bigger role in infectious disease research and response. *Proc. Natl. Acad. Sci. USA* **2016**, *113*, 4–7. [CrossRef]

40. Morse, S.S.; Mazet, J.A.; Woolhouse, M.; Parrish, C.R.; Carroll, D.; Karesh, W.B.; Zambrana-Torrelio, C.; Lipkin, W.I.; Daszak, P. Prediction and prevention of the next pandemic zoonosis. *Lancet* **2012**, *380*, 1956–1965. [CrossRef]

41. Manlove, K.R.; Walker, J.G.; Craft, M.E.; Huyvaert, K.P.; Joseph, M.B.; Miller, R.S.; Nol, P.; Patyk, K.A.; O'Brien, D.; Walsh, D.P. "One Health" or three? Publication silos among the one health disciplines. *PLoS Biol.* **2016**, *14*, e1002448. [CrossRef]

42. Chretien, J.-P.; Riley, S.; George, D.B. Mathematical modeling of the West Africa Ebola epidemic. *eLife* **2015**, *4*, e09186. [CrossRef]

43. Wood, J.L.; Leach, M.; Waldman, L.; Macgregor, H.; Fooks, A.R.; Jones, K.E.; Restif, O.; Dechmann, D.; Hayman, D.T.; Baker, K.S.; et al. A framework for the study of zoonotic disease emergence and its drivers: Spillover of bat pathogens as a case study. *Philos. Trans. R. Soc. Lond. Ser. B Biol. Sci.* **2012**, *367*, 2881–2892. [CrossRef]

44. Restif, O.; Hayman, D.T.; Pulliam, J.R.; Plowright, R.K.; George, D.B.; Luis, A.D.; Cunningham, A.A.; Bowen, R.A.; Fooks, A.R.; O'Shea, T.J. Model-guided fieldwork: practical guidelines for multidisciplinary research on wildlife ecological and epidemiological dynamics. *Ecol. Lett.* **2012**, *15*, 1083–1094. [CrossRef]

45. Brierley, L.; Vonhof, M.J.; Olival, K.J.; Daszak, P.; Jones, K.E. Quantifying global drivers of zoonotic bat viruses: A process-based perspective. *Am. Nat.* **2016**, *187*, E53–E64. [CrossRef]

46. Pigott, D.M.; Golding, N.; Mylne, A.; Huang, Z.; Henry, A.J.; Weiss, D.J.; Brady, O.J.; Kraemer, M.U.; Smith, D.L.; Moyes, C.L. Mapping the zoonotic niche of Ebola virus disease in Africa. *eLife* **2014**, *3*, e04395. [CrossRef]

47. Pigott, D.M.; Golding, N.; Mylne, A.; Huang, Z.; Weiss, D.J.; Brady, O.J.; Kraemer, M.U.; Hay, S.I. Mapping the zoonotic niche of Marburg virus disease in Africa. *Trans. R. Soc. Trop. Med. Hyg.* **2015**, *109*, 366–378. [CrossRef]

48. Peterson, A.; Bauer, J.; Mills, J. Ecologic and geographic distribution of filovirus disease. *Emerg. Infect. Dis.* **2004**, *10*, 40–47. [CrossRef]

49. Monaghan, A.J.; Morin, C.W.; Steinhoff, D.F.; Wilhelmi, O.; Hayden, M.; Quattrochi, D.A.; Reiskind, M.; Lloyd, A.L.; Smith, K.; Schmidt, C.A. On the seasonal occurrence and abundance of the Zika virus vector mosquito *Aedes aegypti* in the contiguous United States. *PLoS Curr.* **2016**, *8*. [CrossRef]

50. Han, B.A.; Schmidt, J.P.; Alexander, L.; Bowden, S.E.; Hayman, D.T.S.; Drake, J.M. Undiscovered bat hosts of filoviruses. *PLoS Negl. Trop. Dis.* **2016**, *10*, e0004815. [CrossRef]

51. Hayman, D.T. Biannual birth pulses allow filoviruses to persist in bat populations. *Proc. R. Soc. Lond. B Biol. Sci.* **2015**, *282*, 20142591. [CrossRef]

52. King, A.A.; de Cellès, M.D.; Magpantay, F.M.; Rohani, P. Avoidable errors in the modelling of outbreaks of emerging pathogens, with special reference to Ebola. *Proc. R. Soc. Lond. B Biol. Sci.* **2015**, *282*, 20150347. [CrossRef]

53.   Plowright, R.K.; Eby, P.; Hudson, P.J.; Smith, I.L.; Westcott, D.; Bryden, W.L.; Middleton, D.; Reid, P.A.; McFarlane, R.A.; Martin, G. Ecological dynamics of emerging bat virus spillover. *Proc. R. Soc. Lond. B Biol. Sci.* **2015**, *282*, 20142124. [CrossRef]

54.   Calvignac-Spencer, S.; Leendertz, S.; Gillespie, T.; Leendertz, F. Wild great apes as sentinels and sources of infectious disease. *Clin. Microbiol. Infect.* **2012**, *18*, 521–527. [CrossRef]

55.   Gillespie, T.R.; Nunn, C.L.; Leendertz, F.H. Integrative approaches to the study of primate infectious disease: Implications for biodiversity conservation and global health. *Am. J. Phys. Anthropol.* **2008**, *137*, 53–69. [CrossRef]

56.   Anti, P.; Owusu, M.; Agbenyega, O.; Annan, A.; Badu, E.K.; Nkrumah, E.E.; Tschapka, M.; Oppong, S.; Adu-Sarkodie, Y.; Drosten, C. Human-bat interactions in rural West Africa. *Emerg. Infect. Dis.* **2015**, *21*, 1418–1421. [CrossRef]

57.   Kamins, A.O.; Restif, O.; Ntiamoa-Baidu, Y.; Suu-Ire, R.; Hayman, D.T.; Cunningham, A.A.; Wood, J.L.; Rowcliffe, J.M. Uncovering the fruit bat bushmeat commodity chain and the true extent of fruit bat hunting in Ghana, West Africa. *Biol. Conserv.* **2011**, *144*, 3000–3008. [CrossRef]

58.   Kamins, A.O.; Rowcliffe, J.M.; Ntiamoa-Baidu, Y.; Cunningham, A.A.; Wood, J.L.; Restif, O. Characteristics and risk perceptions of Ghanaians potentially exposed to bat-borne zoonoses through bushmeat. *EcoHealth* **2014**, *12*, 104–120. [CrossRef]

59.   Kippax, S. Understanding and integrating the structural and biomedical determinants of HIV infection: A way forward for prevention. *Curr. Opin. HIV AIDS* **2008**, *3*, 489–494. [CrossRef]

60.   Mabry, P.L.; Olster, D.H.; Morgan, G.D.; Abrams, D.B. Interdisciplinarity and systems science to improve population health: A view from the NIH office of behavioral and social sciences research. *Am. J. Prev. Med.* **2008**, *35*, S211–S224. [CrossRef]

61.   Jin, J.; Sklar, G.E.; Oh, V.M.S.; Li, S.C. Factors affecting therapeutic compliance: A review from the patient's perspective. *Ther. Clin. Risk Manag.* **2008**, *4*, 269.

62.   Ogilvie, D.; Craig, P.; Griffin, S.; Macintyre, S.; Wareham, N.J. A translational framework for public health research. *BMC Public Health* **2009**, *9*, 116. [CrossRef]

63.   Jephcott, F.L.; Wood, J.L.; Cunningham, A.A. Facility-based surveillance for emerging infectious diseases; diagnostic practices in rural West African hospital settings: Observations from Ghana. *Phil. Trans. R. Soc. B* **2017**, *372*, 20160544. [CrossRef]

64.   Manguvo, A.; Mafuvadze, B. The impact of traditional and religious practices on the spread of Ebola in West Africa: Time for a strategic shift. *Pan. Afr. Med. J.* **2015**, *22* (Suppl. 1), 9.

65.   Carrion Martin, A.I.; Derrough, T.; Honomou, P.; Kolie, N.; Diallo, B.; Kone, M.; Rodier, G.; Kpoghomou, C.; Jansa, J.M. Social and cultural factors behind community resistance during an Ebola outbreak in a village of the Guinean Forest region, February 2015: A field experience. *Int. Health* **2016**, *8*, 227–229. [CrossRef]

66.   Ulin, P.R. African women and AIDS: Negotiating behavioral change. *Soc. Sci. Med.* **1992**, *34*, 63–73. [CrossRef]

67.   De Bruym, M. Women and aids in developing countries: The XIIth international conference on the social sciences and medicine. *Soc. Sci. Med.* **1992**, *34*, 249–262. [CrossRef]

68.   Ventura-Garcia, L.; Roura, M.; Rell, C.; Posada, E.; Gascon, J.; Aldasoro, E.; Munoz, J.; Pool, R. Socio-cultural aspects of chagas disease: A systematic review of qualitative research. *PLoS Negl. Trop. Dis.* **2013**, *7*, e2410. [CrossRef]

69.   Richards, P.; Amara, J.; Ferme, M.C.; Mokuwa, E.; Sheriff, A.I.; Suluku, R.; Voors, M. Social pathways for Ebola virus disease in rural Sierra Leone, and some implications for containment. *PLoS Negl. Trop. Dis.* **2015**, *9*, e0003567. [CrossRef]

70.   Sands, P.; Mundaca-Shah, C.; Dzau, V.J. The neglected dimension of global security—A framework for countering infectious-disease crises. *N. Eng. J. Med.* **2016**, *374*, 1281–1287. [CrossRef]

71.   Global Health Security Agenda. 2024 Framework. Available online: https://www.ghsagenda.org/docs/default-source/default-document-library/ghsa-2024-files/ghsa-2024-framework.pdf?sfvrsn=4 (accessed on 30 March 2019).

72.   Spengler, J.R.; Ervin, E.D.; Towner, J.S.; Rollin, P.E.; Nichol, S.T. Perspectives on West Africa Ebola virus disease outbreak, 2013–2016. *Emerg. Infect. Dis.* **2016**, *22*, 956–963. [CrossRef]

73. Pandey, A.; Atkins, K.E.; Medlock, J.; Wenzel, N.; Townsend, J.P.; Childs, J.E.; Nyenswah, T.G.; Ndeffo-Mbah, M.L.; Galvani, A.P. Strategies for containing Ebola in West Africa. *Science* **2014**, *346*, 991–995. [CrossRef]

74. World Health Organization. *Factors that Contributed to Undetected Spread of the Ebola Virus and Impeded Rapid Containment*; WHO: Geneva, Switzerland, 2015; Available online: https://www.who.int/csr/disease/ebola/one-year-report/factors/en/ (accessed on 17 March 2019).

75. DuBois, M.; Wake, C.; Sturridge, S.; Bennett, C. The Ebola response in West Africa: Exposing the Politics and Culture of International Aid. Available online: http://www.odi.org/publications/9936-ebola-response-west-africa-exposing-politics-culture-international-aid (accessed on 14 February 2019).

76. AlJezeera America. Saudi Arabia Announces 92 more MERS deaths, Sacks Deputy Health Minister. Available online: http://america.aljazeera.com/articles/2014/6/3/saudi-raises-mersdeathtollandcases.html (accessed on 17 March 2018).

77. The Guardian. China Accused of SARS Cover-up. Available online: http://www.theguardian.com/world/2003/apr/09/sars.china (accessed on 17 March 2019).

78. Convention on Biological Diversity. Nagoya Protocol. Available online: https://www.cbd.int/abs/about/ (accessed on 17 March 2019).

79. Institute of Medicine. *Enabling Rapid and Sustainable Public Health Research During Disasters: Summary of a Joint Workshop by the Institute of Medicine and the U.S. Department of Health and Human Services*; The National Academies Press: Washington, DC, USA, 2015; p. 190. [CrossRef]

80. Garrett, L. Ebola is back. And Trump is trying to kill funding for it. Available online: https://foreignpolicy.com/2018/05/09/ebola-is-back-and-trump-is-trying-to-kill-funding-for-it/ (accessed on 17 March 2019).

81. Kaiser Family Foundation. Trump administration requests rescission of $252M in 2015 Ebola funds as Congo addresses new outbreak. Available online: https://www.kff.org/news-summary/trump-administration-requests-rescission-of-252m-in-2015-ebola-funds-as-congo-addresses-new-outbreak/ (accessed on 17 March 2019).

82. Mills, J.N.; Ksiazek, T.G.; Peters, C.; Childs, J.E. Long-term studies of hantavirus reservoir populations in the southwestern United States: A synthesis. *Emerg. Infect. Dis.* **1999**, *5*, 135. [CrossRef]

83. Luis, A.D.; Kuenzi, A.J.; Mills, J.N. Species diversity concurrently dilutes and amplifies transmission in a zoonotic host–pathogen system through competing mechanisms. *Proc. Natl. Acad. Sci. USA* **2018**, *115*, 7979–7984. [CrossRef]

84. Luis, A.D.; Douglass, R.J.; Hudson, P.J.; Mills, J.N.; Bjørnstad, O.N. Sin nombre hantavirus decreases survival of male deer mice. *Oecologia* **2012**, *169*, 431–439. [CrossRef]

85. Bill and Melinda Gates Foundation. How We Work: Information Sharing Approach. Available online: https://www.gatesfoundation.org/How-We-Work/General-Information/Information-Sharing-Approach (accessed on 12 June 2018).

86. Bill and Melinda Gates Foundation. How we work: Open Access Policy. Available online: https://www.gatesfoundation.org/how-we-work/general-information/open-access-policy (accessed on 17 March 2019).

87. Wellcome Trust. Open Access Policy. Available online: https://wellcome.ac.uk/funding/managing-grant/open-access-policy (accessed on 2 February 2018).

88. Berger, K.M.; Schneck, P.A. National and transnational security implications of asymmetric access to and use of biological data. *Front. Bioeng. Biotechnol.* **2019**, *7*, 1–7. [CrossRef]

89. Wellcome Trust. Sharing Data During Zika and Other Global Health Emergencies. Available online: https://wellcome.ac.uk/news/sharing-data-during-zika-and-other-global-health-emergencies (accessed on 20 October 2018).

90. United Nations. About the Nagoya Protocol. Available online: https://www.cbd.int/abs/about/ (accessed on 14 August 2018).

91. World Health Organization. *Pandemic influenza preparedness Framework for sharing of influenza viruses and access to vaccines and other benefits*; WHO: Geneva, Switzerland, 2009. Available online: https://www.who.int/influenza/resources/pip_framework/en/ (accessed on 17 March 2019).

92. Ribeiro, C.D.; Koopmans, M.P.; Haringhuizen, G.B. Threats to timely sharing of pathogen sequence data. *Science* **2018**, *362*, 404–406. [CrossRef]

93. Christopher, M.M. One health, one literature: Weaving together veterinary and medical research. *Sci. Transl. Med.* **2015**, *7*, 303fs36. [CrossRef]

94. Hitziger, M.; Esposito, R.; Canali, M.; Aragrande, M.; Hasler, B.; Ruegg, S.R. Knowledge integration in one health policy formulation, implementation and evaluation. *Bull. World Health Organ.* **2018**, *96*, 211–218. [CrossRef]

95. Wellcome Trust. Sharing Research Findings and Data Relevant to the Ebola Outbreak in the Democratic Republic of Congo. Available online: https://wellcome.ac.uk/what-we-do/our-work/sharing-research-findings-and-data-relevant-ebola-outbreak-drc (accessed on 2 February 2018).

5

Virus–Host Interactions Involved in Lassa Virus Entry and Genome Replication

María Eugenia Loureiro *⬤, Alejandra D'Antuono and Nora López

Centro de Virología Animal (CEVAN), CONICET-SENASA, Av Sir Alexander Fleming 1653, Martínez, Provincia de Buenos Aires B1640CSI, Argentina; adantuono@gmail.com (A.D.); noramlopar@gmail.com (N.L.)
* Correspondence: eugenialoureiro@yahoo.com.ar.

Abstract: Lassa virus (LASV) is the causative agent of Lassa fever, a human hemorrhagic disease associated with high mortality and morbidity rates, particularly prevalent in West Africa. Over the past few years, a significant amount of novel information has been provided on cellular factors that are determinant elements playing a role in arenavirus multiplication. In this review, we focus on host proteins that intersect with the initial steps of the LASV replication cycle: virus entry and genome replication. A better understanding of relevant virus–host interactions essential for sustaining these critical steps may help to identify possible targets for the rational design of novel therapeutic approaches against LASV and other arenaviruses that cause severe human disease.

Keywords: Lassa fever; arenavirus; LASV; virus–host interactions; entry; replication

1. Introduction

The *Arenaviridae* family includes viruses carried by mammalian hosts, classified in the Mammarenavirus genus, and members that infect reptilian hosts, which belong to the Reptarenavirus and Hartmanivirus genera [1]. Mammarenaviruses comprise 35 currently recognized species that are classified into two main groups, Old World (OW) and New World (NW) viruses. Within the NW group, viruses are divided into Clade A, Clade A-recombinant (Clade D), Clade B, and Clade C, according to their phylogenetic relationships. Clade B includes the apathogenic Tacaribe virus (TCRV), along with the known South American pathogens that produce severe hemorrhagic disease in humans: Junín virus (JUNV), the causative agent of Argentine hemorrhagic fever; and Machupo, Chapare, Guanarito, and Sabia viruses. OW mammarenaviruses include the prototypic lymphocytic choriomeningitis virus (LCMV), of worldwide distribution, and other viruses endemic to the African continent such as Mopeia (MOPV), Lujo (LUJV), and Lassa virus (LASV). LASV is the causative agent of Lassa fever (LF), a human hemorrhagic disease transmitted through contact with infected rodents (*Mastomys* spp.) that is particularly prevalent in Nigeria, Liberia, Sierra Leone, and Guinea. After infection, an average incubation time of 10 days is usually followed by general flu-like symptoms, including fever, malaise, and headache. Hemorrhagic and/or neurologic involvement can be associated with severe cases of LF [2]. Up to 500,000 infections and >5000 deaths occur every year, with mortality rates which can rise up to 50% in hospitalized patients, 90% in women in the last month of pregnancy, and nearly 100% mortality in fetuses [3]. Neurological sequelae including deafness are common features in LF survivors [4,5].

Arenaviruses are enveloped viruses with a negative-sense RNA genome, consisting of two single-stranded segments named S (ca. 3.4 kb) and L (ca. 7.2 kb), each encoding two proteins with an ambisense strategy for expression. The S segment encodes the nucleoprotein (NP) and the precursor of the envelope glycoprotein complex (GPC), while the L segment encodes the viral RNA-dependent RNA polymerase (L) and a matrix protein (Z) that is involved in virus assembly and budding [6].

The open reading frames, in opposite orientations, are separated by a noncoding intergenic region predicted to fold into strong stem-loop structures [7].

GPC is expressed as a single precursor polypeptide that is cleaved twice by cellular proteases to generate a stable signal peptide (SSP), a receptor-binding subunit (GP1), and a trans-membrane fusion subunit (GP2). Both the peripheral GP1 and the SSP remain noncovalently associated with GP2, and assemble into the trimeric glycoprotein (GP) complex that mediates receptor recognition and fusion of the viral and host cell membranes [8–10].

NP is the most abundant viral protein both in virions and infected cells, and plays critical roles during arenavirus life cycle. NP associates tightly with the viral genomic and antigenomic RNAs forming ribonucleoprotein (RNP) complexes called nucleocapsids. Nucleocapsids bind the L polymerase, constituting the biologically active units for transcription of subgenomic viral mRNAs and for viral genome replication [11–13]. In addition, NP interacts with the Z matrix protein and contributes to the packaging of RNPs into viral particles during virion morphogenesis [14–16]. Crystallographic studies revealed that LASV NP is organized in two distinct domains [17]. The N-terminal domain contains a basic crevice, initially proposed to be an m7GTP cap binding site and later reported to function in binding RNA [17,18]. The C-terminal domain of NP harbors a functional 3′-5′ exoribonuclease activity of the DExD/H-box protein family that has been shown to oppose the host type I interferon (IFN-I)-mediated immune response during viral infection. In this regard, NP is capable of degrading small viral doubled-stranded RNA fragments that could function as pathogen-associated molecular patterns, to prevent their recognition by cellular pattern recognition receptors (PRRs) [17,19–21]. In addition, the role of NP in the negative regulation of IFN-I production has been linked to its ability to prevent the nuclear translocation and transcriptional activity of the nuclear factor kappa B (NF-kB), and its direct association with the retinoic acid-inducible gene I (RIG-I) and I-kappa-B kinase epsilon (IKKε), thereby inhibiting the activation and nuclear translocation of the interferon regulatory factor 3 (IRF-3) [22–24].

Following arenavirus entry, nucleocapsids are delivered into the cytoplasm of the host cell where transcription and replication of viral RNA segments occur. The arenavirus Z protein directs the assembly and budding of infectious particles from the plasma membrane, co-opting proteins from the endosomal sorting complexes required for transport (ESCRT) that facilitate virus egress [25].

Over the past few years, a significant amount of novel information has accrued regarding cellular proteins that play a role in the arenavirus life cycle, including in pathogenesis, immune evasion and virus entry and egress [25–28]. Here, we summarize current knowledge on host factors that are involved in LASV entry and discuss factors crucial for LASV RNA replication. Deepening the knowledge about relevant virus-host interactions essential for sustaining these early critical steps may help identify possible targets for the rational design of novel therapeutic approaches against LASV and other arenaviruses that cause severe human disease.

2. Virus–Host Interactions Involved in LASV Entry

2.1. α-Dystroglycan (α-DG) Is the Principal Receptor for LASV Entry

Arenaviruses primarily attach to cells by binding of their surface GP to specific receptor/entry factors at the plasma membrane of host cells. α-DG was the first entry receptor discovered for LASV, as well as for other OW and for Clade C NW arenaviruses [29,30], and its interaction with GP has been widely characterized [31]. DG is expressed as a precursor and proteolytically cleaved to generate the mature α and β subunits that together serve as a molecular bridge between the extracellular matrix and the cytoplasm [32–35]. α-DG is found in the extracellular compartment, where it binds components such as laminin, and requires O-glycosylation to perform its biological functions [36,37], whereas the transmembrane β subunit (β-DG) docks to the cytoskeleton by associating to the cytoplasmic adaptor proteins dystrophin and utrophin [35,38,39]. DG is expressed in most cell types, but its expression patterns and glycosylation levels differ depending on the tissue [34,35].

Further reports on arenavirus biology provide evidence that the α-DG receptor requires a specific type of glycosylation for efficient virus attachment; in particular, O-mannosylation, rarely found in mammals [40,41]. LASV tightly binds to the "matriglycan" platform displayed on α-DG, a polymer composed of 3-xylose-α1, 3-glucuronic acid-β1 (Xylα1-3GlcAβ1-3) disaccharide repeats, which is linked to α-DG through phosphorylated O-mannose. Like-acetylglucosaminyltransferase (LARGE) is required for the attachment of ligand-binding moieties to phosphorylated O-mannose on α-DG [42]. Moreover, the recent determination of the crystal structure of the mature LASV and LCMV GPs in prefusion conformation demonstrates that the GP ectodomain engages matriglycan via multiple contacts, with a close similarity to the molecular mechanisms driving α-DG recognition of host extracellular matrix (ECM) proteins [43,44]. Therefore, it is reasonable to conceive that LASV would mimic the behavior of different host ECMs that normally interact with glycosylated membrane receptors to gain access to the cell. Indeed, post-translational modification of α-DG by the glycosyltransferase LARGE is required for both efficient LASV infection and laminin binding [45–47]. Mutagenesis and functional studies further identified two threonine (Thr) residues (Thr317 and Thr319) within a highly conserved amino acid motif in α-DG that play a key role in LARGE-mediated α-DG modification, and are required for recognition by LASV GP and laminin [48]. These findings further support the idea that arenaviruses displaying high affinity for α-DG may be able to compete with host ligands and displace them from the receptor to infiltrate the cell [45,48]. Thereafter, upon receptor recognition, the encounter of cellular α-DG with LASV GP induces tyrosine phosphorylation of β-DG's cytosolic domain as well as it triggers β-DG's dissociation from the cytoskeletal adaptor utrophin [49]. Then, it is envisioned that this later step of detachment of virus-bound DG from the actin-based cytoskeleton may ease subsequent endocytosis of the virus–receptor complex.

2.2. LASV Can Use Phosphatidylserine Receptors to Enter the Cell

The existence of alternative viral receptors was initially suggested by the observations that certain cell-types deficient in functional α-DG, i.e., hepatocytes, could be highly susceptible to LASV infection and that mice lacking the LARGE gene sustain LASV replication at a level comparable to that in wild-type mice [35,50]. cDNA library screening studies from Kawaoka's group singled out the Tyro3/Axl/Mer (TAM) receptor tyrosine kinases Axl and Tyro3/Dtk as potential LASV receptor candidates [51]. TAM family members are tyrosine-kinases which expose tandem immunoglobulin-related domains to the extracellular matrix. These domains interact with host protein S (ProS) and growth arrest-specific gene 6 (Gas6), which are serum proteins that bind the negatively charged phospholipid phosphatidylserine (PtdSer). PtdSer is translocated from the inner leaflet to the external leaflet of the plasma membrane in apoptotic cells, where it acts as a signal for professional phagocytes (macrophages and dendritic cells) as well as non-professional phagocytes (e.g., epithelial cells) [52,53]. TAM receptors have been shown to play a role in virus entry of several RNA viruses such as Ebola (EBOV), dengue (DENV) and Zika, through a mechanism termed "apoptotic mimicry" [54–56]. This mechanism involves recognition of PtdSer exposed on the viral surface, incorporated from the cellular lipid bilayer during the budding process, as a signal for virus uptake [57–59]. Of note, there is evidence that cells infected with the NW arenavirus Pichinde display PtdSer on their plasma membranes; therefore, it is reasonable to conceive that both NW and OW arenaviruses could benefit from PtdSer receptors for viral entry [60]. In the case of LASV, initial studies using a HIV-based lentiviral vector pseudotyped with LASV GP empirically confirmed the capability of Axl to facilitate viral entry to cells lacking optimal carbohydrate modification of α-DG or to DG knockout cells [51]. Experiments from the Choe's group applying alternative lentiviral pseudotyped platforms showed no enhancement of LASV (or LCMV) entry upon overexpression of Axl in human embryonic kidney (HEK-293T) cells [61] and hypothesized that LASV internalization via α-DG may be preferred over

PtdSer receptors. Later, experiments from the Kunz's group using a recombinant LCMV system expressing LASV GP (rLCMV-LASVGP) ultimately confirmed that the endogenous expression of Axl does not actually enhance viral entry in the presence of fully functional α-DG receptor but it strongly augments viral infection in the absence of α-DG [62].

In line with these findings, T-cell immunoglobulin mucin I (TIM-1) has also been recently identified as a PtdSer receptor for LASV entry [63]. TIM receptors are cell surface glycoproteins that display an extracellular immunoglobulin variable-like domain (IgV), bearing a structural pocket with high affinity for PtdSer [64]. Unlike TAM receptors, TIM directly binds PtdSer, without the need for the Gas6 or ProS adaptors. It was demonstrated that TIM-I also mediates entry of vesicular stomatitis virus pseudovirions bearing LASV GP, either in the absence of α-DG or under conditions where it is inadequately glycosylated [63]. This behavior resembles that of Axl, suggesting a similarity between the entry route promoted by TAM and TIM receptors. In this sense, although functional α-DG would be the first LASV receptor of choice, the use of PtdSer receptors could function as a non-canonical GP-independent mechanism exploited by the virus to expand the spectrum of cellular tropism.

2.3. DC-SIGN and LSECtin Lectin Receptors Can Mediate LASV Cell Entry

Two additional receptor candidates were identified in the cDNA screening studies [51]: dendritic cell-specific intercellular adhesion molecule -3 grabbing nonintegrin (DC-SIGN) and liver and lymph node sinusoidal endothelial calcium-dependent lectin (LSECtin), both of which belong to the calcium-dependent (C-type) family of lectins. Of note, there is previous evidence indicating that DC-SIGN can facilitate infection of the NW JUNV and other enveloped viruses, including EBOV and Rift Valley fever virus [65–67]. Likewise, LSECtin has been implicated in entry of EBOV, SARs coronavirus and Japanese encephalitis virus [68–70]. As observed for TAM receptors, both DC-SIGN and LSECtin enhanced the susceptibility of cells to infection by LASV GP-pseudotyped lentivirus and participate in LASV entry independently of α-DG [51]. These lectin receptors were more effective at enhancing virus infection than TAM receptors, but importantly, none of these alternative receptors showed higher efficiency than properly modified α-DG, the principal portal of entry for LASV [51] (Figure 1). It was also shown that DC-SIGN or LSECtin binding to LASV GP is carbohydrate-specific, a fact that is characteristic of this C-type lectins family [51]. Strikingly, experiments using monocyte-derived immature human dendritic cells (MDDCs), which lack expression of Axl and Tyro3, demonstrated that upregulated expression of DC-SIGN correlates with enhanced virus attachment and productive infection, and that highly mannosylated glycans exposed on LASV GP1 surface interact with DC-SIGN during attachment [71]. Thus, DC-SIGN and LSECtin may facilitate LASV entry into dendritic cells, which represent the preferred early targets for arenavirus infection [72,73].

2.4. LASV Entry Involves Macropinocytosis and Intracellular LAMP1 Receptor for Virus Fusion

Upon receptor binding, OW arenaviruses including LASV, enter the host cell by a clathrin-independent endocytic process followed by transport to late endosomal compartments, where pH-dependent fusion of viral and cell membrane takes place [74,75]. Strikingly, sodium hydrogen exchangers (NHEs) have been identified through a genome-wide small interfering RNA screen, as host factors involved in the multiplication of LCMV in human cells [76]. Based on pharmacological and genetic analysis, Iwasaki et al. further validated NHE as entry factors for LCMV and LASV, implicating macropinocytosis in arenavirus entry [77]. Moreover, using the pseudotyped rLCMV-LASVGP and a panel of specific inhibitors for cellular factors involved in the regulation of macropinocytosis, Oppliger et al. showed that DG-mediated LASV entry depends on regulatory factors, including NHE, associated with this pathway [78].

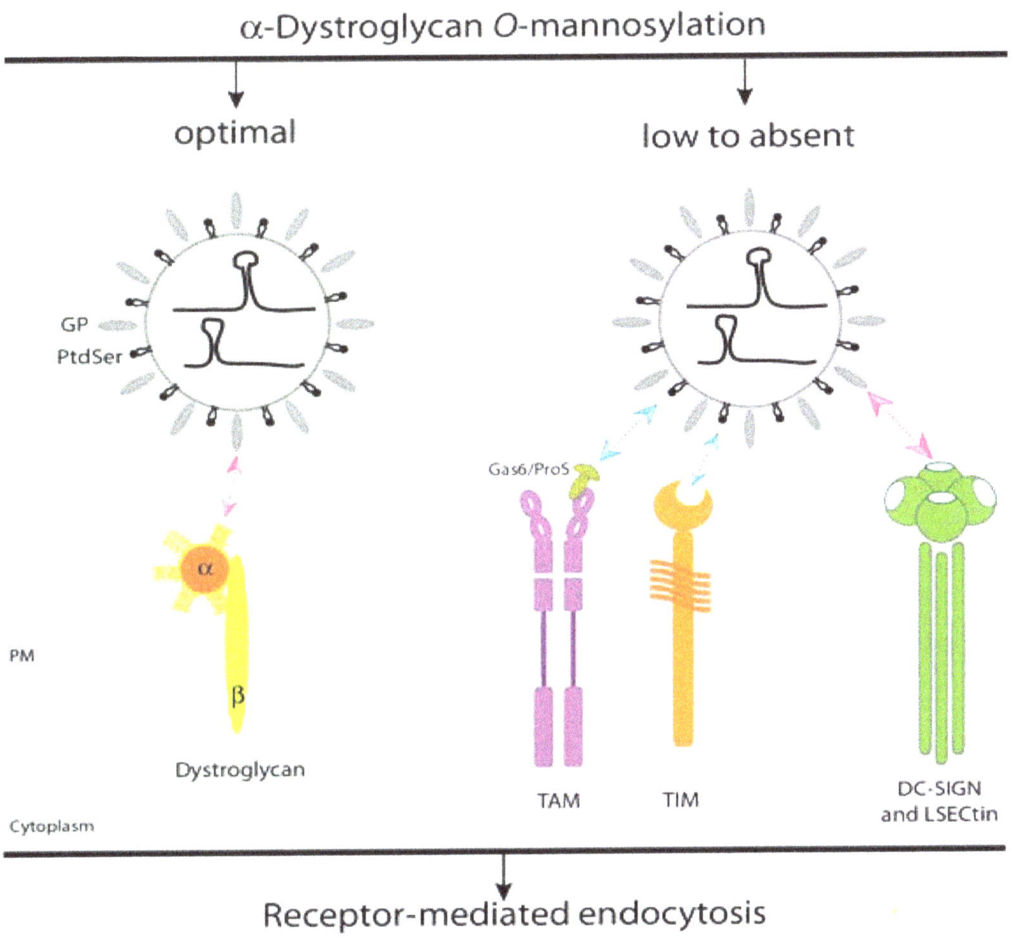

α-Dystroglycan *O*-mannosylation

Figure 1. Model of cell receptor/s recognition by Lassa virus (LASV). Left panel. The α-dystroglycan (α-DG) receptor needs to be *O*-mannosylated for efficient virus attachment. In the presence of a fully functional α-DG receptor, LASV enters host cells after binding to the matriglycan platform displayed on α-DG. Right panel. In the absence of α-DG or in conditions where it is inadequately glycosylated, phosphatidylserine (PtdSer)-binding receptors (TAM; TIM) and C-type lectin receptors (DC-SIGN; LSECtin) can mediate α-DG-independent entry. TAM kinases bind Gas6 or ProS serum proteins, which bind to PtdSer molecules exposed on the viral envelope membrane. TIM directly binds PtdSer, without a need for the Gas6 or ProS adaptors. C-type lectins interact with glycans on the LASV glycoprotein (GP). PM: plasma membrane; TAM: Tyro3/Axl/Mer; TIM: T-cell immunoglobulin mucin; DC-SIGN: dendritic cell-specific intercellular adhesion molecule-3 nonintegrin; LSECtin: liver and lymph node sinusoidal endothelial calcium-dependent lectin. Cartoon diagram not to scale.

An unbiased haploid genetic screening in α-DG-deficient cells pinpointed the lysosome-associated membrane protein 1 (LAMP1) as a late endosomal co-receptor specifically required for efficient LASV entry [79]. LAMP1 is mostly found in lysosomes, but it also locates in other endosomal structures. It is hypothesized that the acidic pH of the late endosome destabilizes the high affinity interaction between LASV GP and α-DG, resulting in a "receptor switch" to LAMP1. In this sense, LAMP1 would work as a secondary intracellular receptor that helps induce the GP conformational changes needed for virus fusion. This interpretation is supported by a series of biochemical studies that demonstrated that LAMP1 directly interacts with LASV GP in a pre-fusion configuration, and which described that the strength of this interaction is modulated by pH conditions, where a drop in pH can destabilize LASV GP affinity for α-DG, thereby inducing potent binding to LAMP1 [79]. Furthermore, structural and functional studies showed that LASV GP1 conformation is stable at low pH conditions, at which it displays a triad of histidine residues that are involved in LAMP1 binding [80,81]. In this regard, LAMP1 facilitates LASV exit from earlier endosomal compartments, avoiding prolonged exposure to a harsh proteolytic environment, increasing the overall efficiency of LASV entry and infection [82]. Besides LAMP1, the haploid genetics screening also pointed out α-2,3-sialyltransferase ST3GAL4, as well as additional factors involved in N-glycosylation and sialylation, as being important for LASV entry. Mutations in ST3GAL4, yielding a specific deficiency in sialylation of LAMP1, totally abrogate its ability to interact with LASV GP [79]. This highlights the strict requirement of a specific glycosylated version of LAMP1 for the biochemical interaction with GP to take place. In sum, it is envisioned that LASV would initially attach to the cell surface via α-DG, a step which would lead to delivery of virions to endosomes. Later, as virus-containing vesicles acidify, LASV would dissociate from the α-DG receptor, gaining affinity for LAMP1, and therefore completing the internalization process in a LASV-unique manner that is distinguishable from a standard endocytic process [83,84].

Altogether, these findings describing virus–host interactions involved in LASV entry disclose the diverse spectrum of mechanisms implemented by the virus to efficiently fulfill its internalization and fusion. On the one hand, the ability to utilize entry strategies alternative to α-DG receptor (such as PtdSer or lectin receptors), provides the virion with versatility to enlarge its cell tropism and promotes access to selected cell-targets such as dendritic cells, which are high privileged sites for early LASV productive infection. On the other side, LASV engagement of the late endosomal receptor LAMP1 likely guarantees the optimal spatial conditions required for virus fusion in close proximity to the endosome membrane. Given that not only α-DG- but also Axl-mediated entry involve LAMP1 co-factor [62], it is conceivable that multiple pathways converge at similar late endosomal compartments to efficiently accomplish LASV entry.

3. Role of Virus–Host Interactions Involving the LASV Replication Complex

3.1. Role of DEAD-Box RNA Helicase 3 (DDX3) in Viral Replication

A series of large-scale proteomic studies applying mass-spectrometry have been undertaken to comprehensively identify novel human protein candidates that could interact with the arenavirus proteins [85–89]. Special attention has been paid to NP-binding partners due to the multifunctional role of NP in the viral cycle, which involves crucial interactions with L and Z viral proteins [12,13,15–17,90], and its ability to hijack host factors to inhibit the antiviral innate immune response [19,22,24,91]. It is believed that identifying essential NP–host cell protein interactions can pave the way in the rational design of novel strategies to tackle arenavirus infections. One of the LASV NP interactors recently identified in human cells is DDX3, a protein belonging to the DEAD (Asp-Glu-Ala-Asp) box RNA helicase family, which harbors ATPase and RNA helicase activities [89]. Of note, DDX3 has also emerged in proteomic studies of virus-infected cells, as a novel interacting partner of the OW LCMV and the NW JUNV NPs [85]. CRISPR/Cas9-mediated deletion of DDX3 gene has been shown to lead to a significant reduction in virus yields of LASV, LCMV or JUNV in cell culture. Subsequently, lentiviral-mediated reconstitution of DDX3 expression resulted in a notable recovery in the infection rate of the three viruses, indicating a relevant role of DDX3 in virus growth as a proviral cellular factor [89].

DDX3 is known to be involved in multiple steps of RNA metabolism, including RNA transcription and the initiation of translation in host cells [92–94]. As other DEAD-box RNA helicases, such as DDX1 and DDX5, DDX3 appears to facilitate replication of different RNA viruses, as the alphavirus Venezuelan equine encephalitis virus and the hepatitis C virus (HCV), among others [95–100]. DDX3 is also required for translation of mRNAs containing a long or structured 5′ untranslated region (UTR), such as human immunodeficiency virus type-1 (HIV-1) genomic RNA (gRNA). Indeed, it was reported that DDX3 interacts with the 5′ region of the target mRNA, binds the eukaryotic translation initiation factor 4G (eIF4G) and poly A-binding protein cytoplasmic 1 (PABP), and interacts with HIV-1 Tat protein to facilitate translation of HIV-1 mRNAs [96,101]. In reference to arenaviruses, it was demonstrated that translation of a synthetic arenavirus mRNA analog was unaffected in DDX3-deficient cells, indicating no critical engagement of DDX3 in viral mRNA translation initiation [89]. In contrast, minireplicon assay-based experiments demonstrated that the pro-arenaviral activity of DDX3 strongly depends on DDX3's ability to promote viral RNA synthesis, involving both previously described DDX3 ATPase and helicase RNA-unwinding activities in this function [89,102].

Strikingly, alternative roles have been ascribed to DDX3 in the context of different viral infections [103,104]. On the one hand, DDX3 is considered an antiviral factor given that it is involved in the innate immune response against some viruses such as HIV-1, DENV and HCV [105–107]. DDX3 has been shown to collaborate in the production of IFN-I, through interaction with components of the RIG-I-mediated IFN-I induction pathway [108–110]. However, in contrast to this IFN-I promoting capacity of DDX3, mechanistic analysis has provided evidence that, in the case of LCMV, DDX3 suppresses the IFN-I response at late times of infection, still it remains to be confirmed whether this IFN-I-suppressive role of DDX3 is sustained in the context of an infection with the pathogenic LASV [89]. Secondly, DDX3 is known to be an essential component for stress granule (SG) assembly, and to interact with other SG proteins, such as eIF4E [111]. Different proteomic approaches based on mass-spectrometry have singled out new arenavirus NP-binding candidates related to the SG biology; including but not limited to the Ras GTPase-activating protein-binding protein 1 (G3BP1), eIF2α, apoptosis-inducing factor mitochondrion-associated 1 (AIFM1) and PABP, yet none of them have been confirmed as LASV interactors by alternative biochemical methods [85,89]. Of note, colocalization experiments have revealed the association of the NW arenavirus TCRV replication–transcription complexes (RTCs), where NP accumulates, with G3BP1 and a non-canonical collection of ribosomal proteins, including the ribosomal proteins RPS6 and RPL10a, as well as translation initiation factors eIF4G and eIF4A [112]. In this regard, the finding that JUNV infection inhibits SG formation [113] might be related to the NP-mediated sequestration of DDX3 and other SG-related proteins, resulting in the lack of availability of essential factors needed for SG nucleation. Similarly, in the case of influenza virus infections, it has been hypothesized that the interaction of DDX3 with the viral NS1 protein prevents DDX3 binding to eIF4E and PABP1 as well as DDX3–NP interaction, thus suppressing SG formation, NP recruitment into SGs, and DDX3 antiviral activity [114]. Therefore, it is possible that in a similar way, LASV NP may counteract DDX3 antiviral function and in turn use DDX3 to enhance its own replication.

3.2. Other RNA Helicases Potentially Involved in LASV Replication

In addition to DDX3, a number of cellular proteins functionally related to RNA biosynthesis and ribonucleoprotein complex assembly, including the DEAD-box helicase 5 (DDX5, also referred to as RNA helicase p68) and RNA helicase A (namely DHX9), members of the DExD/Hbox protein family, have been identified as potential overlapping targets of the LCMV L protein and the NP of LASV, LCMV, and/or JUNV (Figure 2) [85,87,89]. Moreover, they have already been confirmed as interactors of the RNA-dependent RNA polymerase (RdRp) of other RNA viruses. For example, DDX5 has been shown to interact with the C-terminal region of HCV NS5B, and has been suggested to be part of the HCV replicase complex [115]. Similarly, DDX5 associates with the influenza A virus PB1 and PB2 proteins [116] and it is needed for an efficient activity of the viral polymerase [117]. Evidence has been provided that DHX9 interacts with the viral genomic RNA and non-structural protein 3 (nsP3) within active replication complexes in Chikungunya virus (CHIKV)-infected cells, displaying an inhibitory effect on viral RNA synthesis and an enhancing effect on viral genome translation, which may imply a regulatory role in CHIKV life cycle [118]. Porcine reproductive and respiratory syndrome virus (family *Arteriviridae*) nucleocapsid protein interacts with DHX9 polymerase to overcome premature termination of viral RNA synthesis [119]. Overall, DExD/H-box helicases emerge as host factors selectively hijacked by polymerases and nucleocapsid or nonstructural proteins from several viruses to facilitate their multiplication. Further work must be carried out to validate the binding of DDX5 and DHX9 helicases to LASV and/or other arenavirus proteins and provide a mechanistic model that could explain the relevance of these interactions.

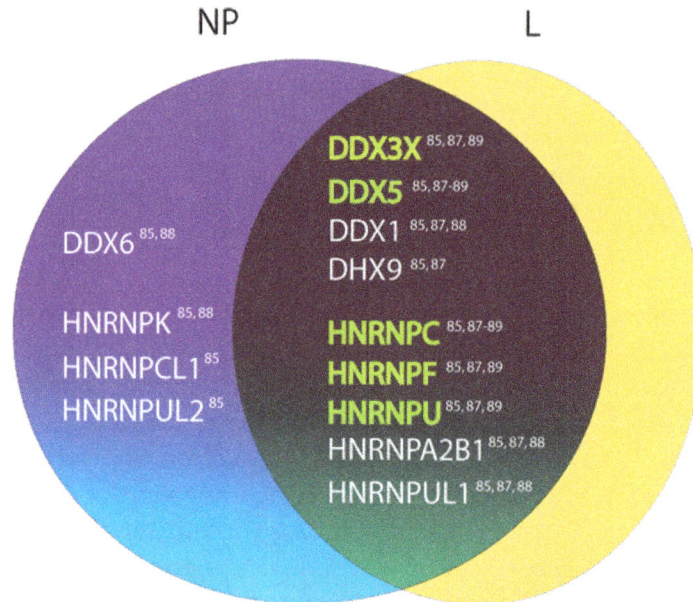

Figure 2. Cellular DExD/H-box helicases and heterogeneous nuclear ribonucleoproteins (hnRNPs) identified among binding partners of the nucleoproteins (NPs) of LASV, lymphocytic choriomeningitis virus (LCMV), and/or Junín virus (JUNV) in different proteomics approaches [85,88,89]. Targets common to the LCMV L polymerase [87] are depicted. LASV NP binding partners are highlighted in green. References are indicated for each target.

Given the observation that many host factors converge as common binding-partners of RNA viruses, it is intriguing whether this is a consequence of the conserved conformational structure shared among proteins from different families of viruses. In particular, segmented negative strand viruses (sNSV) polymerases share key conserved motifs, specifically those corresponding to the fingers, palm and thumb subdomains within the RdRp domain located in the central part of the polypeptide chain. The central ring-like RdRp domain is linked to appendages that would be dedicated to 5′ mRNA capping activities [120–123]. Based on the amino acid sequence motif conservation displayed by sNSV polymerases and the structural similarity between the polymerases of the bunyavirus La Crosse encephalitis virus and influenza virus revealed by crystallographic studies, an overall structural configuration has been proposed for arenavirus L protein. It consists of a canonical RdRp core with N- and C- extensions that form a cavity connected to the exterior by four tunnels (NTP entry, template entry, template exit, and product exit) [124,125]. Structural information has led to a model for sNSV vRNA synthesis in which the L protein would operate in either transcription mode or replication mode, not only during initiation, but also along the whole RNA synthesis process [125,126]. A key question that needs to be addressed is how the polymerase switches from one mode to the other. For arenaviruses, there is genetic and biochemical evidence that L–L interaction is essential for polymerase activity, suggesting that the L polymerase may function in an oligomeric conformation [127]. Thus, as proposed for influenza virus [128,129], a conformational transition of the polymerase from a monomeric state during transcription to an oligomeric state during replication might be hypothesized. In this sense, it is probable that the association with cellular partners may additionally modulate the switch from the transcriptase to the replicase mode of the arenavirus polymerase. To date, DDX3 is the sole NP and L protein interactor for LASV or any other arenavirus that has been demonstrated to contribute in viral RNA synthesis, although the precise underlying mechanism remains to be fully understood. However, it is tempting to speculate that the binding of DDX3 (and eventually other cellular RNA helicases) with NP and L in a replicase complex, may contribute to the unwinding of viral RNA secondary structures such as RNA hairpins within the non-coding intergenic regions, which must be read-through during replication to accomplish full length genome and antigenome RNA synthesis. Likewise, DDX3 and/or other host helicases may facilitate encapsidation of the nascent chain by NP during replication.

3.3. Host Heterogeneous Nuclear Ribonucleoproteins as Candidate Factors Required for the LASV Life Cycle

Other host factors that have recently emerged as potential candidate partners of LASV as well as LCMV and JUNV NP and/or L polymerase are the components of the heterogeneous nuclear ribonucleoprotein (hnRNP) family, including hnRNPA2/B1, one of the most abundant hnRNPs belonging to the A/B type [85,88,89]. HnRNPs are RNA-binding proteins involved in processing pre-mRNAs as well as in mRNA translation, trafficking and stability. Notably, previous reports have already demonstrated the interaction between JUNV NP and hnRNP A1 and that depletion of hnRNP A1 and A2 caused a strong inhibition of virus yield, suggesting a key role of hnRNPs A/B in JUNV multiplication [130]. Additionally, hnRNP K, an LCMV and JUNV NP binding partner detected in the proteomic screening by King et al. [85], has also been reported as a necessary host factor required for JUNV multiplication [131]. Likewise, studies from different groups have similarly ascribed relevant functions to hnRNPs in other viral infections. For example, hnRNP A2/B1 has been proposed to work as a positive regulator in viral RNA synthesis of influenza A virus, hnRNP A2 has been shown to regulate the trafficking of HIV-1 genomic RNA, and hnRNP K has been shown to support vesicular stomatitis virus replication by regulating cell survival and cellular gene expression [132–134]. Altogether, although further research needs to be completed to unveil the importance of hnRNPs in the *Arenaviridae* family, it is intriguing whether any of these proteins would specifically associate with the LASV RNP complex, playing a critical function either in viral genome transcription and/or replication.

3.4. Z Protein Interactors

Arenavirus Z matrix protein has been proposed to drive a mechanism to ensure accurate packaging of all necessary virion components. Apart from its pivotal role in virus assembly and budding [135,136], Z also inhibits viral RNA synthesis by directly binding the L polymerase to trigger its catalytic inactivation, and this can still occur in the absence of host cellular factors [137,138]. Of note, it has been hypothesized that the Z–L complex not only guarantees downregulation of viral gene expression, but also serves as a platform for the functional polymerase to remain locked on the template and be properly packaged into the mature virion [138]. Interestingly, a recent proteomics approach based on JUNV Z has pinpointed a number of targets that were incorporated to Z virus-like particles (VLPs) and purified JUNV particles and which include common interactors of the L and NP proteins, such as DDX3, DDX5, DHX9, hnRNPA2/B1, and PABP [86]. Actually, this is not a totally unexpected observation. For instance, it has been demonstrated for HIV-1 that DHX9 protein stimulates transcription of HIV-1 RNA as well as it associates with the Gag protein to ensure it is adequately recruited into virus particles during the assembly process [139]. In line with this, it is predictable that the association of Z protein with key cellular factors required for viral RNA synthesis may concomitantly facilitate virus packaging and/or make these factors available to complement the activity of viral RNP upon cell entry.

4. Concluding Remarks

LASV is currently considered a top priority emerging pathogen causing severe hemorrhagic fever outbreaks [140]. At this moment, treatment is limited to the nonspecific antiviral ribavirin, shown to be partially effective in LASV infections [141], and the use of favipiravir is still under investigation [142,143]. Moreover, there is no FDA-approved vaccine against LASV or any other arenavirus to date. Therefore, there is an urgent need to develop novel approaches to combat and prevent the infection with these viruses.

In the last years, several reports have provided robust evidence that LASV can utilize alternative entry factors apart from the well-characterized α-DG [144]. Novel lectin and PtdSer receptors have emerged as non-canonical LASV ports of entry, proposed to enhance the viral cell tropism and/or redirect infection to selected cell types.

Studies on virus–host interactions have also improved our understanding of the mechanisms driving LASV replication. A recent series of proteomic approaches oriented to the analysis of the interactome of arenavirus NP, L, and Z proteins in human cells singled out several host factors, such as DExD/H-box helicases and heterogeneous nuclear RNPs, which might be potentially involved in arenavirus RNA synthesis. Particularly, it was demonstrated that the DDX3 ATP-dependent RNA helicase is a LASV target and may be dually exploited to both suppress the host immunity and promote viral replication and/or transcription, since DDX3 ATPase and helicase activities are involved in promoting optimal levels of viral RNA synthesis. Notably, it has recently been reported that a chemical compound directed to an RNA binding site of DDX3 protein displayed broad-spectrum antiviral activity against HIV drug-resistant strains, HCV, DENV, and West Nile virus infection [145]. In this regard, it is intriguing whether the use of DDX3-blocking compounds could be tentatively applied as a novel weapon to battle LASV infections.

Acknowledgments: The authors would like to apologize to all those researchers whose excellent studies were not included in this review due to space limitations.

References

1. Maes, P.; Alkhovsky, S.V.; Bao, Y.; Beer, M.; Birkhead, M.; Briese, T.; Buchmeier, M.J.; Calisher, C.H.; Charrel, R.N.; Choi, I.R.; et al. Taxonomy of the family Arenaviridae and the order Bunyavirales: Update 2018. *Arch. Virol.* **2018**, *163*, 2295–2310. [CrossRef]

2. Basler, C.F. Molecular pathogenesis of viral hemorrhagic fever. *Semin. Immunopathol.* **2017**, *39*, 551–561. [CrossRef] [PubMed]

3. Ogbu, O.; Ajuluchukwu, E.; Uneke, C.J. Lassa fever in West African sub-region: An overview. *J. Vector Borne Dis.* **2007**, *44*, 1–11. [PubMed]

4. Cashman, K.A.; Wilkinson, E.R.; Zeng, X.; Cardile, A.P.; Facemire, P.R.; Bell, T.M.; Bearss, J.J.; Shaia, C.I.; Schmaljohn, C.S. Immune-Mediated Systemic Vasculitis as the Proposed Cause of Sudden-Onset Sensorineural Hearing Loss following Lassa Virus Exposure in Cynomolgus Macaques. *mBio* **2018**, *9*, e01896-18. [CrossRef] [PubMed]

5. Mateer, E.J.; Huang, C.; Shehu, N.Y.; Paessler, S. Lassa fever-induced sensorineural hearing loss: A neglected public health and social burden. *PLoS Negl. Trop. Dis.* **2018**, *12*, e0006187. [CrossRef]

6. Buchmeier, M.J.; De la Torre, J.C.; Peters, C.J. *Arenaviridae: The Viruses and Their Replication*; Wolters Kluwer Health/Lippincott Williams & Wilkins: Philadelphia, PA, USA, 2007.

7. Kiening, M.; Weber, F.; Frishman, D. Conserved RNA structures in the intergenic regions of ambisense viruses. *Sci. Rep.* **2017**, *7*, 16625. [CrossRef]

8. Eschli, B.; Quirin, K.; Wepf, A.; Weber, J.; Zinkernagel, R.; Hengartner, H. Identification of an N-terminal trimeric coiled-coil core within arenavirus glycoprotein 2 permits assignment to class I viral fusion proteins. *J. Virol.* **2006**, *80*, 5897–5907. [CrossRef]

9. Burri, D.J.; da Palma, J.R.; Kunz, S.; Pasquato, A. Envelope glycoprotein of arenaviruses. *Viruses* **2012**, *4*, 2162–2181. [CrossRef]

10. Hastie, K.M.; Saphire, E.O. Lassa virus glycoprotein: Stopping a moving target. *Curr. Opin. Virol.* **2018**, *31*, 52–58. [CrossRef]

11. Hass, M.; Golnitz, U.; Muller, S.; Becker-Ziaja, B.; Gunther, S. Replicon system for Lassa virus. *J. Virol.* **2004**, *78*, 13793–13803. [CrossRef]

12. Lee, K.J.; Novella, I.S.; Teng, M.N.; Oldstone, M.B.; de La Torre, J.C. NP and L proteins of lymphocytic choriomeningitis virus (LCMV) are sufficient for efficient transcription and replication of LCMV genomic RNA analogs. *J. Virol.* **2000**, *74*, 3470–3477. [CrossRef]

13. Lopez, N.; Jacamo, R.; Franze-Fernandez, M.T. Transcription and RNA replication of tacaribe virus genome and antigenome analogs require N and L proteins: Z protein is an inhibitor of these processes. *J. Virol.* **2001**, *75*, 12241–12251. [CrossRef] [PubMed]

14. Casabona, J.C.; Levingston Macleod, J.M.; Loureiro, M.E.; Gomez, G.A.; Lopez, N. The RING domain and the L79 residue of Z protein are involved in both the rescue of nucleocapsids and the incorporation of glycoproteins into infectious chimeric arenavirus-like particles. *J. Virol.* **2009**, *83*, 7029–7039. [CrossRef]

15. Ortiz-Riano, E.; Cheng, B.Y.; de la Torre, J.C.; Martinez-Sobrido, L. The C-terminal region of lymphocytic choriomeningitis virus nucleoprotein contains distinct and segregable functional domains involved in NP-Z interaction and counteraction of the type I interferon response. *J. Virol.* **2011**, *85*, 13038–13048. [CrossRef] [PubMed]

16. Shtanko, O.; Imai, M.; Goto, H.; Lukashevich, I.S.; Neumann, G.; Watanabe, T.; Kawaoka, Y. A role for the C terminus of Mopeia virus nucleoprotein in its incorporation into Z protein-induced virus-like particles. *J. Virol.* **2010**, *84*, 5415–5422. [CrossRef] [PubMed]

17. Qi, X.; Lan, S.; Wang, W.; Schelde, L.M.; Dong, H.; Wallat, G.D.; Ly, H.; Liang, Y.; Dong, C. Cap binding and immune evasion revealed by Lassa nucleoprotein structure. *Nature* **2010**, *468*, 779–783. [CrossRef] [PubMed]

18. Hastie, K.M.; Liu, T.; Li, S.; King, L.B.; Ngo, N.; Zandonatti, M.A.; Woods, V.L.; de la Torre, J.C., Jr.; Saphire, E.O. Crystal structure of the Lassa virus nucleoprotein-RNA complex reveals a gating mechanism for RNA binding. *Proc. Natl. Acad. Sci. USA* **2011**, *108*, 19365–19370. [CrossRef] [PubMed]

19. Carnec, X.; Baize, S.; Reynard, S.; Diancourt, L.; Caro, V.; Tordo, N.; Bouloy, M. Lassa virus nucleoprotein mutants generated by reverse genetics induce a robust type I interferon response in human dendritic cells and macrophages. *J. Virol.* **2011**, *85*, 12093–12097. [CrossRef]

20. Reynard, S.; Russier, M.; Fizet, A.; Carnec, X.; Baize, S. Exonuclease domain of the Lassa virus nucleoprotein is critical to avoid RIG-I signaling and to inhibit the innate immune response. *J. Virol.* **2014**, *88*, 13923–13927. [CrossRef]

21. Huang, Q.; Shao, J.; Lan, S.; Zhou, Y.; Xing, J.; Dong, C.; Liang, Y.; Ly, H. In vitro and in vivo characterizations of the Pichinde viral NP exoribonuclease function. *J. Virol.* **2015**, *89*, 6595–6607. [CrossRef]

22. Pythoud, C.; Rodrigo, W.W.; Pasqual, G.; Rothenberger, S.; Martinez-Sobrido, L.; de la Torre, J.C.; Kunz, S. Arenavirus nucleoprotein targets interferon regulatory factor-activating kinase IKKepsilon. *J. Virol.* **2012**, *86*, 7728–7738. [CrossRef] [PubMed]

23. Rodrigo, W.W.; Ortiz-Riano, E.; Pythoud, C.; Kunz, S.; de la Torre, J.C.; Martinez-Sobrido, L. Arenavirus nucleoproteins prevent activation of nuclear factor kappa B. *J. Virol.* **2012**, *86*, 8185–8197. [CrossRef] [PubMed]

24. Zhou, S.; Cerny, A.M.; Zacharia, A.; Fitzgerald, K.A.; Kurt-Jones, E.A.; Finberg, R.W. Induction and inhibition of type I interferon responses by distinct components of lymphocytic choriomeningitis virus. *J. Virol.* **2010**, *84*, 9452–9462. [CrossRef] [PubMed]

25. Urata, S.; Yasuda, J. Molecular mechanism of arenavirus assembly and budding. *Viruses* **2012**, *4*, 2049–2079. [CrossRef]

26. Shao, J.; Liang, Y.; Ly, H. Human hemorrhagic Fever causing arenaviruses: Molecular mechanisms contributing to virus virulence and disease pathogenesis. *Pathogens* **2015**, *4*, 283–306. [CrossRef] [PubMed]

27. Hayes, M.; Salvato, M. Arenavirus evasion of host anti-viral responses. *Viruses* **2012**, *4*, 2182–2196. [CrossRef]

28. Fedeli, C.; Moreno, H.; Kunz, S. Novel Insights into Cell Entry of Emerging Human Pathogenic Arenaviruses. *J. Mol. Biol.* **2018**, *430*, 1839–1852. [CrossRef] [PubMed]

29. Cao, W.; Henry, M.D.; Borrow, P.; Yamada, H.; Elder, J.H.; Ravkov, E.V.; Nichol, S.T.; Compans, R.W.; Campbell, K.P.; Oldstone, M.B. Identification of alpha-dystroglycan as a receptor for lymphocytic choriomeningitis virus and Lassa fever virus. *Science* **1998**, *282*, 2079–2081. [CrossRef] [PubMed]

30. Spiropoulou, C.F.; Kunz, S.; Rollin, P.E.; Campbell, K.P.; Oldstone, M.B. New World arenavirus clade C, but not clade A and B viruses, utilizes alpha-dystroglycan as its major receptor. *J. Virol.* **2002**, *76*, 5140–51463. [CrossRef]

31. Acciani, M.; Alston, J.T.; Zhao, G.; Reynolds, H.; Ali, A.M.; Xu, B.; Brindley, M. Mutational analysis of Lassa virus glycoprotein highlights regions required for alpha-dystroglycan utilization. *J. Virol.* **2017**, *91*, e00574-17. [CrossRef]

32. Holt, K.H.; Crosbie, R.H.; Venzke, D.P.; Campbell, K.P. Biosynthesis of dystroglycan: Processing of a precursor propeptide. *FEBS Lett.* **2000**, *468*, 79–83. [CrossRef]

33. Ibraghimov-Beskrovnaya, O.; Ervasti, J.M.; Leveille, C.J.; Slaughter, C.A.; Sernett, S.W.; Campbell, K.P. Primary structure of dystrophin-associated glycoproteins linking dystrophin to the extracellular matrix. *Nature* **1992**, *355*, 696–702. [CrossRef]

34. Ibraghimov-Beskrovnaya, O.; Milatovich, A.; Ozcelik, T.; Yang, B.; Koepnick, K.; Francke, U.; Campbell, K.P. Human dystroglycan: Skeletal muscle cDNA, genomic structure, origin of tissue specific isoforms and chromosomal localization. *Hum. Mol. Genet.* **1993**, *2*, 1651–1657. [CrossRef]

35. Barresi, R.; Campbell, K.P. Dystroglycan: From biosynthesis to pathogenesis of human disease. *J. Cell Sci.* **2006**, *119*, 199–207. [CrossRef] [PubMed]

36. Ervasti, J.M.; Campbell, K.P. A role for the dystrophin-glycoprotein complex as a transmembrane linker between laminin and actin. *J. Cell Biol.* **1993**, *122*, 809–823. [CrossRef] [PubMed]

37. Michele, D.E.; Campbell, K.P. Dystrophin-glycoprotein complex: Post-translational processing and dystroglycan function. *J. Biol. Chem.* **2003**, *278*, 15457–15460. [CrossRef] [PubMed]

38. Ervasti, J.M.; Campbell, K.P. Membrane organization of the dystrophin-glycoprotein complex. *Cell* **1991**, *66*, 1121–1131. [CrossRef]

39. Chung, W.; Campanelli, J.T. WW and EF hand domains of dystrophin-family proteins mediate dystroglycan binding. *Mol. Cell Biol. Res. Commun. MCBRC* **1999**, *2*, 162–171. [CrossRef]

40. Imperiali, M.; Thoma, C.; Pavoni, E.; Brancaccio, A.; Callewaert, N.; Oxenius, A. O Mannosylation of alpha-dystroglycan is essential for lymphocytic choriomeningitis virus receptor function. *J. Virol.* **2005**, *79*, 14297–14308. [CrossRef]

41. Kunz, S.; Rojek, J.M.; Kanagawa, M.; Spiropoulou, C.F.; Barresi, R.; Campbell, K.P.; Oldstone, M.B. Posttranslational modification of alpha-dystroglycan, the cellular receptor for arenaviruses, by the glycosyltransferase LARGE is critical for virus binding. *J. Virol.* **2005**, *79*, 14282–14296. [CrossRef]

42. Yoshida-Moriguchi, T.; Campbell, K.P. Matriglycan: A novel polysaccharide that links dystroglycan to the basement membrane. *Glycobiology* **2015**, *25*, 702–713. [CrossRef] [PubMed]

43. Hastie, K.M.; Igonet, S.; Sullivan, B.M.; Legrand, P.; Zandonatti, M.A.; Robinson, J.E.; Garry, R.F.; Rey, F.A.; Oldstone, M.B.; Saphire, E.O. Crystal structure of the prefusion surface glycoprotein of the prototypic arenavirus LCMV. *Nat. Struct. Mol. Biol.* **2016**, *23*, 513–521. [CrossRef]

44. Hastie, K.M.; Zandonatti, M.A.; Kleinfelter, L.M.; Heinrich, M.L.; Rowland, M.M.; Chandran, K.; Branco, L.M.; Robinson, J.E.; Garry, R.F.; Saphire, E.O. Structural basis for antibody-mediated neutralization of Lassa virus. *Science* **2017**, *356*, 923–928. [CrossRef] [PubMed]

45. Kunz, S.; Rojek, J.M.; Perez, M.; Spiropoulou, C.F.; Oldstone, M.B. Characterization of the interaction of lassa fever virus with its cellular receptor alpha-dystroglycan. *J. Virol.* **2005**, *79*, 5979–5987. [CrossRef] [PubMed]

46. Rojek, J.M.; Spiropoulou, C.F.; Campbell, K.P.; Kunz, S. Old World and clade C New World arenaviruses mimic the molecular mechanism of receptor recognition used by alpha-dystroglycan's host-derived ligands. *J. Virol.* **2007**, *81*, 5685–5695. [CrossRef] [PubMed]

47. Kanagawa, M.; Saito, F.; Kunz, S.; Yoshida-Moriguchi, T.; Barresi, R.; Kobayashi, Y.M.; Muschler, J.; Dumanski, J.P.; Michele, D.E.; Oldstone, M.B.; et al. Molecular recognition by LARGE is essential for expression of functional dystroglycan. *Cell* **2004**, *117*, 953–964. [CrossRef]

48. Hara, Y.; Kanagawa, M.; Kunz, S.; Yoshida-Moriguchi, T.; Satz, J.S.; Kobayashi, Y.M.; Zhu, Z.; Burden, S.J.; Oldstone, M.B.; Campbell, K.P. Like-acetylglucosaminyltransferase (LARGE)-dependent modification of dystroglycan at Thr-317/319 is required for laminin binding and arenavirus infection. *Proc. Natl. Acad. Sci. USA* **2011**, *108*, 17426–17431. [CrossRef]

49. Moraz, M.L.; Pythoud, C.; Turk, R.; Rothenberger, S.; Pasquato, A.; Campbell, K.P.; Kunz, S. Cell entry of Lassa virus induces tyrosine phosphorylation of dystroglycan. *Cell. Microbiol.* **2013**, *15*, 689–700. [CrossRef] [PubMed]

50. Imperiali, M.; Sporri, R.; Hewitt, J.; Oxenius, A. Post-translational modification of {alpha}-dystroglycan is not critical for lymphocytic choriomeningitis virus receptor function in vivo. *J. Gen. Virol.* **2008**, *89*, 2713–2722. [CrossRef]

51. Shimojima, M.; Stroher, U.; Ebihara, H.; Feldmann, H.; Kawaoka, Y. Identification of cell surface molecules involved in dystroglycan-independent Lassa virus cell entry. *J. Virol.* **2012**, *86*, 2067–2078. [CrossRef]

52. Lemke, G.; Rothlin, C.V. Immunobiology of the TAM receptors. *Nat. Rev. Immunol.* **2008**, *8*, 327–336. [CrossRef] [PubMed]

53. Lemke, G. Biology of the TAM receptors. *Cold Spring Harb. Perspect. Biol.* **2013**, *5*, a009076. [CrossRef] [PubMed]

54. Shimojima, M.; Takada, A.; Ebihara, H.; Neumann, G.; Fujioka, K.; Irimura, T.; Jones, S.; Feldmann, H.; Kawaoka, Y. Tyro3 family-mediated cell entry of Ebola and Marburg viruses. *J. Virol.* **2006**, *80*, 10109–10116. [CrossRef] [PubMed]

55. Meertens, L.; Carnec, X.; Lecoin, M.P.; Ramdasi, R.; Guivel-Benhassine, F.; Lew, E.; Lemke, G.; Schwartz, O.; Amara, A. The TIM and TAM families of phosphatidylserine receptors mediate dengue virus entry. *Cell Host Microbe* **2012**, *12*, 544–557. [CrossRef] [PubMed]

56. Meertens, L.; Labeau, A.; Dejarnac, O.; Cipriani, S.; Sinigaglia, L.; Bonnet-Madin, L.; Le Charpentier, T.; Hafirassou, M.L.; Zamborlini, A.; Cao-Lormeau, V.M.; et al. Axl Mediates ZIKA Virus Entry in Human Glial Cells and Modulates Innate Immune Responses. *Cell Rep.* **2017**, *18*, 324–333. [CrossRef] [PubMed]

57. Morizono, K.; Xie, Y.; Olafsen, T.; Lee, B.; Dasgupta, A.; Wu, A.M.; Chen, I.S. The soluble serum protein Gas6 bridges virion envelope phosphatidylserine to the TAM receptor tyrosine kinase Axl to mediate viral entry. *Cell Host Microbe* **2011**, *9*, 286–298. [CrossRef] [PubMed]

58. Mercer, J.; Helenius, A. Vaccinia virus uses macropinocytosis and apoptotic mimicry to enter host cells. *Science* **2008**, *320*, 531–535. [CrossRef]

59. Amara, A.; Mercer, J. Viral apoptotic mimicry. *Nat. Rev. Microbiol.* **2015**, *13*, 461–469. [CrossRef]

60. Soares, M.M.; King, S.W.; Thorpe, P.E. Targeting inside-out phosphatidylserine as a therapeutic strategy for viral diseases. *Nat. Med.* **2008**, *14*, 1357–1362. [CrossRef]

61. Jemielity, S.; Wang, J.J.; Chan, Y.K.; Ahmed, A.A.; Li, W.; Monahan, S.; Bu, X.; Farzan, M.; Freeman, G.J.; Umetsu, D.T.; et al. TIM-family proteins promote infection of multiple enveloped viruses through virion-associated phosphatidylserine. *PLoS Pathog.* **2013**, *9*, e1003232. [CrossRef]

62. Fedeli, C.; Torriani, G.; Galan-Navarro, C.; Moraz, M.L.; Moreno, H.; Gerold, G.; Kunz, S. Axl Can Serve as Entry Factor for Lassa Virus Depending on the Functional Glycosylation of Dystroglycan. *J. Virol.* **2018**, *92*, e01613-17. [CrossRef] [PubMed]

63. Brouillette, R.B.; Phillips, E.K.; Patel, R.; Mahauad-Fernandez, W.; Moller-Tank, S.; Rogers, K.J.; Dillard, J.A.; Cooney, A.L.; Martinez-Sobrido, L.; Okeoma, C.; et al. TIM-1 Mediates Dystroglycan-Independent Entry of Lassa Virus. *J. Virol.* **2018**, *92*, e00093-18. [CrossRef] [PubMed]

64. Freeman, G.J.; Casasnovas, J.M.; Umetsu, D.T.; DeKruyff, R.H. TIM genes: A family of cell surface phosphatidylserine receptors that regulate innate and adaptive immunity. *Immunol. Rev.* **2010**, *235*, 172–189. [CrossRef] [PubMed]

65. Martinez, M.G.; Bialecki, M.A.; Belouzard, S.; Cordo, S.M.; Candurra, N.A.; Whittaker, G.R. Utilization of human DC-SIGN and L-SIGN for entry and infection of host cells by the New World arenavirus, Junin virus. *Biochem. Biophys. Res. Commun.* **2013**, *441*, 612–617. [CrossRef]

66. Leger, P.; Tetard, M.; Youness, B.; Cordes, N.; Rouxel, R.N.; Flamand, M.; Lozach, P.Y. Differential Use of the C-Type Lectins L-SIGN and DC-SIGN for Phlebovirus Endocytosis. *Traffic* **2016**, *17*, 639–656. [CrossRef]

67. Alvarez, C.P.; Lasala, F.; Carrillo, J.; Muniz, O.; Corbi, A.L.; Delgado, R. C-type lectins DC-SIGN and L-SIGN mediate cellular entry by Ebola virus in cis and in trans. *J. Virol.* **2002**, *76*, 6841–6844. [CrossRef]

68. Powlesland, A.S.; Fisch, T.; Taylor, M.E.; Smith, D.F.; Tissot, B.; Dell, A.; Pohlmann, S.; Drickamer, K. A novel mechanism for LSECtin binding to Ebola virus surface glycoprotein through truncated glycans. *J. Biol. Chem.* **2008**, *283*, 593–602. [CrossRef]

69. Gramberg, T.; Hofmann, H.; Moller, P.; Lalor, P.F.; Marzi, A.; Geier, M.; Krumbiegel, M.; Winkler, T.; Kirchhoff, F.; Adams, D.H.; et al. LSECtin interacts with filovirus glycoproteins and the spike protein of SARS coronavirus. *Virology* **2005**, *340*, 224–236. [CrossRef]

70. Shimojima, M.; Takenouchi, A.; Shimoda, H.; Kimura, N.; Maeda, K. Distinct usage of three C-type lectins by Japanese encephalitis virus: DC-SIGN, DC-SIGNR, and LSECtin. *Arch. Virol.* **2014**, *159*, 2023–2031. [CrossRef]

71. Goncalves, A.R.; Moraz, M.L.; Pasquato, A.; Helenius, A.; Lozach, P.Y.; Kunz, S. Role of DC-SIGN in Lassa virus entry into human dendritic cells. *J. Virol.* **2013**, *87*, 11504–11515. [CrossRef]

72. Baize, S.; Kaplon, J.; Faure, C.; Pannetier, D.; Georges-Courbot, M.C.; Deubel, V. Lassa virus infection of human dendritic cells and macrophages is productive but fails to activate cells. *J. Immunol.* **2004**, *172*, 2861–2869. [CrossRef]

73. Macal, M.; Lewis, G.M.; Kunz, S.; Flavell, R.; Harker, J.A.; Zuniga, E.I. Plasmacytoid dendritic cells are productively infected and activated through TLR-7 early after arenavirus infection. *Cell Host Microbe* **2012**, *11*, 617–630. [CrossRef] [PubMed]

74. Quirin, K.; Eschli, B.; Scheu, I.; Poort, L.; Kartenbeck, J.; Helenius, A. Lymphocytic choriomeningitis virus uses a novel endocytic pathway for infectious entry via late endosomes. *Virology* **2008**, *378*, 21–33. [CrossRef] [PubMed]

75. Rojek, J.M.; Sanchez, A.B.; Nguyen, N.T.; de la Torre, J.C.; Kunz, S. Different mechanisms of cell entry by human-pathogenic Old World and New World arenaviruses. *J. Virol.* **2008**, *82*, 7677–7687. [CrossRef] [PubMed]

76. Panda, D.; Das, A.; Dinh, P.X.; Subramaniam, S.; Nayak, D.; Barrows, N.J.; Pearson, J.L.; Thompson, J.; Kelly, D.L.; Ladunga, I.; et al. RNAi screening reveals requirement for host cell secretory pathway in infection by diverse families of negative-strand RNA viruses. *Proc. Natl. Acad. Sci. USA* **2011**, *108*, 19036–19041. [CrossRef] [PubMed]

77. Iwasaki, M.; Ngo, N.; de la Torre, J.C. Sodium hydrogen exchangers contribute to arenavirus cell entry. *J. Virol.* **2014**, *88*, 643–654. [CrossRef]

78. Oppliger, J.; Torriani, G.; Herrador, A.; Kunz, S. Lassa Virus Cell Entry via Dystroglycan Involves an Unusual Pathway of Macropinocytosis. *J. Virol.* **2016**, *90*, 6412–6429. [CrossRef] [PubMed]

79. Jae, L.T.; Raaben, M.; Herbert, A.S.; Kuehne, A.I.; Wirchnianski, A.S.; Soh, T.K.; Stubbs, S.H.; Janssen, H.; Damme, M.; Saftig, P.; et al. Virus entry. Lassa virus entry requires a trigger-induced receptor switch. *Science* **2014**, *344*, 1506–1510. [CrossRef]

80. Cohen-Dvashi, H.; Cohen, N.; Israeli, H.; Diskin, R. Molecular mechanism for LAMP1 recognition by Lassa Virus. *J. Virol.* **2015**, *89*, 7584–7592. [CrossRef]

81. Li, S.; Sun, Z.; Pryce, R.; Parsy, M.L.; Fehling, S.K.; Schlie, K.; Siebert, C.A.; Garten, W.; Bowden, T.A.; Strecker, T.; et al. Acidic pH-Induced conformations and LAMP1 binding of the Lassa Virus glycoprotein spike. *PLoS Pathog.* **2016**, *12*, e1005418. [CrossRef]

82. Hulseberg, C.E.; Fénéant, L.; Szymańska, K.M.; White, J.M. LAMP1 increases the efficiency of Lassa Virus infection by promoting fusion in less acidic endosomal compartments. *MBio* **2018**, *2*, e01818-17. [CrossRef] [PubMed]

83. Cohen-Dvashi, H.; Israeli, H.; Shani, O.; Katz, A.; Diskin, R. Role of LAMP1 Binding and pH Sensing by the Spike Complex of Lassa Virus. *J. Virol.* **2016**, *90*, 10329–10338. [CrossRef] [PubMed]

84. Israeli, H.; Cohen-Dvashi, H.; Shulman, A.; Shimon, A.; Diskin, R. Mapping of the Lassa virus LAMP1 binding site reveals unique determinants not shared by other old world arenaviruses. *PLoS Pathog.* **2017**, *13*, e1006337. [CrossRef] [PubMed]

85. King, B.R.; Hershkowitz, D.; Eisenhauer, P.L.; Weir, M.E.; Ziegler, C.M.; Russo, J.; Bruce, E.A.; Ballif, B.A.; Botten, J. A Map of the Arenavirus Nucleoprotein-Host Protein Interactome Reveals that Junin Virus Selectively Impairs the Antiviral Activity of Double-Stranded RNA-Activated Protein Kinase (PKR). *J. Virol.* **2017**, *91*, e00763-17. [CrossRef] [PubMed]

86. Ziegler, C.M.; Eisenhauer, P.; Kelly, J.A.; Dang, L.N.; Beganovic, V.; Bruce, E.A.; King, B.R.; Shirley, D.J.; Weir, M.E.; Ballif, B.A.; et al. A proteomic survey of Junin virus interactions with human proteins reveals host factors required for arenavirus replication. *J. Virol.* **2018**, *92*, e01565-17. [CrossRef]

87. Khamina, K.; Lercher, A.; Caldera, M.; Schliehe, C.; Vilagos, B.; Sahin, M.; Kosack, L.; Bhattacharya, A.; Majek, P.; Stukalov, A.; et al. Characterization of host proteins interacting with the lymphocytic choriomeningitis virus L protein. *PLoS Pathog.* **2017**, *13*, e1006758. [CrossRef]

88. Iwasaki, M.; Minder, P.; Cai, Y.; Kuhn, J.H.; Yates, J.R., 3rd; Torbett, B.E.; de la Torre, J.C. Interactome analysis of the lymphocytic choriomeningitis virus nucleoprotein in infected cells reveals ATPase Na+/K+ transporting subunit Alpha 1 and prohibitin as host-cell factors involved in the life cycle of mammarenaviruses. *PLoS Pathog.* **2018**, *14*, e1006892. [CrossRef]

89. Loureiro, M.E.; Zorzetto-Fernandes, A.L.; Radoshitzky, S.; Chi, X.; Dallari, S.; Marooki, N.; Leger, P.; Foscaldi, S.; Harjono, V.; Sharma, S.; et al. DDX3 suppresses type I interferons and favors viral replication during Arenavirus infection. *PLoS Pathog.* **2018**, *14*, e1007125. [CrossRef]

90. Loureiro, M.E.; D'Antuono, A.; Levingston Macleod, J.M.; Lopez, N. Uncovering viral protein-protein interactions and their role in arenavirus life cycle. *Viruses* **2012**, *4*, 1651–1667. [CrossRef]

91. Martinez-Sobrido, L.; Zuniga, E.I.; Rosario, D.; Garcia-Sastre, A.; de la Torre, J.C. Inhibition of the type I interferon response by the nucleoprotein of the prototypic arenavirus lymphocytic choriomeningitis virus. *J. Virol.* **2006**, *80*, 9192–9199. [CrossRef]

92. Chang, P.C.; Chi, C.W.; Chau, G.Y.; Li, F.Y.; Tsai, Y.H.; Wu, J.C.; Wu Lee, Y.H. DDX3, a DEAD box RNA helicase, is deregulated in hepatitis virus-associated hepatocellular carcinoma and is involved in cell growth control. *Oncogene* **2006**, *25*, 1991–2003. [CrossRef] [PubMed]

93. Lai, M.C.; Chang, W.C.; Shieh, S.Y.; Tarn, W.Y. DDX3 regulates cell growth through translational control of cyclin E1. *Mol. Cell. Biol.* **2010**, *30*, 5444–5453. [CrossRef]

94. Cruciat, C.M.; Dolde, C.; de Groot, R.E.; Ohkawara, B.; Reinhard, C.; Korswagen, H.C.; Niehrs, C. RNA helicase DDX3 is a regulatory subunit of casein kinase 1 in Wnt-beta-catenin signaling. *Science* **2013**, *339*, 1436–1441. [CrossRef] [PubMed]

95. Ariumi, Y.; Kuroki, M.; Abe, K.; Dansako, H.; Ikeda, M.; Wakita, T.; Kato, N. DDX3 DEAD-box RNA helicase is required for hepatitis C virus RNA replication. *J. Virol.* **2007**, *81*, 13922–13926. [CrossRef]

96. Lai, M.C.; Wang, S.W.; Cheng, L.; Tarn, W.Y.; Tsai, S.J.; Sun, H.S. Human DDX3 interacts with the HIV-1 Tat protein to facilitate viral mRNA translation. *PLoS ONE* **2013**, *8*, e68665. [CrossRef]

97. Yasuda-Inoue, M.; Kuroki, M.; Ariumi, Y. Distinct DDX DEAD-box RNA helicases cooperate to modulate the HIV-1 Rev function. *Biochem. Biophys. Res. Commun.* **2013**, *434*, 803–808. [CrossRef]

98. Chahar, H.S.; Chen, S.; Manjunath, N. P-body components LSM1, GW182, DDX3, DDX6 and XRN1 are recruited to WNV replication sites and positively regulate viral replication. *Virology* **2013**, *436*, 1–7. [CrossRef]

99. Amaya, M.; Brooks-Faulconer, T.; Lark, T.; Keck, F.; Bailey, C.; Raman, V.; Narayanan, A. Venezuelan equine encephalitis virus non-structural protein 3 (nsP3) interacts with RNA helicases DDX1 and DDX3 in infected cells. *Antivir. Res.* **2016**, *131*, 49–60. [CrossRef] [PubMed]

100. Shih, J.W.; Tsai, T.Y.; Chao, C.H.; Wu Lee, Y.H. Candidate tumor suppressor DDX3 RNA helicase specifically represses cap-dependent translation by acting as an eIF4E inhibitory protein. *Oncogene* **2008**, *27*, 700–714. [CrossRef]

101. Soto-Rifo, R.; Rubilar, P.S.; Limousin, T.; de Breyne, S.; Decimo, D.; Ohlmann, T. DEAD-box protein DDX3 associates with eIF4F to promote translation of selected mRNAs. *EMBO J.* **2012**, *31*, 3745–3756. [CrossRef] [PubMed]

102. Garbelli, A.; Beermann, S.; Di Cicco, G.; Dietrich, U.; Maga, G. A motif unique to the human DEAD-box protein DDX3 is important for nucleic acid binding, ATP hydrolysis, RNA/DNA unwinding and HIV-1 replication. *PLoS ONE* **2011**, *6*, e19810. [CrossRef]

103. Ariumi, Y. Multiple functions of DDX3 RNA helicase in gene regulation, tumorigenesis, and viral infection. *Front. Genet.* **2014**, *5*, 423. [CrossRef] [PubMed]

104. Valiente-Echeverria, F.; Hermoso, M.A.; Soto-Rifo, R. RNA helicase DDX3: At the crossroad of viral replication and antiviral immunity. *Rev. Med. Virol.* **2015**, *25*, 286–299. [CrossRef] [PubMed]

105. Gringhuis, S.I.; Hertoghs, N.; Kaptein, T.M.; Zijlstra-Willems, E.M.; Sarrami-Forooshani, R.; Sprokholt, J.K.; van Teijlingen, N.H.; Kootstra, N.A.; Booiman, T.; van Dort, K.A.; et al. HIV-1 blocks the signaling adaptor MAVS to evade antiviral host defense after sensing of abortive HIV-1 RNA by the host helicase DDX3. *Nat. Immunol.* **2017**, *18*, 225–235. [CrossRef]

106. Li, G.; Feng, T.; Pan, W.; Shi, X.; Dai, J. DEAD-box RNA helicase DDX3X inhibits DENV replication via regulating type one interferon pathway. *Biochem. Biophys. Res. Commun.* **2015**, *456*, 327–332. [CrossRef] [PubMed]

107. Oshiumi, H.; Ikeda, M.; Matsumoto, M.; Watanabe, A.; Takeuchi, O.; Akira, S.; Kato, N.; Shimotohno, K.; Seya, T. Hepatitis C virus core protein abrogates the DDX3 function that enhances IPS-1-mediated IFN-beta induction. *PLoS ONE* **2010**, *5*, e14258. [CrossRef] [PubMed]

108. Schroder, M.; Baran, M.; Bowie, A.G. Viral targeting of DEAD box protein 3 reveals its role in TBK1/IKKepsilon-mediated IRF activation. *EMBO J.* **2008**, *27*, 2147–2157. [CrossRef]

109. Soulat, D.; Burckstummer, T.; Westermayer, S.; Goncalves, A.; Bauch, A.; Stefanovic, A.; Hantschel, O.; Bennett, K.L.; Decker, T.; Superti-Furga, G. The DEAD-box helicase DDX3X is a critical component of the TANK-binding kinase 1-dependent innate immune response. *EMBO J.* **2008**, *27*, 2135–2146. [CrossRef] [PubMed]

110. Gu, L.; Fullam, A.; Brennan, R.; Schroder, M. Human DEAD box helicase 3 couples IkappaB kinase epsilon to interferon regulatory factor 3 activation. *Mol. Cell. Biol.* **2013**, *33*, 2004–2015. [CrossRef]

111. Shih, J.W.; Wang, W.T.; Tsai, T.Y.; Kuo, C.Y.; Li, H.K.; Wu Lee, Y.H. Critical roles of RNA helicase DDX3 and its interactions with eIF4E/PABP1 in stress granule assembly and stress response. *Biochem. J.* **2012**, *441*, 119–129. [CrossRef]

112. Baird, N.L.; York, J.; Nunberg, J.H. Arenavirus infection induces discrete cytosolic structures for RNA replication. *J. Virol.* **2012**, *86*, 11301–11310. [CrossRef]

113. Linero, F.N.; Thomas, M.G.; Boccaccio, G.L.; Scolaro, L.A. Junin virus infection impairs stress-granule formation in Vero cells treated with arsenite via inhibition of eIF2alpha phosphorylation. *J. Gen. Virol.* **2011**, *92*, 2889–2899. [CrossRef] [PubMed]

114. Thulasi Raman, S.N.; Liu, G.; Pyo, H.M.; Cui, Y.C.; Xu, F.; Ayalew, L.E.; Tikoo, S.K.; Zhou, Y. DDX3 Interacts with Influenza A Virus NS1 and NP Proteins and Exerts Antiviral Function through Regulation of Stress Granule Formation. *J. Virol.* **2016**, *90*, 3661–3675. [CrossRef] [PubMed]

115. Goh, P.Y.; Tan, Y.J.; Lim, S.P.; Tan, Y.H.; Lim, S.G.; Fuller-Pace, F.; Hong, W. Cellular RNA helicase p68 relocalization and interaction with the hepatitis C virus (HCV) NS5B protein and the potential role of p68 in HCV RNA replication. *J. Virol.* **2004**, *78*, 5288–5298. [CrossRef] [PubMed]

116. Jorba, N.; Juarez, S.; Torreira, E.; Gastaminza, P.; Zamarreno, N.; Albar, J.P.; Ortin, J. Analysis of the interaction of influenza virus polymerase complex with human cell factors. *Proteomics* **2008**, *8*, 2077–2088. [CrossRef]

117. Bortz, E.; Westera, L.; Maamary, J.; Steel, J.; Albrecht, R.A.; Manicassamy, B.; Chase, G.; Martinez-Sobrido, L.; Schwemmle, M.; Garcia-Sastre, A. Host- and strain-specific regulation of influenza virus polymerase activity by interacting cellular proteins. *mBio* **2011**, *16*, e00151-11. [CrossRef] [PubMed]

118. Matkovic, R.; Bernard, E.; Fontanel, S.; Eldin, P.; Chazal, N.; Hassan Hersi, D.; Merits, A.; Peloponese, J.M., Jr.; Briant, L. The host DHX9 DExH Box helicase is recruited to Chikungunya virus replication complexes for optimal genomic RNA translation. *J. Virol.* **2018**, JVI.01764. [CrossRef]

119. Liu, L.; Tian, J.; Nan, H.; Tian, M.; Li, Y.; Xu, X.; Huang, B.; Zhou, E.; Hiscox, J.A.; Chen, H. Porcine Reproductive and Respiratory Syndrome Virus Nucleocapsid Protein Interacts with Nsp9 and Cellular DHX9 To Regulate Viral RNA Synthesis. *J. Virol.* **2016**, *90*, 5384–5398. [CrossRef]

120. Wilda, M.; Lopez, N.; Casabona, J.C.; Franze-Fernandez, M.T. Mapping of the tacaribe arenavirus Z-protein binding sites on the L protein identified both amino acids within the putative polymerase domain and a region at the N terminus of L that are critically involved in binding. *J. Virol.* **2008**, *82*, 11454–11460. [CrossRef]

121. Kranzusch, P.J.; Schenk, A.D.; Rahmeh, A.A.; Radoshitzky, S.R.; Bavari, S.; Walz, T.; Whelan, S.P. Assembly of a functional Machupo virus polymerase complex. *Proc. Natl. Acad. Sci. USA* **2010**, *107*, 20069–20074. [CrossRef]

122. Morin, B.; Coutard, B.; Lelke, M.; Ferron, F.; Kerber, R.; Jamal, S.; Frangeul, A.; Baronti, C.; Charrel, R.; de Lamballerie, X.; et al. The N-terminal domain of the arenavirus L protein is an RNA endonuclease essential in mRNA transcription. *PLoS Pathog.* **2010**, *6*, e1001038. [CrossRef] [PubMed]

123. Brunotte, L.; Lelke, M.; Hass, M.; Kleinsteuber, K.; Becker-Ziaja, B.; Gunther, S. Domain structure of Lassa virus L protein. *J. Virol.* **2011**, *85*, 324–333. [CrossRef] [PubMed]

124. Reguera, J.; Gerlach, P.; Cusack, S. Towards a structural understanding of RNA synthesis by negative strand RNA viral polymerases. *Curr. Opin. Struct. Biol.* **2016**, *36*, 75–84. [CrossRef] [PubMed]

125. Ferron, F.; Weber, F.; de la Torre, J.C.; Reguera, J. Transcription and replication mechanisms of Bunyaviridae and Arenaviridae L proteins. *Virus Res.* **2017**, *234*, 118–134. [CrossRef]

126. Gerlach, P.; Malet, H.; Cusack, S.; Reguera, J. Structural Insights into Bunyavirus Replication and Its Regulation by the vRNA Promoter. *Cell* **2015**, *161*, 1267–1279. [CrossRef]

127. Sanchez, A.B.; de la Torre, J.C. Genetic and biochemical evidence for an oligomeric structure of the functional L polymerase of the prototypic arenavirus lymphocytic choriomeningitis virus. *J. Virol.* **2005**, *79*, 7262–7268. [CrossRef]

128. Chang, S.; Sun, D.; Liang, H.; Wang, J.; Li, J.; Guo, L.; Wang, X.; Guan, C.; Boruah, B.M.; Yuan, L.; et al. Cryo-EM structure of influenza virus RNA polymerase complex at 4.3 A resolution. *Mol. Cell* **2015**, *57*, 925–935. [CrossRef]

129. Ortin, J.; Martin-Benito, J. The RNA synthesis machinery of negative-stranded RNA viruses. *Virology* **2015**, *479–480*, 532–544. [CrossRef]

130. Maeto, C.A.; Knott, M.E.; Linero, F.N.; Ellenberg, P.C.; Scolaro, L.A.; Castilla, V. Differential effect of acute and persistent Junin virus infections on the nucleo-cytoplasmic trafficking and expression of heterogeneous nuclear ribonucleoproteins type A and B. *J. Gen. Virol.* **2011**, *92*, 2181–2190. [CrossRef]

131. Brunetti, J.E.; Scolaro, L.A.; Castilla, V. The heterogeneous nuclear ribonucleoprotein K (hnRNP K) is a host factor required for dengue virus and Junin virus multiplication. *Virus Res.* **2015**, *203*, 84–91. [CrossRef]

132. Chang, C.K.; Chen, C.J.; Wu, C.C.; Chen, S.W.; Shih, S.R.; Kuo, R.L. Cellular hnRNP A2/B1 interacts with the NP of influenza A virus and impacts viral replication. *PLoS ONE* **2017**, *12*, e0188214. [CrossRef] [PubMed]

133. Levesque, K.; Halvorsen, M.; Abrahamyan, L.; Chatel-Chaix, L.; Poupon, V.; Gordon, H.; DesGroseillers, L.; Gatignol, A.; Mouland, A.J. Trafficking of HIV-1 RNA is mediated by heterogeneous nuclear ribonucleoprotein A2 expression and impacts on viral assembly. *Traffic* **2006**, *7*, 1177–1193. [CrossRef] [PubMed]

134. Dinh, P.X.; Das, A.; Franco, R.; Pattnaik, A.K. Heterogeneous nuclear ribonucleoprotein K supports vesicular stomatitis virus replication by regulating cell survival and cellular gene expression. *J. Virol.* **2013**, *87*, 10059–10069. [CrossRef] [PubMed]

135. Strecker, T.; Eichler, R.; Meulen, J.; Weissenhorn, W.; Dieter Klenk, H.; Garten, W.; Lenz, O. Lassa virus Z protein is a matrix protein and sufficient for the release of virus-like particles [corrected]. *J. Virol.* **2003**, *77*, 10700–10705. [CrossRef] [PubMed]

136. Fehling, S.K.; Lennartz, F.; Strecker, T. Multifunctional nature of the arenavirus RING finger protein Z. *Viruses* **2012**, *4*, 2973–3011. [CrossRef] [PubMed]

137. Loureiro, M.E.; Wilda, M.; Levingston Macleod, J.M.; D'Antuono, A.; Foscaldi, S.; Marino Buslje, C.; Lopez, N. Molecular determinants of arenavirus Z protein homo-oligomerization and L polymerase binding. *J. Virol.* **2011**, *85*, 12304–12314. [CrossRef] [PubMed]

138. Kranzusch, P.J.; Whelan, S.P. Arenavirus Z protein controls viral RNA synthesis by locking a polymerase-promoter complex. *Proc. Natl. Acad. Sci. USA* **2011**, *108*, 19743–19748. [CrossRef]

139. Roy, B.B.; Hu, J.; Guo, X.; Russell, R.S.; Guo, F.; Kleiman, L.; Liang, C. Association of RNA helicase a with human immunodeficiency virus type 1 particles. *J. Biol. Chem.* **2006**, *281*, 12625–12635. [CrossRef]

140. WHO. List of Blueprint Priority Diseases. Available online: https://www.who.int/blueprint/priority-diseases/en/ (accessed on 28 January 2019).

141. McCormick, J.B.; King, I.J.; Webb, P.A.; Scribner, C.L.; Craven, R.B.; Johnson, K.M.; Elliott, L.H.; Belmont-Williams, R. Lassa fever. Effective therapy with ribavirin. *N. Engl. J. Med.* **1986**, *314*, 20–26. [CrossRef]

142. Safronetz, D.; Rosenke, K.; Westover, J.B.; Martellaro, C.; Okumura, A.; Furuta, Y.; Geisbert, J.; Saturday, G.; Komeno, T.; Geisbert, T.W.; et al. The broad-spectrum antiviral favipiravir protects guinea pigs from lethal Lassa virus infection post-disease onset. *Sci. Rep.* **2015**, *12*, 14775. [CrossRef]

143. Raabe, V.N.; Kann, G.; Ribner, B.S.; Morales, A.; Varkey, J.B.; Mehta, A.K.; Lyon, G.M.; Vanairsdale, S.; Faber, K.; Becker, S.; et al. Favipiravir and Ribavirin Treatment of Epidemiologically Linked Cases of Lassa Fever. *Clin. Infect. Dis.* **2017**, *1*, 855–859. [CrossRef] [PubMed]

144. Torriani, G.; Galan-Navarro, C.; Kunz, S. Lassa Virus Cell Entry Reveals New Aspects of Virus-Host Cell Interaction. *J. Virol.* **2017**, *91*, 1–8. [CrossRef] [PubMed]

145. Brai, A.; Fazi, R.; Tintori, C.; Zamperini, C.; Bugli, F.; Sanguinetti, M.; Stigliano, E.; Este, J.; Badia, R.; Franco, S.; et al. Human DDX3 protein is a valuable target to develop broad spectrum antiviral agents. *Proc. Natl. Acad. Sci. USA* **2016**, *113*, 5388–5393. [CrossRef] [PubMed]

6

A Short Report on the Lack of a Pyrogenic Response of Australian Genomic Group IV Isolates of *Coxiella burnetii* in Guinea Pigs

Aminul Islam [1],*, John Stenos [1], Gemma Vincent [1] and Stephen Graves [1,2]

[1] Australian Rickettsial Reference Laboratory, University Hospital Geelong, Geelong, VIC 3220, Australia; johns@barwonhealth.org.au (J.S.); gvince@barwonhealth.org.au (G.V.); graves.rickettsia@gmail.com (S.G.)

[2] New South Wales Health Pathology, Nepean Hospital, Penrith, NSW 2751, Australia

* Correspondence: aislam.islam@gmail.com.

Abstract: This small study reports on a non-pyrogenic response of five different Australian isolates of *Coxiella burnetii* (*C. burnetii*). They were all members of Genomic Group IV and obtained from three cases of acute human infection, one case of chronic human infection and one case of goat abortion. The guinea pigs infected with these isolates did not develop fever (temperature $\geq 40.0\ ^\circ$C), which is consistent with other members of this genomic group that were isolated from elsewhere in the world. In contrast, guinea pigs infected with the classical USA tick isolate, Nine Mile phase 1 (RSA 493) of Genomic Group I, experienced a four-day febrile period.

Keywords: *C. burnetii*; Q fever; Australia; pyrogenicity; guinea pigs

1. Introduction

Guinea pigs are an excellent small animal model of acute Q fever (infection with *Coxiella burnetii* or *C. burnetii*) in humans [1–3]. However, not all isolates of *C. burnetii* will cause fever (pyrogenicity) in guinea pigs. This feature of the bacterium appears to be related to the genomic group to which the isolate belongs, with group IV and VI known to be non-pyrogenic [4].

Recent Australian isolates of *C. burnetii* belong to a unique subset of genomic group IV; however, most were isolated from patients with acute Q fever, many of whom had presented with fever [5]. The question investigated in this small study was whether a selection of these Australian isolates were pyrogenic in guinea pigs.

2. Materials and Methods

2.1. Animal Ethics

This study was approved by the Australian Rickettsial Reference Laboratory Animal Care and Ethics Committee (ACEC/010). All experimental works were performed in a biosafety level 3 laboratory at the Department of Microbiology, John Hunter Hospital, Newcastle, New South Wales, Australia.

2.2. Coxiella Burnetii Isolates

Five Australian isolates of *C. burnetii* were selected for use in this study, with a range of molecular and epidemiological features (Table 1). All were members of genomic group IV, but represented three different genotypes (CbAu01, CbAu04 and CbAu06) according to a multi-locus variable number of tandem repeats (VNTR) analysis (MLVA). These genotypes were shown to be unique to Australia [5]. There were four human isolates that came from three cases of acute infection (AuQ01, AuQ10 and

AuQ43) and one case of chronic infection (AuQ04). There was also one isolate from an aborting goat (AuQ57), which was associated with a number of human cases [6].

C. burnetii Nine Mile phase 1 (RSA493), originally obtained from a tick in the USA and belonging to Genomic Group I, was used as a positive control, as it was known to be pyrogenic in guinea pigs. Sterile cell culture medium (RPMI-1640) was used as a negative control.

Table 1. Brief molecular and epidemiological features of the five Australian isolates of *Coxiella burnetii* (*C. burnetii*) used in the pyrogenicity study.

C. burnetii Isolates	MLVA * Genotype	Epidemiological Features					
		Type of Q Fever	Year	Location	Animal Contact	Symptoms	Source of Isolate
AuQ01 (Human)	CbAu01	Acute	2005	Armidale, Northern NSW	Goat	Fever, Jaundice	Blood
AuQ04 (Human)	CbAu04	Chronic	2007	Swan Hill, Northern VIC	Unknown	Fever, Endocarditis/ Aortic valve incompetence	Surgically removed tissue
AuQ10 (Human)	CbAu06	Acute	2011	Coffs Harbour, Northern NSW	Unknown	Fever, Haemophagocytic Syndrome	Blood
AuQ43 (Human)	CbAu01	Acute	2012	Mt Louisa, Northern QLD	Unknown	Fever	Blood
AuQ57 (Animal)	CbAu01	Goat coxiello-sis	2012	Meredith, Central VIC	Goat	Abortion	Aborted foetus

* MLVA-multiple locus variable number of tandem repeats analysis.

2.3. Culture and Quantification of C. burnetii in VERO Cell Line and Wild Mice

Vero cells were grown in 10ml RPMI (Gibco, Australia) supplemented with 10% new born calf serum (NBCS) (Gibco, Australia) and 1% L-glutamine (Gibco, Australia). The five *C. burnetii* isolates were inoculated into Vero cell monolayer and grown at 37 °C with 5% CO_2 for 14 days. The infected monolayer was removed by scrapping and each preparation inoculated intraperitoneally into a single outbred mouse. This was done to ensure that all *C. burnetii* cells were in phase 1 (virulent) for the later guinea pig infection [7]. Each infected mouse was euthanized seven days later and its enlarged spleen removed aseptically. Each spleen was separately homogenized in 5 mL of Hank's Balanced Salt Solution and the concentration of *C. burnetii* DNA measured by quantitative real-time PCR (qPCR) using an assay targeting the single-copy com1 gene [8]. Each spleen suspension was adjusted to contain between 10^6 and 10^7 *C. burnetii* per 0.2 mL.

2.4. Experimental Guinea Pig Infection

Outbred breeds of adult male guinea pigs were used in this study ($n = 24$). One week prior to the start of the experiment, an IPTT300 temperature transponder (Biomedic Data Systems, Inc., Seaford, DE, USA) was implanted into the sub-cutaneous tissue on the flank of each guinea pig.

Each guinea pig was anaesthetized with a 0.2 mL intramuscular injection of 9.5 mL of ketamine (100 mg/mL) and 0.5 mL of xylazine (100 mg/mL). Each anaesthetized guinea pig had 0.2 mL of the infected mouse spleen suspension introduced slowly into its nostrils via a fine-bore plastic Pasteur pipette. The guinea pigs inhaled the liquid slowly and the *C. burnetii* presumably entered the animals' lungs.

2.5. Monitoring Guinea Pig Temperature with Probe

Guinea pig temperatures were recorded daily for 21 days using an IPTT-300 Smart Probe held over the location of the subcutaneous temperature transponder in the guinea pig.

A temperature at or above 40 °C was defined as a fever and the guinea pig considered to be febrile. The experiment was terminated at day 21 post-infection by which time all guinea pig temperatures had returned to normal.

3. Results

The temperature changes in the 24 guinea pigs (grouped according to the isolate of *C. burnetii* used to infect them) are shown in the Figure 1. The four guinea pigs given only Roswell Park Memorial Institute (RPMI) medium intranasally (negative controls) did not develop a fever at any stage.

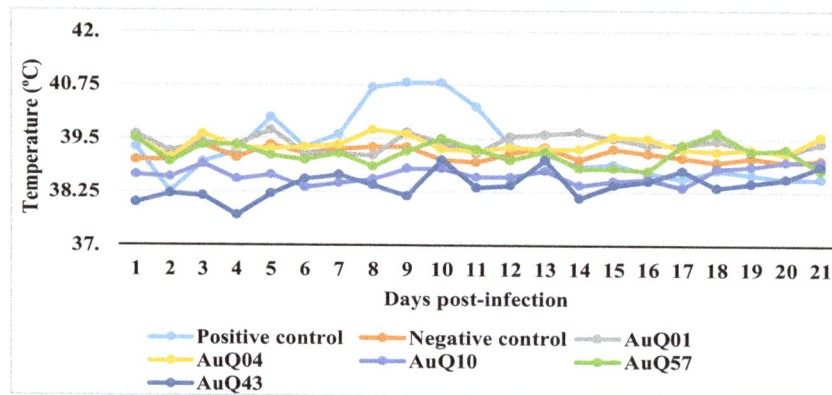

Figure 1. The temperature pattern of guinea pigs infected with five different Australian isolates of *C. burnetii*, with the positive (NM1) and negative (sterile RPMI 1640 media) controls over a period of 21 days post-infection. Febrile response (temperature $\geq$ 40.0 °C) in positive controls sustained from days 8–11 with an early onset at day 5. Throughout the experimental period, the five Australian isolates and negative control did not show febrile response and remained under 40.0 °C. The average value of temperature in each group is shown in the graph.

The four guinea pigs given *C. burnetii* Nine Mile phase 1 (positive control), developed fever (40.6 ± 0.3) from days 8–11 after infection (four-day duration). None of the five Australian *C. burnetii* isolates, inoculated into 16 guinea pigs, resulted in fever (38.6 ± 1.0). They were all non-pyrogenic.

4. Discussion

The best small animal model for studying Q fever is the guinea pig, as it develops a fever of limited duration, similar to infected humans [3]. However, not all isolates of *C. burnetii* are pyrogenic in the guinea pig. Studies of non-Australian isolates show that those from genomic groups IV and VI are non-pyrogenic [4]. This study has now demonstrated the same phenomenon of non-pyrogenicity in five Australian isolates, which all belong to genomic group IV, albeit to a unique subgroup. The four human isolates used in this study caused fever in the human patients from whom the bacteria were obtained. However, they did not cause fever in the guinea pigs. While the pathological basis for this difference is not known, there is a practical significance to it. When using guinea pigs to test new vaccines for use against Q fever and using abrogation of fever as a clinical indicator of vaccine success, it is necessary to use a challenge isolate of *C. burnetii* that causes fever in the non-immunized guinea pigs. On the basis of this small study it will not be possible to use Australian isolates of *C. burnetii* for challenge in Q fever vaccine studies, if abrogation of fever is used as a clinical marker of vaccine protection. It appears that the Nine Mile phase 1 isolate of *C. burnetii* is required for this purpose.

5. Conclusions

Australian isolates of *C. burnetii* do not cause fever in experimentally infected guinea pigs, confirming what has been shown in other genomic group IV isolates elsewhere in the world.

Author Contributions: A.I., G.V. and S.G. designed and carried out the experiments. J.S. provided scientific guidance and administrative support.

Acknowledgments: The financial support of Anne Crotty and the administrative support of Stephen Braye, both of NSW Health Pathology, Newcastle, Australia, is appreciated.

References

1. Scott, G.H.; Burger, G.T.; Kishimoto, R.A. Experimental *Coxiella burnetii* infection of guinea pigs and mice. *Lab. Anim. Sci.* **1978**, *28*, 673–675. [PubMed]
2. Russell-Lodrigue, K.E.; Zhang, G.Q.; McMurray, D.N.; Samuel, J.E. Clinical and pathologic changes in a guinea pig aerosol challenge model of acute Q fever. *Infect. Immun.* **2006**, *74*, 6085–6091. [CrossRef] [PubMed]
3. Bewley, K.R. Animal models of Q fever (*Coxiella burnetii*). *Comp. Med.* **2013**, *63*, 469–476.
4. Russell-Lodrigue, K.E.; Andoh, M.; Poels, W.J.; Shive, H.R.; Weeks, B.R.; Zhang, G.Q.; Tersteeg, C.; Masegi, T.; Hotta, A.; Yamaguchi, Y.; et al. *Coxiella burnetii* isolates cause genogroup-specific virulence in mice and guinea pig models of acute Q fever. *Infect. Immun.* **2009**, *77*, 5640–5650. [CrossRef] [PubMed]
5. Vincent, G.; Stenos, J.; Latham, J.; Fenwick, S.; Graves, S. Novel genotypes of *Coxiella burnetii* identified in isolates from Australian Q fever patients. *Int. J Med. Micro.* **2016**, *306*, 463–470. [CrossRef]
6. Bond, K.A.; Vincent, G.; Wilks, C.R.; Franklin, L.; Sutton, B.; Stenos, J.; Cowan, R.; Lim, K.; Athan, E.; Harris, O.; et al. One health approach to controlling a Q fever outbreak on an Australian goat farm. *Epidemiol. Infect.* **2016**, *144*, 1129–1141. [CrossRef]
7. Ormsbee, R.A.; Bell, E.J.; Lackman, D.B.; Tallent, G. The influence of phase on the protective potency of Q fever vaccine. *J. Immunol.* **1964**, *92*, 404–412. [PubMed]
8. Lockhart, M.G.; Graves, S.R.; Banazis, M.J.; Fenwick, S.G.; Stenos, J. A comparison of methods for extracting DNA from *Coxiella burnetii* as measured by a duplex qPCR assay. *Lett. Appl. Microbiol.* **2011**, *52*, 513–520. [CrossRef] [PubMed]

7

Antimicrobial Resistance (AMR) in the Food Chain: Trade, One Health and Codex

Anna George [1,2]

[1]   Centre on Global Health Security, Chatham House, London SW1Y 4LE, UK; anna.george.c@gmail.com or
     Anna.George@murdoch.edu.au

[2]   Public Policy and International Affairs, Murdoch University, Murdoch, WA 6150, Australia

Abstract: Strategies that take on a One Health approach to addressing antimicrobial resistance (AMR) focused on reducing human use of antimicrobials, but policy-makers now have to grapple with a different set of political, economic, and highly sensitive trade interests less amenable to government direction, to tackle AMR in the food chain. Understanding the importance and influence of the intergovernmental Codex negotiations underway on AMR in the Food Chain is very weak but essential for AMR public policy experts. National and global food producing industries are already under pressure as consumers learn about the use of antimicrobials in food production and more so when the full impact of AMR microorganisms in the food chain and on the human microbiome is better understood. Governments will be expected to respond. Trade-related negotiations on access and use made of antimicrobials is political: the relevance of AMR 'evidence' is already contested and not all food producers or users of antimicrobials in the food chain are prepared to, or capable of, moving at the same pace. In trade negotiations governments defend their interpretation of national interest. Given AMR in the global food chain threatens national interest, both AMR One Health and zoonotic disease experts should understand and participate in all trade-related AMR negotiations to protect One Health priorities. To help facilitate this an overview and analysis of Codex negotiations is provided.

Keywords: AMR; One Health; food chain; trade; Codex; WHO; World Trade Organization (WTO)

---

1. Background: Access to and Use of Antimicrobials

A global political consensus has been reached confirming antimicrobials underpin human health security so access and use of these miracle products has to be wound back across all sectors of the economy [1]. One key agenda slow to emerge is antimicrobial resistance in the food chain with consequences for food safety, food security and significant implications for trade policy.

The complex integrated strategies needed to reign-in the use of antimicrobials in the food, agricultural and associated industry sectors have the capacity to transform the somewhat benign and logical 'AMR (antimicrobial resistance) One Health Framework' into a quagmire of competing interests—as not all producers and users of antimicrobials are prepared to, and some not yet capable of, limiting their use of antimicrobials. But to preserve the AMR One Health global consensus much will depend on how these trade related issues are handled and will require significant leadership and clear recognition of the health security implications of failure.

The UK 2016 O'Neil AMR Report [2] mapped out possible consequences of not safeguarding these precious antimicrobials and analyzed the capacity of this AMR phenomena to economically disrupt and negatively impact on many industry sectors. On the human costs, more accurate research and analysis recording actual numbers of AMR related deaths and the exponential growth of health/productivity costs is emerging that will better reflect the consequences from AMR events [3,4]. This sensitive data is likely to reverberate politically.

Such politically sensitive data and revelations from research on AMR in the food chain will inevitably place 'food trade' firmly in the spotlight. Trade policy, at its best, can help induce higher safety standards, better quality food, and safer products. But the spread of AMR microorganisms could represent one of the biggest challenges to trade in safe food and may lead to trade disruption and financial loss.

Existing trade frameworks and obligations may be capable of addressing this issue but only if sensitized and adapted to prioritize safeguarding health security by providing the flexibility for governments to implement measures to safeguard their food-chain and help preserve antimicrobials, particularly those important for human medicine.

AMR is an economic and global trade issue, so criticism of government action or regulatory changes perceived as running counter to concepts of 'free trade' will need to be managed. But this is also an opportunity for those who have extolled the benefits of trade to step up and deliver on this crucial AMR agenda.

There are after all several precedents where similar large and economically painful transformations have been deemed necessary linked to 'access and use'—sometimes for the public or global good and often to facilitate trade in new technologies or facilitate new forms of production and accumulation. For example, intellectual property and copyright provisions extended through WTO Trade-Related Aspects of Intellectual Property (TRIPS) [5]; reducing chemical toxicity in domestic products—EU REACH Legislation (Registration, Evaluation, Authorization and Restrictions of Chemicals) [6], and promoting health objectives—Tobacco Plain Packaging Policy [7].

With such complex trade agendas, it was inevitably these transformations created economic disruption by altering access and or use provisions which redistributed costs, benefits, investments and profits. All involved high levels of political contestation as access provisions and/or regulations were redefined at the national level or through multilateral negotiations. Interestingly, lessons and tactics used to support or block these transformations are beginning to resonate in the AMR debates and some have been picked up by media [8].

Implementing effective AMR One Health strategies will require a similar level of political commitment and leadership to transform access and use provisions to preserve the efficacy of antimicrobials, particularly for human medicine.

2. Policy Coherence—Are Trade Policies Understood and Integrated into AMR One Health Strategies?

National AMR One Health Strategies already focus on altering both access provisions and use made of antimicrobials for human use. The other major area of antibiotic use—food production—is yet to be as systematically adapted to achieve national one health objectives. Unlike reducing human use which is negotiated and conducted entirely at the national level usually by government health authorities, but to influence the access and use of antimicrobials in food production (domestic and imported) is more complex. And involves many more interested parties. The 2006 EU ban on the use of antibiotics as growth promotors is an example of the complex legal, trade and political implications that can flow from such decisions.

A fundamental understanding how national trade policies harmonize/comply with international trade rules and obligations is essential. This includes understanding the technical and legal structures that enable and legitimize the use of antimicrobials in the food chain as well as the capacity to exclude them in specific circumstances from imported food.

This will require AMR public health experts to be active in setting AMR government priorities in these trade-related negotiations to ensure AMR policy coherence: The international standard setting body for food safety, Codex Alimentarius Commission (Codex); the World Trade Organization (WTO); and also Bilateral and Regional Free Trade Agreements.

The rational for engaging in such esoteric areas of trade policy is that any new interpretations, obligations, rules, procedures/guidelines evolving from, for example, Codex negotiations on 'AMR in the food chain' have the capacity to impact on the access to and use made of antimicrobials. But of equal importance, such multilateral decisions could also circumscribe the regulatory and legal options available to national governments in implementing their AMR strategies and their domestic export/import policies if national legislation/regulations are not introduced or adapted to reflect One Health priorities. One example to be aware of is introducing the capacity to develop 'national lists' of antimicrobials as discussed in Codex TFAMR Report REP 19/AMR.

An overview of negotiations currently underway in the Codex food standard setting body may help make transparent the complex political and legal obligations linked to international trade. Understanding the food/trade linkage is critical especially if national inter-agency policy cohesion has not fully integrated these trade-related elements. And introducing new regulations on AMR may be problematic if political commitment or bureaucratic capacity to regulate is weak.

For example, the technical and scientific complexity of the AMR/food subject matter and navigating the huge number of Codex standards and guidelines [9] is challenging so these negotiations are usually left to 'expert' bodies responsible for Codex, or, decisions driven by broader national trade objectives managed through foreign/trade policy negotiators.

Bureaucratically integrating the trade agenda into One Health Action Plans may be difficult but is essential. These trade-related linkages should be comprehensively understood for their effect and appropriately responded to in-line with national AMR One Health security priorities.

3. Codex Alimentarius Commission (Codex): Current Negotiations on AMR in the Food Chain and Understanding the Political Context

AMR in the food chain was earlier addressed through the Taskforce on Antimicrobial Resistance (TFAMR) from 2007–2011. In 2016 Governments agreed to re-convene the TFAMR with a broader mandate to address the entire food chain and to report back to the Codex Commission by 2020 [10]. The Terms of Reference are: to revise the *Code of Practice to Minimize and Contain Antimicrobial Resistance* and to develop new *Guidelines on integrated monitoring and surveillance of antimicrobial resistance*.

Gaining consensus agreement through this Codex/TFAMR process may not be easy, particularly as these two documents will also be directly and indirectly endorsing the use of antimicrobials in the food chain. Which antimicrobials can be used in the food chain and in what circumstances represents a highly contested political agenda, particularly antimicrobials used for growth promotion and those deemed essential for human medicine. Codex Guidelines endorsed by Member States may also provide direct or indirect legitimacy for the use of these antimicrobials.

Unlike WTO negotiations, Codex/TFAMR negotiations enable participation and active input from non-government entities. A reading of the open-source negotiating draft documents with input from governments, industry and consumer representatives provide insights into some of the more contentious areas [11]. While few would argue the need for global collaboration (such as the TFAMR process) to minimize the spread of AMR microorganisms is important but if significant differences arise over containing the use of antimicrobials in the food chain this could in-effect serve to hinder government action to proactively protect consumers.

The question of consistency with WTO rules is often a good excuse for government inaction. And an added factor to be cognizant of—given the 'standard setting' role of Codex which links directly into related WTO obligations—is that Codex standards can, and are, often used to justify positions taken in WTO Trade Dispute cases. Or trade disagreements arising when Sanitary and Phytosanitary (SPS) or Technical Barriers to Trade (TBT) agreements are enacted to restrict or place conditionality on imports.

The use of antimicrobials in the food chain is a politically and scientifically contested agenda. And, despite the UN General Assembly 'public health security' framing and political endorsement of the WHO AMR One Health framework and the Global Action Plan (GAP) [12], the Codex/TFAMR parameters open for discussion may not sufficiently prioritize or be consistent with 'human health' priorities. Given that a key human health priority is to maintain the efficacy of medically important antimicrobials, so the veracity of action taken to achieve this will be a significant indicator. AMR policy makers should monitor this agenda closely.

For example, to date, neither of the TFAMR draft negotiation texts refer to the WHO Guidelines on Use of Medically Important Antimicrobials in Food-producing Animals biocides appear to now be excluded; and, altering Codex Maximum Residue Limits (MRL) to consider MRLs for medically important antimicrobials do not seem to be open for discussion.

4. AMR One Health Policies: Role of the World Trade Organization (WTO)

The WTO along with other international agencies has responded to the United Nations General Assembly Resolution on AMR. WTO Director General, Azevedo, has stated the existing WTO framework provides non-discriminatory measures and flexibility for governments to address AMR One Health policies especially around food safety [13]. Azevedo is stating the obvious—it is government's responsibility to activate the legal and regulatory framework to protect their citizens.

AMR in the food chain is a new and complex challenge but implementing such legal and regulatory policies referred to by the WTO DG may not be simply. The international trade environment has expanded considerable since the WTO was established and is more legally complex. National trade policy and the governance framework often have to account for both WTO obligations and broader more intrusive obligations imbedded in new FTAs which may limit the scope for independent national based policy development.

Also, some important structural and capacity issues may be relevant. For example, governments who have lost some in-house regulatory and governance capacity through adopting neo-liberal market based self-regulation strategies and some regulatory limitations flowing from harmonization and trade facilitation policies. Public health experts are often not sufficiently involved in these trade negotiations.

Azevedo's view that the WTO enables implementation of AMR One Health strategies rests on government's commitment at the national level to manage/protect the domestic and export food chain in line with WTO obligations. For food-related imports the Sanitary and Phytosanitary (SPS) or Technical Barriers to Trade (TBT) agreements can be activated but have a relatively narrow interpretive space unless backed up by national regulations.

This WTO report to Codex/TFAMR also records individual governments' input on AMR issues linked to SPS reporting and illustrates some sensitive trade access issues yet to be tested, particularly related to proposed EU regulations [14] (pp. 8–12) The TBT provisions are also likely to be a strong focus as consumers demand of governments more accurate labelling information on antimicrobial use [15].

Implementing longer term SPS measures may rely on specific 'scientific evidence-based data' i.e., directly linking food to human transfer of AMR microorganisms. Emergency measures to contain contaminated food imports are generally considered to be short-term temporary measures. In implementing national regulations that are compliant with WTO obligations the key concept is 'non-discrimination' (in trade parlance—national treatment provisions). This FAO/WTO 'toolkit' is an excellent guide to comprehend these trade rules and obligations for both policy makers and non-WTO experts [16] (pp. 12–17).

5. State of Play: Codex TFAMR Negotiations on AMR in the Food Chain

The health concerns linked to AMR in the food chain encompass both the pathogenic and non-pathogenic AMR microorganisms as both can have serious health consequences [17] (pp. 7–10). It is not yet clear how the 'non-pathogenic' AMR microorganisms in the food chain will be dealt with in the Codex TFAMR process.

Those involved in AMR research, media and consumers may be surprised to know that there are major gaps in monitoring/surveillance and proactive testing for AMR microorganisms in the food chain. Only in 2016 was the draft proposal from the specially convened London Meeting forwarded to Codex and integrated into TFAMR's mandate to develop surveillance guidelines [18] (p. 5). Few if any countries currently systematically test food imports for the presence of AMR microorganisms (whether immediately harmful or not). The rational for lack of action is often circular—based on claims of not enough scientific evidence and/or on the need to first comply with WTO trade obligations [19].

Even in countries with sophisticated governance processes and reliable economic and trade statistics there are considerable gaps in understanding the volume and use made of antimicrobials in animal production and the AMR consequences flowing from this use.

Antimicrobials used in agriculture and aquaculture production are not well understood and even less is known of the effects of AMR in the environment, wildlife, water, or soil etc. [20] Addressing the largely unknown environmental factors, that link to broader forms of AMR contagion has been particularly slow to receive substantive oversight or policy/regulatory focus [17,20,21]. Only some of these aspects may actually be considered in the Codex TFAMR process.

Always in multilateral negotiations, language, and agreed text describing the terms and definitions of the problem areas and the scope of issues, principles, and definitions that can be legitimately addressed are fundamental. And these definitions will impact on the capacity to agree on meaningful outcomes to address the issues at hand.

The formal intergovernmental negotiations remain non-transparent to the broader public and media but the open-source TFAMR working draft texts to revise the AMR Code of Practice (CRD20) [22] and develop new Surveillance Guidelines (CRD18) [23] are available and convey the complexity and political sensitivity of these negotiations. Most useful in providing a sense of negotiations is the formal reporting prepared for the July 2019 Codex Alimentarius Commission, which synthesizes TFAMR outcomes indicating consensus language and points of difference [24]. Several of these outstanding and contested issues will be worked through intersessionally by the two drafting groups led by US and Netherlands and reported to the next TFAMR negotiations in December 2019.

6. Codex/TFAMR Political Sensitivities and Contentious Issues

The current work program of the Codex TFAMR negotiations indicates a considerable amount of work has yet to be undertaken, particularly on the new issues being addressed. It may also be difficult to meet the 2020 deadline. The following three issues are included below as 'Case Studies' for those who wish to delve further into the negotiating dynamics. These Case Studies illustrate some of the complex issues yet to be dealt with and deserve the attention and active engagement by governments, consumers, media and public health experts.

(1)   The scope of the 'food chain'—new issues to be included;
(2)   Securing antimicrobials of importance for human medicine;
(3)   Interpretation attached to evidence—scientific evidence-based versus precautionary principle.

7. Conclusions

The global transition to safeguard antimicrobials is underway but care will have to be taken to ensure that health security is not derailed by narrow interpretations or vested interests. No doubt, particularly at this stage of the negotiations many of the parameters for discussion have ambiguity built-in and while this might placate some concerns there is always the danger these limitations can become in-built into the decisions eventually evolving from the TFAMR [22] (pp. 3–7).

The many but yet little known consequences of AMR in the food chain will emerge as research efforts intensify and unravel the complex AMR effects on the broader ecosystem, including wildlife, water, and soil. Highly dangerous zoonotic diseases are already impacted by AMR affecting large populations so ongoing threats from zoonotic diseases cannot be neatly compartmentalized or insulated from the effects of AMR microorganisms originating from the food chain [25,26].

Information of actual and possible spread of AMR identified in the Expert Report—including to wildlife, insects, and parasites—are yet to be revealed and some but not all aspects will be examined in the TFAMR discussions. This raises questions of which international organization will take responsibility. Infectious and zoonotic disease experts, with their established links to national security frameworks, should obviously have an interest in how this AMR gap will be addressed. These experts should also be actively inputting into the Codex TFAMR negotiations.

Other interesting developments are emerging alongside the Codex/TFAMR negotiations. Leadership on AMR policy is evolving from investors, finance industry and some in the food sectors with potential to be a powerful force for change. Their strategies are now in advance of many government policies and also the current approach being taken in Codex TFAMR negotiations.

And the 73rd UN General Assembly will convene to consider progress made on AMR and the recommendations developed through its Interagency Coordination Group on Antimicrobial Resistance (IACG) [27]. These deliberations should provide a broader overarching model to drive AMR One Health strategies and provide clearer direction to trade-related AMR negotiations such as the Codex TFAMR.

Achieving consensus on a global approach to minimize the spread of AMR is essential but will require significant leadership and incentives to develop the necessary technical capacity to transition away from relying on antimicrobials. But ultimately it is the responsibility of national governments to maintain public confidence in their food chain and to implement governance and regulatory changes needed to address this global health security threat and protect citizens.

Case Study 1. Defining the Scope of AMR in the Food Chain More Broadly

The TFAMR tasked the Codex Secretariat [28] (provided by FAO/WHO) to develop 'scientific advice' on the scope of AMR in the food chain. The FAO/WHO convened an expert meeting and produced this Summary Report on foodborne antimicrobial resistance—Role of environment, crops and biocides [20]. The primary purpose was to synthesize current scientific literature concerning the transmission of AMR from environmental sources—including from water, soil, wildlife, humans, and equipment.

This Expert Group Report, distributed in advance of the meeting, initially was not formally registered on the TFAMR Website [11] but the FAO representative summarized some findings under the item: Scientific Advice to Codex [24], (pp. 1–2): Recording widespread reports of AMR bacteria contamination of foods of plant origin, numerous documented outbreaks of AMR foodborne infections traced to foods of plant origin clearly indicate the potential of these products to transmit AMR microorganisms to human contaminated from multiple sources: water, soil, wildlife, humans, and equipment, and that "Steps should be taken to reduce the likelihood of antimicrobial agents and antimicrobial-resistant bacteria entering the environment from agriculture practices and agricultural food production should be protected from environmental sources of contamination." [24] (p. 1)

Also, reference made to Good Agricultural Practices—to reduce microbial contamination; and, Integrated Pest Management practices to help reduce the need for antimicrobials; on the use of biocides " … there was strong theoretical and laboratory evidence to indicate biocides select for increased resistance to antimicrobials through cross or co-resistance, but empirical evidence is limited" [24] (p. 2). The expert group recommended biocides should be used according to manufacturers' recommendations.

Closing off some issues around biocides the Codex/TFAMR Report now records this agreement: "Antimicrobials used as biocides, including disinfectants, are excluded from the scope of these guidelines" [24] (p. 10).

Some issues raised in the Expert Group Report [20] will be addressed at the next TFAMR meeting in December 2019 and other elements now integrated for further consideration. For example, the draft Code of Conduct definition of 'the food chain' was endorsed by the TFAMR as: *"Production to consumption continuum including, primary production (food producing animals, plants/crops), harvest/slaughter, packing, processing, storage, transport, and retail distribution to the point of consumption"* [22] (p. 4).

Many very sensitive issues, including defining principles are yet to be settled—use of growth promotors and the introduction of government's developing 'national lists' could be usefully developed (but concerns expressed at the potential of such 'lists' to impact trade) [24] (p. 6).

Also worth noting is the WHO/FAO/OIE Report to the TFAMR contains a long list of forthcoming expert meetings to research/analyze outstanding AMR issues including many raised by the Expert Group [20]. But this will be a lengthy process before relevant data and advice will be available [29].

Given the threat to public health of AMR already affecting the food chain and the broader environment, any delay in taking counter-measures to actively protect citizens from such exposure is highly problematic. Especially if reasons for inaction are predicated on the basis that 'evidence' is not available when screening and testing has not been actively pursued by governments or the food industries responsible, or, data is not made transparently available for research.

Case Study 2: Securing Antimicrobials of Importance for Human Medicine—The WHO CIA List

The WHO has already defined the *List of Critically Important Antimicrobials for Human Medicine* (WHO CIA List) [30] which ranks antimicrobials used in human medicine based on two criteria—importance to human health and the likelihood of resistance transmission through the food chain. The WHO also developed and released what could be described as guidance for implementing this CIA List—*The WHO Guidelines on Use of Medically Important Antimicrobials in Food-producing Animals* (WHO Guidelines) [31].

Given the logical progression of these two WHO documents, which essentially provides important implementation guidance to help preserve the antimicrobials most important for human health, but this appears to be a step too far for some countries not yet ready or prepared to take these steps. This resistance was reflected in the Codex/TFAMR documents which excludes any endorsement of these WHO Guidelines. This is an important issue that will not simply disappear, so some background may be useful.

In 2017 after a two year process the WHO Guidelines were released and immediately drew criticism from the U.S. including in this media release from USDA Acting Chief Scientist questioned the legitimacy of the 'evidence' underpinning them as well as the role of the WHO in developing guidelines over subject matter perceived as being the preserve of the Codex and the OIE [32]. This information document from the WHO clarifies the background to the development of the WHO Guidelines and reiterating its role is to protect public health and the antimicrobials important for human medicine. Antibiotics used only in Animals were not included in the WHO Guidelines [33].

Some business-focused media coverage provided this commentary on the politics behind this unusual public criticism of the WHO's mandate to develop such guidance [34]. A later contrary response from some key US Lawmakers on the Codex/TFAMR negotiations regarding the use of 'growth promoters' demonstrated the level of internal contestation that can arise [35].

This difference in opinion over the WHO Guidelines was carried through to Codex TFAMR negotiations with the WHO representative being asked to clarify the 'status' of the WHO CIA List and its Guidelines. A summary of WHO's response is below but the full explanation should be understood as it clearly defines the WHO's mandate to develop these two reports, the governance and operational procedures underpinning them, and the political flexibility accorded to governments [24].

The WHO's statement appears to clarify that both WHO documents have the same status and includes the following points: Both reports are science based, the primary focus is to protect public health and they are not open to negotiations. Their adoption by the World Health Assembly is not required under WHO rules and implementation by Member States is voluntary [24] (p. 2).

With the WHO Guidelines now a source of political contention and questioning the legitimacy of decision making will prove disruptive. But in this important health security agenda questioning the legitimacy of data also has the potential to create a significant fracturing of the global consensus on AMR One Health Policy. Consumer and Health non-government organization's input to TFAMR indicated their full support for the WHO Guidelines.

This dispute over politically endorsing the WHO Guidelines will not be resolved easily or quickly as it signals implementing these WHO Guidelines to preserve the WHO CIA List may be politically problematic or too difficult for some countries.

However, in stark contrast, the recommendations outlined in the OIE List of Antimicrobial Agents of Veterinary Importance [36] and the WHO CIA List [30] are being simultaneously supported. But there are obvious significant compatibility problems that run counter to the objectives of the WHO CIA List. Endorsement of the OIE List sanctions the use of many of the medically important antimicrobials listed in the WHO's CIA List.

The two documents may be individually internally consistent according to the guidance for developing them, but not compatible for delivering the objective of preserving the effectiveness of medically important antimicrobials for human use—the WHO CIA List.

This, of course, is not the only difference in approach, and it would be naïve to expect that such political differences would not arise when significant economic interests are at stake. But questioning the legitimacy of the WHO Guidelines, particularly by such a powerful player as the U.S. could put a break on measures to reduce using medically important antimicrobials that are currently extensively used in food production. Other interested parties may welcome this dispute to delay transitioning away from antimicrobial use. Worth noting, the TFAMR has not yet substantially focused on antimicrobials important for humans also used in crop production or the broader environment [20,37]. These issues will also be highly relevant for zoonotic and infectious disease experts.

Interestingly, asset managers of large investments in the global food industry are moving well ahead of the deliberations in Codex (and many governments). Their agenda links into the WHO CIA list and supports many of the implementation elements contained in the WHO Guidelines [38]. These corporate bodies are aware and expecting AMR trade regulations to be enacted [39] to preserve antimicrobials important for human health. The EU being the most advanced and its One Health Strategy includes commitment to act to protect citizens, food producers and that the efforts made by EU farmers " ... are not compromised by the non-prudent use of antimicrobials in EU trading partners" [40]. The U.S. FDA Strategy for the Safety of Imported Food also indicates a strategic focus on consumer safety [41].

Case Study 3: The Political Agenda: Scientific-Evidence Based Data versus Precautionary Principle

For a complex subject such as 'AMR in the food chain' the interpretation of what constitutes 'evidence' and the legitimacy this conveys matters—particularly in Codex [42], OIE [43], and the WTO [44] trade-related deliberations. To state the obvious, scientific evidence-based data matters but there are numerous examples of scientific evidence-based claims being overturned as so narrow to be almost meaningless or totally unjustifiable, including many attached to controversial health and food issues i.e. tobacco use, and obesity issues.

AMR also shines a light on the need to implement and develop basic hygiene and public health infrastructure. Developing countries' technical capacity/resources to minimize the dangers of AMR in the food chain are yet to be sufficiently addressed [45]. From an economic and development perspective, those countries relying on export earnings from food production are particularly vulnerable. But for those with well-developed public health systems there remains considerable resistance to transparently collect or test the basic data needed to analyze consequences of antibiotic use in their food producing animals and agriculture.

A reading of the many submissions made into the TFAMR negotiations by government, industry and consumer representatives should leave the reader in no doubt of the underlying sensitivities and interpretations of 'valid' scientific data and risk. Some of these positions may however be overtaken by other events. For example, the WTO Secretariat's Report to the TFAMR demonstrates that multilateral dialogue on trade and AMR in the food chain is being opened up to further scrutiny outside of Codex. WTO Members engaged in a substantive dialogue on AMR issues in the SPS Committee for the first time, primarily focused on EU legislative intentions to address AMR in the food chain [14].

This EU regulatory information provided is important and covers a range of issues and given the response from several countries will be politically sensitive and played out in both Codex and WTO forums. Topics worth noting being developed by the EU include legislative measures: Addressing public health risk of AMR; reserving certain antimicrobials for treatment of infections in humans only; misuse of antimicrobials in medicated feed for prophylaxis and limiting treatment duration. The report records interesting responses and questions to the EU representative from several governments. The report also includes a list of 'regular and emergency' SPS and TBT Notifications submitted by Member States.

The debate opened up in the WTO SPS Committee may not yet have fully registered at the December Codex/TFAMR meeting but is significant. These new inputs now formally expressed to the SPS Committee illustrate further the importance of fully integrating WTO and Codex policy into national AMR One Health strategic planning.

For an observer of the Codex/TFAMR negotiations it is interesting to note that national-based AMR One Health implementation policies are actively reducing human access to antimicrobials. And at the global level, governments have politically endorsed the position that antimicrobials need to be protected and treated as a global public good. Contrasting this, reaching agreement on action to stop or reduce the non-therapeutic use of antimicrobials for food-producing animals and also to preserve medically important antimicrobials for humans, seem to require a much higher standard of scientific evidence-based data. As consumers' understanding of the AMR One Health agenda develops, they may not support such reticence to act on this important health security issue.

References

1. United Nations Seventy-First Session of the General Assembly—Political Declaration of the High-Level Meeting on Antimicrobial Resistance, A/RES/71/3 held on 21 September 2016, Resolution Adopted 5 October 2016. Available online: http://www.un.org/en/ga/search/view_doc.asp?symbol=A/RES/71/3 (accessed on 4 February 2019).
2. Review of Antimicrobial Resistance. Available online: https://amr-review.org/ (accessed on 14 February 2019).
3. Burnham, J.P.; Olsen, M.A.; Kollef, M.H. Re-Estimating Annual Deaths Due to Multidrug-Resistant Organism Infections. Available online: https://www.cambridge.org/core/journals/infection-control-and-hospital-epidemiology/article/reestimating-annual-deaths-due-to-multidrugresistant-organism-infections/C9B09A787FCCA1EA992AF45066F3FF7C (accessed on 15 February 2019).
4. CIDRAP. New Estimates Aim to Define the True Burden of Superbug Infections. Available online: http://www.cidrap.umn.edu/news-perspective/2019/02/new-estimates-aim-define-true-burden-superbug-infections (accessed on 14 February 2019).
5. WTO. Overview: The TRIPS Agreement. Available online: https://www.wto.org/english/tratop_e/trips_e/intel2_e.htm (accessed on 10 February 2019).
6. European Union. Understanding EU Reach. Available online: https://echa.europa.eu/regulations/reach/understanding-reach (accessed on 10 February 2019).
7. WTO. Panel Upholds Australia Plain Packaging Policy for Tobacco Products. Available online: https://www.ictsd.org/bridges-news/bridges/news/wto-panel-upholds-australia-plain-packaging-policy-for-tobacco-products (accessed on 10 February 2019).
8. Guardian. Diversion tactics: How Big Pharma is Muddying the Waters on Animal Antibiotics. Available online: https://www.theguardian.com/environment/2018/jun/19/animal-antibiotics-calm-down-about-your-chicken-says-big-pharma (accessed on 5 March 2019).
9. Codex Scorecard. Available online: http://www.fao.org/fao-who-codexalimentarius/thematic-areas/antimicrobial-resistance/en/-c437070 (accessed on 14 February 2019).

10. Ad hoc Codex. Intergovernmental Task Force on Antimicrobial Resistance (TFAMR). Available online: http://www.fao.org/fao-who-codexalimentarius/committees/committee/en/?committee=TFAMR (accessed on 4 February 2019).

11. Ad Hoc Codex. Intergovernmental Task force on Antimicrobial Resistance—TFAMR 6th Session, 10/12/2018-14/12/2018 Busan, Republic of Korea. Available online: http://www.fao.org/fao-who-codexalimentarius/meetings/detail/en/?meeting=TFAMR&session=6 (accessed on 4 February 2019).

12. WHO. Global Action Plan on Antimicrobial Resistance. Available online: https://www.who.int/antimicrobial-resistance/global-action-plan/en/ (accessed on 5 March 2019).

13. WTO. Director General, Azevêdo. A. Statement to Trilateral meeting with WHO, WIPO and WTO, How WTO. Can Help to Meet Challenge of Antimicrobial Resistance, Geneva, 16 October 2016. Available online: https://www.wto.org/english/news_e/spra_e/spra142_e.htm (accessed on 4 February 2019).

14. Ad Hoc Codex. Intergovernmental Task force on Antimicrobial Resistance: Matters Arising from Other Relevant International Organizations (OECD, World Bank, World Customs Organization, WTO). Available online: http://www.fao.org/fao-who-codexalimentarius/sh-proxy/en/?lnk=1&url=https%3A%2F%2Fworkspace.fao.org%2Fsites%2Fcodex%2FMeetings%2FCX-804-06%2FWD%2Famr06_04e.pdf (accessed on 27 February 2019).

15. ReAct. Antibiotic Footprint: Change the Way Food is Labeled? Available online: https://www.reactgroup.org/news-and-views/news-and-opinions/year-2019/antibiotic-footprint-change-the-way-food-is-labelled/ (accessed on 27 February 2019).

16. The Food and Agriculture Organization of the UN; World Trade Organization. Trade and Food Standards 2017. Available online: http://www.fao.org/3/a-i7407e.pdf (accessed on 4 February 2019).

17. UK Science and Innovation Network. Wellcome Trust and USA CDC. Initiatives for Addressing Antimicrobial Resistance in the Environment. Available online: https://wellcome.ac.uk/sites/default/files/antimicrobial-resistance-environment-report.pdf (accessed on 21 February 2019).

18. Codex. Report of the Physical Working Group on AMR, London December 2016. Available online: http://www.fao.org/fao-who-codexalimentarius/sh-proxy/en/?lnk=1&url=https%253A%252F%252Fworkspace.fao.org%252Fsites%252Fcodex%252FMeetings%252FCX-701-40%252FWD%252Fcac40_12_Add2e.pdf (accessed on 5 March 2019).

19. George, A.; George. Antimicrobial Resistance, Trade, Food Safety and Security. One Health 2018, 5, 6–8. [CrossRef] [PubMed]

20. FAO; WHO. Expert Meeting on Foodborne Antimicrobial Resistance: Role of Environment, Crop and Biocides. 2018. Available online: https://www.who.int/foodsafety/areas_work/antimicrobial-resistance/FAO_WHO_AMR_Summary_Report_June2018.pdf?ua=1 (accessed on 6 February 2019).

21. Collignon, P.; Beggs, J.J.; Walsh, T.R.; Gandra, S.; Laxminarayan, R. Anthropological and Socioeconomic Factors Contributing to Global Antimicrobial Resistance: A Univariate and Multivariable Analysis. Lancet Planet. Health 2018, 2, e398–e405. [CrossRef]

22. Codex TFAMR. Proposed Draft Revision of the Code of Practice to Minimize and Contain Foodborne Antibiotic Resistance. Available online: http://www.fao.org/fao-who-codexalimentarius/sh-proxy/en/?lnk=1&url=https%253A%252F%252Fworkspace.fao.org%252Fsites%252Fcodex%252FMeetings%252FCX-804-06%252FCRDs%252Famr6_CRD20x.pdf (accessed on 9 February 2019).

23. Codex TFAMR. Proposed Draft Guidelines on Integrated Monitoring and Surveillance of Foodborne Antimicrobial Resistance. Available online: http://www.fao.org/fao-who-codexalimentarius/sh-proxy/en/?lnk=1&url=https%253A%252F%252Fworkspace.fao.org%252Fsites%252Fcodex%252FMeetings%252FCX-804-06%252FCRDs%252Famr6_CRD18x.pdf (accessed on 9 February 2019).

24. Report of the Sixth Session of the Codex Ad Hoc Intergovernmental Task Force on Antimicrobial Resistance, Busan, Korea, 10–14 December 2018. Available online: http://www.fao.org/fao-who-codexalimentarius/sh-proxy/en/?lnk=1&url=https%253A%252F%252Fworkspace.fao.org%252Fsites%252Fcodex%252FMeetings%252FCX-804-06%252FREPORT%252FFINAL+REPORT%252FREP19_AMRe.pdf (accessed on 24 January 2019).

25. Cantas, L.; Suer, K. Review: The Important Bacterial Zoonoses in "One Health' Concept. Available online: https://www.ncbi.nlm.nih.gov/pmc/articles/PMC4196475/ (accessed on 13 February 2019).

26. European Centre for Disease Prevention and Control (ECDC). Antimicrobial Resistance in Zoonotic Bacteria Still High in Humans, Animals and Food Say ECDC and EFSA. Available online: https://ecdc.europa.eu/sites/portal/files/documents/Pressrelease_ECDCEFSA_AMRzoonoses2016.pdf (accessed on 13 February 2019).

27. Interagency Coordination Group on Antimicrobial Resistance: Draft Recommendations. Available online: https://www.who.int/antimicrobial-resistance/interagency-coordination-group/Draft_IACG_recommendations_for_public_discussion_290119.pdf (accessed on 23 February 2019).

28. Codex Secretariat. Available online: http://www.fao.org/fao-who-codexalimentarius/about-codex/codex-secretariat/en/ (accessed on 20 February 2019).

29. Codex TFAMR. Matters Arising from FAO, WHO and OIE Including The Report of the Joint FAO/WHO Expert Meeting (in Collaboration with OIE) on Foodborne Antimicrobial Resistance. Available online: http://www.fao.org/fao-who-codexalimentarius/sh-proxy/en/?lnk=1&url=https%253A%252F%252Fworkspace.fao.org%252Fsites%252Fcodex%252FMeetings%252FCX-804-06%252FWD%252Famr06_03e.pdf (accessed on 9 February 2019).

30. WHO. List of Critically Important Antimicrobials (WHO CIA List). Available online: https://www.who.int/foodsafety/areas_work/antimicrobial-resistance/cia/en/ (accessed on 10 February 2019).

31. WHO. Guidelines on Use of Medically Important Antimicrobials in Food-Producing Animals. Available online: https://www.who.int/foodsafety/publications/cia_guidelines/en/ (accessed on 8 February 2019).

32. USDA. Chief Scientist Statement on WHO Guidelines on Antibiotics. Available online: https://www.usda.gov/media/press-releases/2017/11/07/usda-chief-scientist-statement-who-guidelines-antibiotics (accessed on 8 February 2019).

33. WHO. Food Safety Antimicrobial Resistance in the Food Chain. Available online: https://www.who.int/foodsafety/areas_work/antimicrobial-resistance/amrfoodchain/en/ (accessed on 20 February 2019).

34. Martin, A.; Hopkins, J.S. *Bloomberg. Trump's USDA Fight Global Guidelines on Livestock Antibiotics*; Bloomberg: New York, NY, USA, 24 July 2018; Available online: https://www.bloomberg.com/news/articles/2018-07-23/trump-s-usda-fights-global-guidelines-on-livestock-antibiotics (accessed on 8 February 2019).

35. Martin, A. Bloomberg, Lawmakers Questions USA > Position on Antimicrobial Use in Livestock 8 December 2018. Available online: https://www.bloomberg.com/news/articles/2018-12-07/lawmakers-question-u-s-position-on-antibiotic-use-in-livestock (accessed on 10 February 2019).

36. OIE. List of Antimicrobial Agents of Veterinary Importance. Available online: http://www.oie.int/fileadmin/Home/eng/Our_scientific_expertise/docs/pdf/AMR/A_OIE_List_antimicrobials_May2018.pdf (accessed on 10 February 2019).

37. Codex TFAMR. Matters Referred by the Codex Alimentarius Commission and other Subsidiary bodies. Available online: http://www.fao.org/fao-who-codexalimentarius/sh-proxy/en/?lnk=1&url=https%253A%252F%252Fworkspace.fao.org%252Fsites%252Fcodex%252FMeetings%252FCX-804-06%252FWD%252Fam06_02e.pdf (accessed on 20 February 2019).

38. FAIRR. Farm Animal Investment Risk and Return: Investor Statement on Antibiotics Stewardship. Available online: https://www.neiinvestments.com/documents/PublicPolicyAndStandards/2017/InvestorStatementonAntibioticsStewardship.pdf (accessed on 8 February 2019).

39. Reducing Agricultural Antibiotics, Can Resistance in Farm Animals be Prevented from Spreading to Humans? Available online: https://www.gbm.hsbc.com/insights/global-research/reducing-agricultural-antibiotics (accessed on 21 February 2019).

40. A European One Health Action Plan Against Antimicrobial Resistance (AMR). Available online: https://ec.europa.eu/health/amr/sites/amr/files/amr_action_plan_2017_en.pdf (accessed on 20 February 2019).

41. USA Food and Drug Administration. (FDA) for the Safety of Imported Food. Available online: https://www.fda.gov/Food/GuidanceRegulation/ImportsExports/Importing/ucm631747.htm (accessed on 27 February 2019).

42. Codex and Science. Available online: http://www.fao.org/fao-who-codexalimentarius/about-codex/science/en/ (accessed on 9 February 2019).

43. OIE Standards and International Trade. Available online: http://www.oie.int/animal-welfare/oie-standards-and-international-trade (accessed on 9 February 2019).

44. WTO Agreements and Public Health. Available online: https://www.wto.org/english/res_e/booksp_e/who_wto_e.pdf (accessed on 9 February 2019).

45. World Bank. Drug-Resistant Infections: A Threat to Our Economic Future (vol2) Final Report. Available online: http://documents.worldbank.org/curated/en/323311493396993758/final-report (accessed on 10 February 2019).

8

Host-Driven Phosphorylation Appears to Regulate the Budding Activity of the Lassa Virus Matrix Protein

Christopher M. Ziegler [1], Philip Eisenhauer [1], Inessa Manuelyan [1,2], Marion E. Weir [3,†], Emily A. Bruce [1], Bryan A. Ballif [3] and Jason Botten [1,4,*]

[1] Department of Medicine, Division of Immunobiology, University of Vermont, Burlington, VT 05405, USA; cziegler@uvm.edu (C.M.Z.); philip.eisenhauer@med.uvm.edu (P.E.); Inessa.Manuelyan@uvm.edu (I.M.); Emily.Bruce@med.uvm.edu (E.A.B.)

[2] Cellular, Molecular and Biomedical Sciences Graduate Program, University of Vermont, Burlington, VT 05405, USA

[3] Department of Biology, University of Vermont, Burlington, VT 05405, USA; marion.weir@cellsignal.com (M.E.W.); bballif@uvm.edu (B.A.B.)

[4] Department of Microbiology and Molecular Genetics, University of Vermont, Burlington, VT 05405, USA

* Correspondence: jbotten@uvm.edu.

† Current address: Cell Signaling Technology, 32 Tozer Rd, Beverly, MA 01915, USA

Abstract: Lassa mammarenavirus (LASV) is an enveloped RNA virus that can cause Lassa fever, an acute hemorrhagic fever syndrome associated with significant morbidity and high rates of fatality in endemic regions of western Africa. The arenavirus matrix protein Z has several functions during the virus life cycle, including coordinating viral assembly, driving the release of new virus particles, regulating viral polymerase activity, and antagonizing the host antiviral response. There is limited knowledge regarding how the various functions of Z are regulated. To investigate possible means of regulation, mass spectrometry was used to identify potential sites of phosphorylation in the LASV Z protein. This analysis revealed that two serines (S18, S98) and one tyrosine (Y97) are phosphorylated in the flexible N- and C-terminal regions of the protein. Notably, two of these sites, Y97 and S98, are located in (Y97) or directly adjacent to (S98) the PPXY late domain, an important motif for virus release. Studies with non-phosphorylatable and phosphomimetic Z proteins revealed that these sites are important regulators of the release of LASV particles and that host-driven, reversible phosphorylation may play an important role in the regulation of LASV Z protein function.

Keywords: Lassa virus; Z protein; late domain; PPXY; budding; release; matrix protein; phosphorylation; arenavirus; mass spectrometry

1. Introduction

The *Mammarenavirus* genus is comprised primarily of rodent-borne viruses, several of which are capable of causing severe hemorrhagic fever syndromes in humans [1]. Lassa virus (LASV), the causative agent of Lassa fever, is carried primarily by the multimammate rat, *Mastomys natalensis*, but other carrier rodents have been identified recently [2–4]. LASV infects up to an estimated 300,000 people each year in western Africa following exposure to rodent excreta or through hunting and consumption of infected rats [2,5–8]. Lassa virus can also spread person-to-person through direct contact with infected bodily fluids, and this pattern of transmission has occurred repeatedly in hospital workers caring for Lassa fever patients since its discovery in 1969 [9–11]. Overall, the case fatality rate is estimated at 1–2%, but significantly higher rates of fatality occur in hospitalized patients [5]. Since 2008, outbreaks in Sierra Leone have resulted in an overall case fatality rate of 69% in hospitalized patients [12]. LASV infection results in fetal loss in most cases [13]. Further, pregnancy greatly increases the risk of fatality from Lassa fever for the mother [13]. Of Lassa fever survivors who were hospitalized, approximately one-third developed hearing loss, and in two-thirds of those patients, the hearing deficit was permanent [14]. Intravenous ribavirin treatment has been shown to reduce mortality from Lassa fever, particularly if administered during the first six days of fever onset, but there is a clear need for more effective therapies [5]. No United States Food and Drug Administration (FDA)-approved vaccines exist for the prevention of LASV infection.

Arenaviruses have a simple, negative-strand RNA genome that encodes a total of four proteins on two segments. The small (S) segment encodes both the nucleoprotein (NP), which encapsidates the viral genome and is required for its replication, and the envelope glycoprotein (GP), which interacts with cell surface receptors to mediate cell entry and membrane fusion [15–20]. The large (L) genome segment encodes the viral RNA-dependent RNA polymerase (L), which replicates and transcribes the genome, and the viral matrix protein (Z) [19–22]. The Z protein is a structural component of the virion, forming a matrix layer on the inner leaflet of the viral envelope, and carries out an array of important functions during viral propagation [23,24]. The Z protein of pathogenic arenaviruses antagonizes interferon production by binding to retinoic acid-inducible gene I (RIG-I) and melanoma differentiation-associated protein 5 (MDA5) to disrupt interactions between RIG-I-like receptors and mitochondrial antiviral signaling (MAVS) [25]. Z can inhibit the translation of capped cellular mRNAs and also regulate the activity of the viral polymerase [26–28]. Z is also an important coordinator of virus particle assembly by interacting with each of the other three viral proteins [29,30].

In addition to these functions, the Z protein is both necessary and sufficient for driving the efficient release of nascent virus particles [23,31,32]. However, minimal levels of virus can be recovered without Z [33]. Two major motifs in the Z protein mediate the efficient release of virus particles. First, a myristoylation modification of the second residue in Z, a glycine, mediates Z's interaction with cellular membranes, a requirement for efficient release [34,35]. Second, all arenavirus Z proteins, with the exception of the Tacaribe virus Z protein, contain one or two proline-rich, late domains near the C-terminus [23,32]. These viral late domains are presumably responsible for recruiting the cellular endosomal sorting complex required for transport (ESCRT) pathway to mediate membrane scission, which is the final step in the virus budding process [36]. New World arenavirus Z proteins contain a P(S/T)AP-type late domain, which can bind the ESCRT-I protein Tsg101, while the Old World Z proteins of the lymphocytic choriomeningitis virus (LCMV) and Dandenong virus contain only a PPXY late domain, which can bind Nedd4-family E3 ubiquitin ligases [23,24,32,37]. Additionally, the Z proteins of several Old World arenaviruses, including Lassa, Mobala, Mopeia, and Ippy viruses, encode both the PPXY and the P(S/T)AP late domains [23,24,32]. In the case of LASV, decreased virus-like particle (VLP) release occurs following mutation of either of LASV Z's PTAP and PPXY late domains, disruption of Z's recruitment of Nedd4-family proteins, and/or loss of specific ESCRT components [23,24,32,37–39]. The release of VLPs for the related Old World arenavirus LCMV is similarly impacted by PPXY late domain or ESCRT component disruption [32]. However, recent work from our lab demonstrated that in a whole virus system, the sole late domain in the LCMV Z protein and the ESCRT pathway it recruits were specifically required for the production of defective interfering particles but not of infectious virus [40]. This illustrates the complexity and diversity in arenavirus release and highlights the need for a greater understanding of the factors involved in this process.

Protein phosphorylation is a reversible post-translational modification that can regulate the activity of enzymes, mediate protein–protein interactions, alter the subcellular localization, conformation, and/or oligomeric state of proteins, as well as regulate the addition or removal of other types of post-translation modifications [41]. This important type of modification is not limited to cellular proteins; a growing body of literature has demonstrated that phosphorylation of viral proteins has important consequences for different viral processes [42–45]. Phosphorylation sites of functional significance have been identified on the matrix proteins in an array of RNA viruses, including the Z protein of the Old World arenavirus LCMV [40,46–51]. Accordingly, we hypothesized that the functionality of the LASV Z protein may be regulated by phosphorylation. To address this hypothesis, mass spectrometry was used to identify phosphorylated residues in LASV Z. This approach revealed three sites of phosphorylation, including two phosphorylated serines and one tyrosine. A VLP release assay demonstrated that serine phosphorylation may negatively impact virus release. These findings are an important first step toward understanding how various functions of the LASV Z protein can be regulated by post-translational modifications.

2. Results and Discussion

To identify sites of phosphorylation, LASV Z protein was affinity purified from VLPs produced from plasmid-transfected cells and subjected to protein gel electrophoresis (Figure 1A). The gel band corresponding to LASV Z was excised and proteolytically digested. The resulting peptides were analyzed by liquid chromatography–tandem mass spectrometry. Three phosphorylated residues in the LASV Z protein were identified: two serine residues (S18 and S98) and one tyrosine residue (Y97) (Figure 1B, Figures S1 and S2). Representative mass spectra and the accompanying fragment ion tables for peptides harboring phosphorylated Y97 (Figure S1A), phosphorylated S98 (Figure S1C), as well as corresponding unphosphorylated peptides are shown (Figure S1B). Representative mass spectra and corresponding fragment ion tables of the peptides harboring phosphorylated S18 (Figure S2A) and unphosphorylated S18 (Figure S2B) are shown.

Each phosphorylation site was mapped onto the NMR structure of LASV Z (Figure 1B) [52]. The arenavirus Z protein is comprised of a central zinc-binding, really interesting new gene (RING) domain flanked by N- and C-terminal domains that appear to be flexible and relatively unstructured [52–57]. All three phosphorylation sites identified are located in these flexible N-terminal (S18) or C-terminal (Y97 and S98) domains of the Z protein (Figure 1B,C) [52]. The N-terminal domain of Z is known to mediate several important functions. It contains a myristoylation site at the second glycine residue which is required for virus budding as well as Z's interaction with the plasma membrane and with the envelope glycoprotein [30,34,35]. Other conserved residues in the N-terminal domain contribute to the production of infectious virus-like particles [58]. Additionally, the N-terminal domain of pathogenic arenaviruses, including LASV, but not of non-pathogenic arenaviruses, can directly bind to and inhibit the function of retinoic acid-inducible gene 1-like receptors (RLRs), which results in decreased macrophage activation [25,59]. The Clustal Omega multiple sequence alignment tool was used to align select mammarenavirus Z proteins (Figure 1C) [60]. This revealed that the S18 phosphorylation site is conserved across LASV strains representing lineages III–VI, as well as in Mobala virus and the New World Oliveros virus (Figure 1C) [61–63]. Notably, a histidine residue is found at this position in multiple lineage II LASV isolates that have recently been sequenced [64]. Interestingly, aspartic acid and glutamic acid, which are negatively charged at a physiological pH similar to phosphate, are substituted for S18 in a number of other New and Old World arenavirus Z proteins, suggesting that a negative charge at this position may be important for Z functionality (Figure 1C).

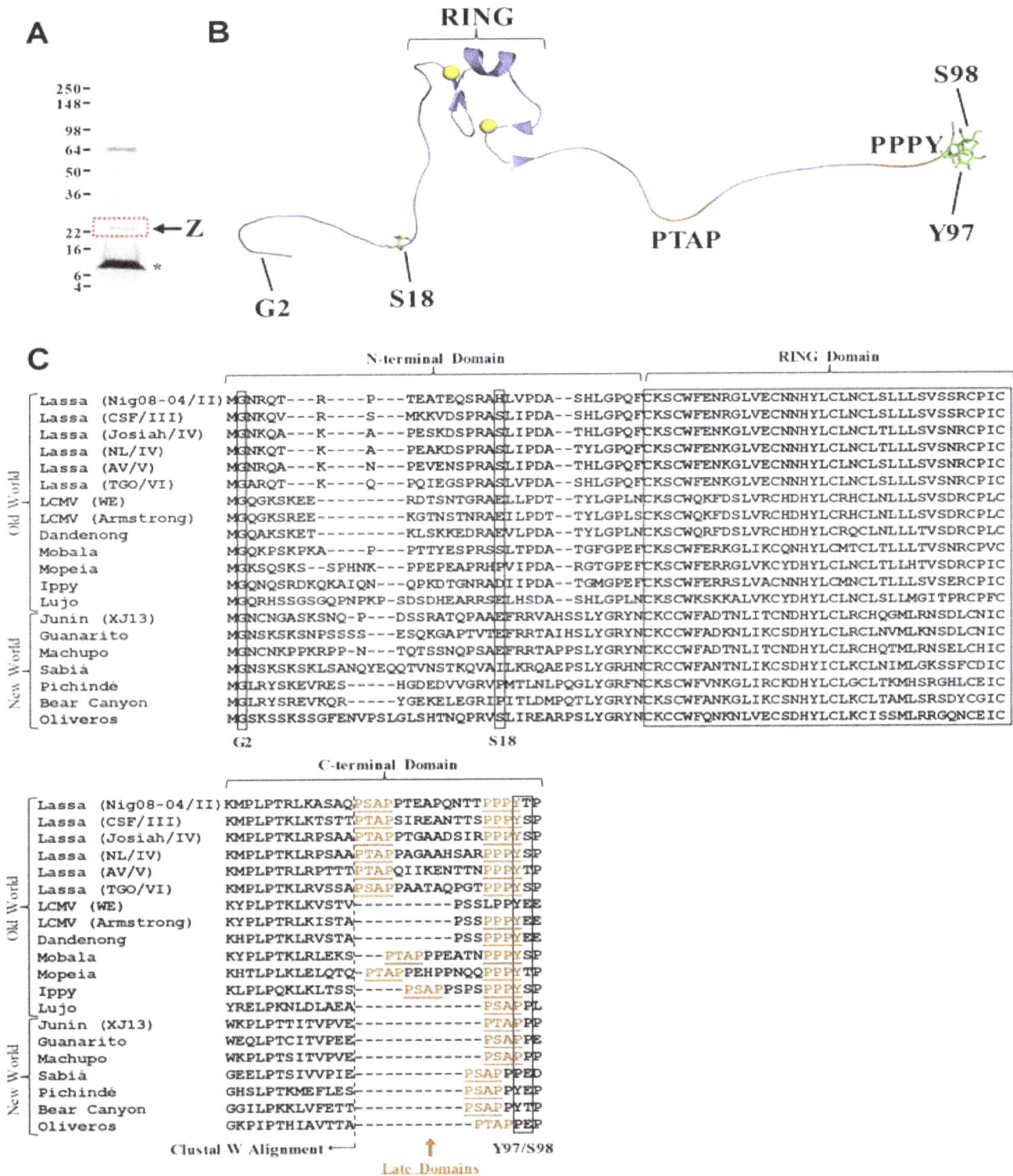

Figure 1. Identification of phosphorylation sites in the Lassa mammarenavirus (LASV) Z matrix protein. (**A**) Coomassie-stained polyacrylamide gel of affinity-purified LASV Z. Streptavidin-coated magnetic beads were used to affinity purify Z from virus-like particles (VLPs) released from cells co-transfected with plasmids encoding a biotin ligase and LASV Z C-terminally tagged with a biotin acceptor peptide (BAP). The band corresponding to the LASV Z protein (indicated by the red box) was excised from the gel and subjected to proteolytic digestion with trypsin or a combination of trypsin and chymotrypsin.

The resultant peptides were extracted and subjected to liquid chromatography–tandem mass spectrometry analysis. The asterisk denotes the band of monomeric streptavidin that is eluted from streptavidin beads following boiling. (**B**) The protein nuclear magnetic resonance structure of the Josiah strain of the LASV Z matrix (PDB 2M1S) is shown. The side chains of the phosphorylated residues (S18, Y97, and S98) are highlighted in green on the protein structure. The two late domains found in LASV Z, PTAP and PPPY, are colored orange. Zinc ions, which are coordinated by the central really interesting new gene (RING) domain of Z, are shown as yellow spheres in the protein structure. The myristoylated glycine residue (at position 2) is also indicated. (**C**) Protein sequence alignment of select mammarenavirus Z proteins. The Clustal Omega multiple sequence alignment tool was used to align the sequences of selected mammarenavirus Z proteins. The portion of the C-terminal region of each Z protein (the amino acids to the right of the dashed vertical line) containing the late domains (designated as orange, underlined amino acids) was aligned with LASV Z strain Josiah, starting with the most C-terminal amino acid. The following accession numbers were used: GU481069.1 (Lassa mammarenavirus, strain Nig08-04), AAO59514.1 (Lassa mammarenavirus, strain CSF), NP_694871.1 (Lassa mammarenavirus, strain Josiah), AAO59510.1 (Lassa mammarenavirus, strain NL), AAO59508.1 (Lassa mammarenavirus, strain AV), MF990887.1 (Lassa mammarenavirus, strain TGO) AAD03395.1 (Lymphocytic choriomeningitis mammarenavirus, strain WE), ABC96003.1 (Lymphocytic choriomeningitis mammarenavirus, strain Armstrong 53b), ABY20731.1 (Dandenong virus), ABC71138.1 (Mobala mammarenavirus), ABC71136.1 (Mopeia mammarenavirus, strain Mozambique), ABC71142.1 (Ippy mammarenavirus), YP_002929492.1 (Lujo mammarenavirus), NP_899216.1 (Junín mammarenavirus, strain XJ13), NP_899220.1 (Guanarito mammarenavirus), NP_899214.1 (Machupo mammarenavirus), ABY59837.1 (Brazilian mammarenavirus), YP_138535.1 (Pichindé mammarenavirus), YP_001649224.1 (Bear Canyon mammarenavirus), YP_001649215.1 (Oliveros mammarenavirus). For each LASV isolate, the corresponding lineage is listed after the strain.

The Y97 and S98 phosphorylation sites lie within the C-terminal tail of the LASV Z protein, a region which contains two proline-rich late domains, PTAP and PPPY (Figure 1B,C). The C-terminal amino acids containing the late domains of selected mammarenavirus Z proteins were aligned (Figure 1C). This analysis showed that Y97 is conserved across the majority of Old World mammarenaviruses (except for Lujo virus) and aligns with Pichindé and Bear Canyon New World mammarenaviruses (Figure 1C). Conservation of a serine or threonine at residues that align with LASV Z S98 is fairly common among Old World mammarenaviruses (Figure 1C). Notably, LCMV possesses a glutamic acid at this position which could substitute for the negative charge of a phosphorylated serine (Figure 1C). However, LASV Z S98 is directly followed by a proline residue. Interestingly, phosphorylated serine or threonine residues directly preceding a proline (pS/T–P) constitute a type of motif that can be recognized by class IV WW domains, including the peptidylprolyl cis/trans isomerase, NIMA-interacting 1 protein (Pin1) [65,66]. Pin1 can mediate conformational changes in substrate proteins that result in altered protein stability or phosphorylation state [67]. Because Pin1 has been implicated in different viral infections and has been shown to bind pS/T–P motifs within viral proteins from hepatitis B virus [68], human T-cell leukemia virus type 1 [69,70], human immunodeficiency virus 1 [71–73], Epstein–Barr virus [74], and Kaposi's sarcoma-associated herpesvirus [75], it may represent an interesting host target for further study in the context of the arenavirus Z protein.

The Y97 phosphorylation site lies within the PPXY late domain, which is conserved across the majority of Old World arenavirus Z proteins (Figure 1C). Our lab recently showed that the homologous tyrosine residue (Y88) in LCMV Z is also phosphorylated [40]. Treating cells with H_2O_2 to block tyrosine phosphatases and permit the accumulation of tyrosines phosphorylated by endogenous kinases demonstrated that both LCMV and LASV Z are phosphorylated on a tyrosine residue (Figure 2A) [76]. This strategy further showed that the phosphotyrosine levels of LASV Z were significantly reduced in the Y97F mutant of LASV Z, indicating that this late domain-embedded tyrosine is likely the major tyrosine phosphorylation site (Figure 2B), similar to what we observed for the PPXY-embedded Y88 in the case of LCMV [40].

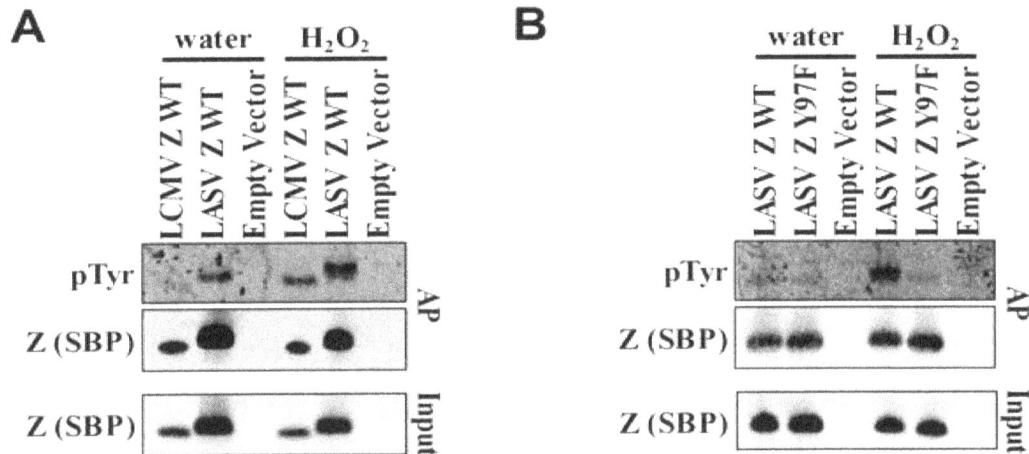

Figure 2. Confirmation of Y97 phosphorylation site in LASV Z. (**A**,**B**) HEK293T cells were transfected with plasmids encoding the indicated streptavidin-binding peptide (SBP)-tagged lymphocytic choriomeningitis virus (LCMV) Z or LASV Z, and two days later streptavidin-coated magnetic beads were used to affinity purify (AP) intracellular Z from cells that had been treated with water or hydrogen peroxide (H_2O_2). Levels of phosphotyrosine and Z-SBP in affinity-purified samples (and unpurified cellular input for Z-SBP) were determined by western blotting with anti-phosphotyrosine or anti-SBP antibodies, respectively. Levels of phosphotyrosine are shown for wild-type (WT) LCMV Z and LASV Z (**A**) as well as for WT and phosphosite-mutant (Y97F) LASV Z proteins (**B**). Western blots are representative of five (**A**) or four (**B**) independent experiments.

A prominent function of the arenavirus Z protein is to drive the release of virus particles. We next sought to determine whether any of the three phosphorylation sites might contribute to the ability of Z to drive virus budding using a VLP release assay (Figure 3A–C). For the phosphoserine residues at S18 or S98, LASV Z protein mutants encoding either an alanine or an aspartic acid substitution at these positions were made in order to prevent or to possibly mimic phosphorylation at the site in question, respectively. Phosphomimetic substitution did not result in a significant change in VLP release for either S18 or S98 (Figure 3A,C). However, substitution with alanine to either phosphoserine site resulted in levels of VLP release that were 1.5- or 2-fold greater than in the WT, suggesting that serine phosphorylation may negatively regulate the release of virus particles (Figure 3A). It is important to note that, in many cases, aspartic acid and glutamic acid do not functionally mimic phosphorylation, particularly when a phosphorylated residue is recognized by an adaptor protein [77]. Our results here could be explained if cellular kinases impinged on viral budding by promoting a phosphoserine-dependent protein–protein interaction, one which cannot be mimicked by the shape or charge afforded by aspartic acid.

For the Y97 phosphosite, phenylalanine and glutamic acid mutants were generated, again to prevent or mimic phosphorylation, respectively. Release of VLPs from cells transfected with LASV Z containing either the non-phosphorylatable (F) or phosphomimetic (E) amino acid at residue 97 was decreased by roughly 50% compared to wild-type Z-containing cells (Figure 3B,C). Given that Y97 lies within the PPXY late domain, which has been previously shown to be required for efficient release of LCMV and LASV VLPs, the results were not surprising [23,32,40] and may indicate a cellular mechanism at play to regulate viral budding. Mutation of the canonical PPXY motif in LASV results in a loss of binding to Nedd4-family E3 ubiquitin ligases, which have been implicated in the release of several other viruses that have a PPXY domain in their matrix protein [24,36]. However, in earlier work with LCMV, despite a reduction in VLP release, disruption of the PPXY late domain did not block the efficient release of infectious virus particles but rather that of defective interfering (DI) particles [40]. Furthermore, greater levels of DI particles were released with recombinant LCMV containing a glutamic acid substitution at its Y88 phosphorylation site relative to the Y88F-mutant virus, suggesting that phosphorylation may positively regulate the release of DI particles [40]. These data raise the intriguing question of whether a similar phenomenon (e.g., whereby phosphorylation of the PPXY late domain regulates the release of a specific class of viral particles) may be occurring with the LASV Z protein. There is currently little data confirming the presence of LASV DI particles. However, it is thought that most animal viruses produce some level of DI particles, and some arenaviruses in particular are known to produce significant levels of DI particles [78,79]. More specifically, a high multiplicity of infection with LASV virus yields lower infectious titers and higher ratios of viral genomic RNA to particles compared with low-multiplicity infections [80]. These findings are consistent with a virus that produces appreciable levels of DI particles [81,82].

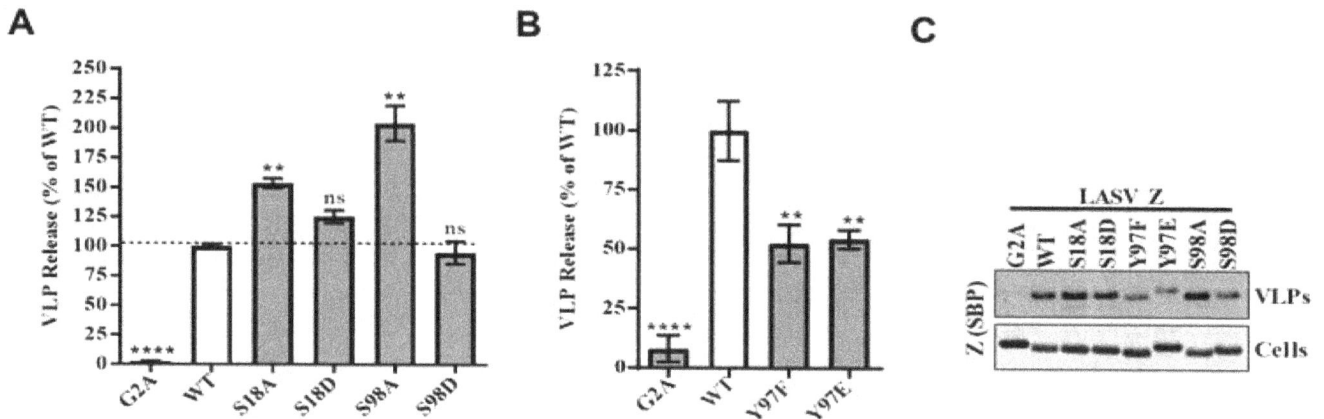

Figure 3. VLP release assay of WT and phosphomutant LASV Z proteins. (A–C) HEK293T cells were transfected with plasmids encoding the WT LASV Z protein or the LASV Z containing mutations that prevent (S to A; Y to F) or mimic (S to D; Y to E) phosphorylation at the serine phosphorylation sites (**A**) or the tyrosine phosphorylation site (**B**). The glycine-to-alanine mutant (G2A) served as a negative control as it prevents myristoylation of Z, resulting in drastic inhibition of Z's budding activity. Quantitative, fluorescent western blotting was used to quantify the amount of intracellular and VLP-derived Z protein. A representative western blot of intracellular or VLP-derived SBP-tagged Z protein is shown in (**C**). The VLP release activity was determined by dividing the quantity of Z in VLPs by the quantity of intracellular Z, then normalized to the amount of wild-type Z. The values represent the mean $\pm$ standard error of the mean from three (**A**) or four (**B**) independent experiments. Mean values were compared using a one-way ANOVA with the Holm–Sidak's test for multiple comparisons. (**A,B**), n.s. (not significant), ** $p < 0.01$, **** $p < 0.0001$.

The discovery of these phosphorylation sites opens up several new avenues for inquiry, including identifying the host kinases involved as well as any phosphosite-binding proteins that may regulate Z protein function. Kinase prediction algorithms could be used to narrow the possible candidate kinases, but empirical screens will be required to determine the kinase(s) that contribute most substantially to Z phosphorylation. Kinase identification for the LASV Z Y97 phosphosite may be aided by evidence in the literature implicating Src family or Abl tyrosine kinases in the phosphorylation of PPXY domains in other proteins—specifically, the Ebola virus matrix protein and the cellular proteins dystroglycan and IFITM3 [46,83,84]. It has also been shown for dystroglycan and IFITM3 that phosphorylation of PPXY motifs can regulate the binding of proteins that contain SH2 domains as well as of the Nedd4-family ubiquitin ligases that bind PPXY domains through their WW domain [83–85]. It is plausible that Old World mammarenavirus Z proteins are regulated in a similar fashion. It will also be important to identify phosphoserine-specific binding proteins (e.g., perhaps Pin1) or proteins containing other phosphoserine-binding domains in order to understand the mechanism by which serine phosphorylation regulates Z protein function [66]. Furthermore, it will be important to determine whether the S18 phosphorylation site or other residues in the N-terminal domain, that are more highly conserved among pathogenic arenaviruses, are involved in the inhibition of RLR signaling and macrophage activation [25,59]. Finally, the clustering of two phosphorylation sites at the C-terminus of the LASV Z protein, spanning two distinct WW domain-binding motifs, contributes to the idea that this region of Z and its corresponding functions may be intricately regulated by a network of distinct host protein partners.

3. Materials and Methods

3.1. Cells and Plasmids

Human embryonic kidney cells (HEK-293T/17, CRL-11268), purchased from American Type Culture Collection (Manassas, VA, USA), were cultured in Dulbecco's Modified Eagle Medium (DMEM) (11965-092) supplemented with 10% fetal bovine serum (FBS) (16140-071) and 1% of penicillin/streptomycin (15140-122), MEM Non-Essential Amino Acids Solution (11140-050), HEPES Buffer Solution (15630-130), and GlutaMAX (35050-061) purchased from Thermo Fisher Scientific (Carlsbad, CA, USA).

Plasmid LASV Z HA-BAP expresses the LASV Z gene from strain Josiah (GenBank #HQ688675.1) with a C-terminal hemagglutinin (HA) affinity tag followed by a tobacco etch virus cleavage site and a biotinylation acceptor peptide in a modified pCAGGS expression vector, as previously described [86, 87]. Plasmid LASV Z WT SBP is comprised of the LASV Z gene C-terminally fused to a six-amino acid linker (AAGGGG) followed by the streptavidin-binding peptide (SBP) affinity tag in a modified pCAGGS vector, as previously described [88]. Genes encoding point mutants of LASV Z (S18A, S18D, Y97F, Y97E, S98A, and S98D) were synthesized and subcloned into the LASV Z WT SBP vector by BioBasic, Inc. (Markham, ON, Canada). Plasmids expressing the Armstrong 53b strain of LCMV Z (GenBank #AY847351.1) with a C-terminal SBP tag have been described previously [40], as has the plasmid encoding the biotin ligase (BirA) [87].

3.2. Identification of Phosphorylation Sites by Mass Spectrometry

To identify potential phosphorylation sites in LASV Z, 1×10^6 HEK293T cells/well were seeded into two six-well plates. After 24 h, each well was transfected with 100 μL DMEM containing 1 μg of LASV Z HA-BAP, 1 μg of plasmid BirA, and 10 μg of polyethyleneinimine (23966, Polysciences, Inc., Warrington, PA, USA). After 48 h, the VLP-containing culture media was collected and clarified by centrifugation, then a solution of 1x Triton lysis buffer (0.5% NP40, 1% Triton X-100 (BP151-100, Fisher Scientific), 140 mM NaCl, 25 mM Tris HCl) with protease (04693159001, Roche, Indianapolis, IN, USA) and phosphatase inhibitor cocktails (4906837001, Roche) was added to lyse the VLPs. Biotin-modified LASV Z protein was affinity purified by incubating the VLP lysate with Dynabeads MyOne Streptavidin T1 beads (65602, Thermo Fisher Scientific) for 2 h at 4 °C while rotating. Following incubation, the beads were washed with 1x Triton lysis buffer and then were eluted in 4x Laemmli sample buffer (250 mM Tris-HCl, 40% glycerol, 8% sodium dodecyl sulfate, and 0.04% bromophenol blue) diluted to 1x in Triton lysis buffer with a final concentration of 5% 2-mercaptoethanol by heating at 100 °C for 10 min. The protein eluate was subjected to electrophoresis on a 4–20% Tris-glycine polyacrylamide gel (EC60285BOX, Invitrogen, Carlsbad, CA, USA). This gel was then stained overnight with Coomassie (40% methanol, 20% acetic acid, and 0.1% Brilliant Blue R (B7920, Sigma-Aldrich, St. Louis, MI, USA) followed by de-staining with a solution of 30% methanol and 10% acetic acid and was imaged on a Canon Canoscan 8800F scanner. The region of the gel lane containing the Z protein was excised and either directly reduced and alkylated with iodoacetamide or not, prior to being subjected to in-gel digestion with a solution of sequencing-grade modified trypsin (V5111, Promega, Madison, WI, USA) or a mixture of trypsin and sequencing-grade chymotrypsin (V1061, Promega), as described previously [40,51]. The resultant peptides were extracted from the gel slice using 2.5% formic acid in 50% acetonitrile and centrifugation. This supernatant was collected, and the gel slice was further dehydrated by incubating with 100% acetonitrile, centrifuging, and collecting the supernatant twice. The solvent was evaporated using a vacuum centrifuge at 37 °C, and the peptides were resuspended in 2.5% acetonitrile and 2.5% formic acid. Liquid chromatography was conducted using a microcapillary column packed with 12 cm Magic C18, 200 Å, 5 µm material (PM5/66100/00, Michrom Bioresources, Auburn, CA, USA) using a MicroAS autosampler (Thermo Scientific, Pittsburgh, PA, USA). The peptides were eluted with a gradient of 5−35% acetonitrile (0.15% formic acid) using a Surveyor Pump Plus HPLC (Thermo Scientific) over 40 min after a 15 min isocratic loading at 2.5% acetonitrile and 0.15% formic acid. Data were acquired in both a stand-alone linear ion trap mass spectrometer (LTQ-XL) and a linear ion trap–orbitrap (LTQ–Orbitrap) hybrid mass spectrometer (both instruments from Thermo Scientific). Ten MS/MS scans in the LTQ followed each linear ion trap or orbitrap survey scan over the entire run. A concatenated database of the LASV Z protein sequence including affinity tags in forward and reverse orientation was queried with SEQUEST software with no enzyme requirement and a 20 PPM precursor mass tolerance (or 2 Da for data collected in the stand-alone LTQ). The following differential modifications were allowed: +79.96633 Da for phosphorylation of serine, threonine, and tyrosine; +15.99492 Da for methionine oxidation; and either 71.0371 Da for cysteine acrylamidation or +57.02146 for cysteine carbamidomethylation.

3.3. Detection of Phosphoproteins by Western Blotting

In order to confirm the presence of phosphorylated LASV Z protein, 5×10^5 HEK293T cells per well were seeded in six-well plates and then transfected 24 h later with 2 µg of the corresponding Z protein plasmids using 8 µg of 1 mg/mL polyethyleneimine. Two days after transfection, the cells were treated with 8.8 mM hydrogen peroxide, or water as a control, for 20 min (min) for phosphotyrosine detection. The cells were then lysed with 1x Triton lysis buffer containing both protease and phosphatase inhibitor cocktails. SBP-tagged Z was affinity purified by incubating with streptavidin-coated magnetic beads for 2 h, followed by elution in 2x Laemmli sample buffer (125 mM Tris-HCl, 20% glycerol, 4% sodium dodecyl sulfate, and 0.02% bromophenol blue) with 5% 2-mercaptoethanol by heating at 100 °C for 10 min. The purified samples or cell input prepared in Laemmli sample buffer were separated by electrophoresis using NuPAGE 4–12% Bis-Tris gels (Thermo Fisher Scientific) with MES buffer (B000202, Thermo Fisher Scientific). Western blotting was carried out using nitrocellulose iBlot 2 gel transfer stacks (IB23001, Thermo Fisher Scientific) and the Invitrogen iBlot 2 transfer apparatus. Membranes for phosphotyrosine detection were blocked for 1 h in protein-free blocking buffer (37572, Thermo Fisher Scientific), and then a mouse anti-phosphotyrosine antibody (clone 4G10, Millipore) diluted (0.2 µg/mL) in protein-free blocking buffer was added to the membrane and incubated overnight at room temperature. The membrane was washed five times with Tris-buffered saline containing 0.1% Tween 20 (BP337, Fisher Scientific, Pittsburgh, PA, USA) (TBST), incubated for 1 h with goat anti-mouse 800 secondary antibody (926-32210, Licor, Lincoln, NE, USA) diluted 1:20,000 in 5% milk, 0.2% Tween 20 (BP337, Fisher Scientific), and 0.02% sodium dodecyl sulfate in phosphate buffered saline (PBS), and then imaged using a Licor Odyssey CLx imaging system. Immunoblotting for the Z protein was conducted by incubating the membrane with an anti-SBP tag antibody (MAB10764, Millipore, Billerica, MA, USA) diluted 1:10,000 and an anti-mouse 800 secondary antibody (926-32210, Licor) diluted 1:3000 in iBind fluorescent detection solution (SLF2019, Thermo Fisher Scientific) in an iBind Flex western device.

3.4. Virus-Like Particle Release Assay

To measure VLP release, 2×10^5 HEK293T cells per well were seeded in 12-well plates and then transfected 24 h later with 0.8 µg of the designated SBP-tagged LASV Z protein-expressing plasmids, using 3.2 µg of polyethyleneimine. One day later, the VLP-containing cell culture media was collected, clarified by centrifugation, and then mixed with 10x Triton lysis buffer with a protease inhibitor cocktail to a final concentration of 1x. The cells were scraped into phosphate-buffered saline, pelleted by centrifugation, and then lysed with 1x Triton lysis buffer containing a protease inhibitor cocktail. The samples were subjected to SDS-PAGE and western blotting as described above. The SBP-tagged Z protein was detected using an anti-SBP tag antibody (MAB10764, Millipore), diluted 1:10,000 in 5% nonfat milk and 0.2% Tween 20 in PBS, and the anti-mouse 800 secondary antibody (926-32210, Licor), diluted 1:20,000 in 5% nonfat milk, 0.02% sodium dodecyl sulfate, and 0.2% Tween 20 in PBS. In order to determine the percent VLP release, the value of each Z protein band on a particular blot was first divided by the sum of the values of all the Z protein bands on that particular blot (normalization by summation as described in [89]). This normalized Z protein quantity in VLPs was divided by the normalized Z quantity in cells for each mutant, and these values were then normalized to the corresponding quotient of Z WT, as described previously [40]. A one-way ANOVA with Holm–Sidak's test for multiple comparisons in GraphPad Prism software was used to analyze differences in VLP release.

Author Contributions: Conceptualization, C.M.Z., B.A.B., J.B.; Funding Acquisition, B.A.B. and J.B.; Investigation, C.M.Z., P.E., and M.E.W.; Project Administration, B.A.B. and J.B.; Visualization, C.M.Z., I.M., M.E.W., and B.A.B., and Writing—original draft preparation and review and editing, C.M.Z., E.A.B., B.A.B., and J.B.

Acknowledgments: The authors gratefully acknowledge NIH grants T32 AI055402 and T32 HL076122 (C.M.Z.), R21 AI088059 (J.B.), 3R41AI132047-01S1 (E.B.), and P20RR021905 and P30GM118228 (Immunobiology and Infectious Disease COBRE) (J.B.). Support for mass spectrometry analysis was provided by the Vermont Genetics Network through NIH grant 8P20GM103449 from the INBRE program and of the NIGMS.

References

1. Charrel, R.N.; Lamballerie, X.D. Arenaviruses other than lassa virus. *Antivir. Res.* **2003**, *57*, 89–100. [CrossRef]

2. Monath, T.P.; Newhouse, V.F.; Kemp, G.E.; Setzer, H.W.; Cacciapuoti, A. Lassa virus isolation from mastomys natalensis rodents during an epidemic in sierra leone. *Science* **1974**, *185*, 263–265. [CrossRef] [PubMed]

3. Lecompte, E.; Fichet-Calvet, E.; Daffis, S.; Koulemou, K.; Sylla, O.; Kourouma, F.; Dore, A.; Soropogui, B.; Aniskin, V.; Allali, B.; et al. Mastomys natalensis and lassa fever, west africa. *Emerg. Infect. Dis.* **2006**, *12*, 1971–1974. [CrossRef] [PubMed]

4. Olayemi, A.; Cadar, D.; Magassouba, N.F.; Obadare, A.; Kourouma, F.; Oyeyiola, A.; Fasogbon, S.; Igbokwe, J.; Rieger, T.; Bockholt, S.; et al. New hosts of the lassa virus. *Sci. Rep.* **2016**, *6*, 25280. [CrossRef] [PubMed]

5. McCormick, J.B.; King, I.J.; Webb, P.A.; Scribner, C.L.; Craven, R.B.; Johnson, K.M.; Elliott, L.H.; Belmont-Williams, R. Lassa fever. *N. Engl. J. Med.* **1986**, *314*, 20–26. [CrossRef]

6. Bonwitt, J.; Kelly, A.H.; Ansumana, R.; Agbla, S.; Sahr, F.; Saez, A.M.; Borchert, M.; Kock, R.; Fichet-Calvet, E. Rat-atouille: A mixed method study to characterize rodent hunting and consumption in the context of lassa fever. *Ecohealth* **2016**, *13*, 234–247. [CrossRef] [PubMed]

7. Monath, T.P. Lassa fever: Review of epidemiology and epizootiology. *Bull. World Health Organ.* **1975**, *52*, 577–592.

8. McCormick, J.B.; Webb, P.A.; Krebs, J.W.; Johnson, K.M.; Smith, E.S. A prospective study of the epidemiology and ecology of lassa fever. *J. Infect. Dis.* **1987**, *155*, 437–444. [CrossRef] [PubMed]

9. Frame, J.D.; Baldwin, J.M.; Gocke, D.J.; Troup, J.M. Lassa fever, a new virus disease of man from west africa: I. Clinical description and pathological findings. *Am. J. Trop. Med. Hyg.* **1970**, *19*, 670–676. [CrossRef]

10. Fisher-Hoch, S.P.; Tomori, O.; Nasidi, A.; Perez-Oronoz, G.I.; Fakile, Y.; Hutwagner, L.; McCormick, J.B. Review of cases of nosocomial lassa fever in nigeria: The high price of poor medical practice. *Br. Med. J.* **1995**, *311*, 857–859. [CrossRef]

11. Ajayi, N.A.; Nwigwe, C.G.; Azuogu, B.N.; Onyire, B.N.; Nwonwu, E.U.; Ogbonnaya, L.U.; Onwe, F.I.; Ekaete, T.; Günther, S.; Ukwaja, K.N. Containing a lassa fever epidemic in a resource-limited setting: Outbreak description and lessons learned from abakaliki, nigeria (January–March 2012). *Int. J. Infect. Dis.* **2013**, *17*, e1011–e1016. [CrossRef]

12. Shaffer, J.G.; Grant, D.S.; Schieffelin, J.S.; Boisen, M.L.; Goba, A.; Hartnett, J.N.; Levy, D.C.; Yenni, R.E.; Moses, L.M.; Fullah, M.; et al. Lassa fever in post-conflict sierra leone. *PLOS Negl. Trop. Dis.* **2014**, *8*, e2748. [CrossRef]

13. Price, M.E.; Fisher-Hoch, S.P.; Craven, R.B.; McCormick, J.B. A prospective study of maternal and fetal outcome in acute lassa fever infection during pregnancy. *Br. Med. J.* **1988**, *297*, 584–587. [CrossRef]

14. Cummins, D.; McCormick, J.B.; Bennett, D.; Samba, J.A.; Farrar, B.; Machin, S.J.; Fisher-Hoch, S.P. Acute sensorineural deafness in lassa fever. *JAMA* **1990**, *264*, 2093–2096. [CrossRef] [PubMed]

15. Clegg, J.C.S.; Wilson, S.M.; Oram, J.D. Nucleotide sequence of the s rna of lassa virus (nigerian strain) and comparative analysis of arenavirus gene products. *Virus Res.* **1991**, *18*, 151–164. [CrossRef]

16. Cao, W.; Henry, M.D.; Borrow, P.; Yamada, H.; Elder, J.H.; Ravkov, E.V.; Nichol, S.T.; Compans, R.W.; Campbell, K.P.; Oldstone, M.B.A. Identification of α-dystroglycan as a receptor for lymphocytic choriomeningitis virus and lassa fever virus. *Science* **1998**, *282*, 2079–2081. [CrossRef] [PubMed]

17. Kunz, S. Receptor binding and cell entry of old world arenaviruses reveal novel aspects of virus-host interaction. *Virology* **2009**, *387*, 245–249. [CrossRef]

18. Klewitz, C.; Klenk, H.-D.; ter Meulen, J. Amino acids from both n-terminal hydrophobic regions of the lassa virus envelope glycoprotein gp-2 are critical for ph-dependent membrane fusion and infectivity. *J. Gen. Virol.* **2007**, *88*, 2320–2328. [CrossRef]

19. Lee, K.J.; Novella, I.S.; Teng, M.N.; Oldstone, M.B.A.; de la Torre, J.C. Np and l proteins of lymphocytic choriomeningitis virus (lcmv) are sufficient for efficient transcription and replication of lcmv genomic RNA analogs. *J. Virol.* **2000**, *74*, 3470–3477. [CrossRef]

20. Lopez, N.; Jacamo, R.; Franze-Fernandez, M.T. Transcription and rna replication of tacaribe virus genome and antigenome analogs require n and l proteins: Z protein is an inhibitor of these processes. *J. Virol.* **2001**, *75*, 12241–12251. [CrossRef]

21. Djavani, M.; Lukashevich, I.S.; Sanchez, A.; Nichol, S.T.; Salvato, M.S. Completion of the lassa fever virus sequence and identification of a ring finger open reading frame at the l rna 5′ end. *Virology* **1997**, *235*, 414–418. [CrossRef] [PubMed]

22. Lukashevich, I.S.; Djavani, M.; Shapiro, K.; Sanchez, A.; Ravkov, E.; Nichol, S.T.; Salvato, M.S. The lassa fever virus l gene: Nucleotide sequence, comparison, and precipitation of a predicted 250 kda protein with monospecific antiserum. *J. Gen. Virol.* **1997**, *78*, 547–551. [CrossRef]

23. Strecker, T.; Eichler, R.; Meulen, J.t.; Weissenhorn, W.; Dieter Klenk, H.; Garten, W.; Lenz, O. Lassa virus z protein is a matrix protein sufficient for the release of virus-like particles. *J. Virol.* **2003**, *77*, 10700–10705. [CrossRef] [PubMed]

24. Fehling, S.; Lennartz, F.; Strecker, T. Multifunctional nature of the arenavirus ring finger protein z. *Viruses* **2012**, *4*, 2973–3011. [CrossRef] [PubMed]

25. Xing, J.; Ly, H.; Liang, Y. The z proteins of pathogenic but not nonpathogenic arenaviruses inhibit rig-i-like receptor-dependent interferon production. *J. Virol.* **2015**, *89*, 2944–2955. [CrossRef] [PubMed]

26. Cornu, T.I.; de la Torre, J.C. Ring finger z protein of lymphocytic choriomeningitis virus (lcmv) inhibits transcription and rna replication of an lcmv s-segment minigenome. *J. Virol.* **2001**, *75*, 9415–9426. [CrossRef] [PubMed]

27. Jacamo, R.; Lopez, N.; Wilda, M.; Franze-Fernández, M.T. Tacaribe virus z protein interacts with the l polymerase protein to inhibit viral rna synthesis. *J Virol* **2003**, *77*. [CrossRef]

28. Kranzusch, P.J.; Whelan, S.P.J. Arenavirus z protein controls viral rna synthesis by locking a polymerase–promoter complex. Kranzusch, P.J.; Whelan, S.P.J. Arenavirus z protein controls viral rna synthesis by locking a polymerase–promoter complex. *Proc. Natl. Acad. Sci. USA* **2011**, *108*, 19743–19748. [CrossRef]

29. Schlie, K.; Maisa, A.; Freiberg, F.; Groseth, A.; Strecker, T.; Garten, W. Viral protein determinants of lassa virus entry and release from polarized epithelial cells. *J. Virol.* **2010**, *84*, 3178–3188. [CrossRef]

30. Capul, A.A.; Perez, M.; Burke, E.; Kunz, S.; Buchmeier, M.J.; de la Torre, J.C. Arenavirus z-glycoprotein association requires z myristoylation but not functional ring or late domains. *J. Virol.* **2007**, *81*, 9451–9460. [CrossRef]

31. Eichler, R.; Strecker, T.; Kolesnikova, L.; ter Meulen, J.; Weissenhorn, W.; Becker, S.; Klenk, H.D.; Garten, W.; Lenz, O. Characterization of the lassa virus matrix protein z: Electron microscopic study of virus-like particles and interaction with the nucleoprotein (np). *Virus Res.* **2004**, *100*, 249–255. [CrossRef] [PubMed]

32. Perez, M.; Craven, R.C.; de la Torre, J.C. The small ring finger protein z drives arenavirus budding: Implications for antiviral strategies. *Proc. Natl. Acad. Sci. USA* **2003**, *100*, 12978–12983. [CrossRef] [PubMed]

33. Zaza, A.D.; Herbreteau, C.H.; Peyrefitte, C.N.; Emonet, S.F. Mammarenaviruses deleted from their z gene are replicative and produce an infectious progeny in bhk-21 cells. *Virology* **2018**, *518*, 34–44. [CrossRef] [PubMed]

34. Strecker, T.; Maisa, A.; Daffis, S.; Eichler, R.; Lenz, O.; Garten, W. The role of myristoylation in the membrane association of the lassa virus matrix protein z. *Virol. J.* **2006**, *3*, 93. [CrossRef] [PubMed]

35. Perez, M.; Greenwald, D.L.; de La Torre, J.C. Myristoylation of the ring finger z protein is essential for arenavirus budding. *J. Virol.* **2004**, *78*, 11443–11448. [CrossRef] [PubMed]

36. Votteler, J.; Sundquist, W.I. Virus budding and the escrt pathway. *Cell Host Microbe* **2013**, *14*, 232–241. [CrossRef] [PubMed]

37. Wang, J.; Danzy, S.; Kumar, N.; Ly, H.; Liang, Y. Biological roles and functional mechanisms of arenavirus z protein in viral replication. *J. Virol.* **2012**, *86*, 9794–9801. [CrossRef]

38. Urata, S.; Noda, T.; Kawaoka, Y.; Yokosawa, H.; Yasuda, J. Cellular factors required for lassa virus budding. *J. Virol.* **2006**, *80*, 4191–4195. [CrossRef]

39. Han, Z.; Lu, J.; Liu, Y.; Davis, B.; Lee, M.S.; Olson, M.A.; Ruthel, G.; Freedman, B.D.; Schnell, M.J.; Wrobel, J.E.; et al. Small-molecule probes targeting the viral ppxy-host nedd4 interface block egress of a broad range of rna viruses. *J Virol* **2014**, *88*. [CrossRef]

40. Ziegler, C.M.; Eisenhauer, P.; Bruce, E.A.; Weir, M.E.; King, B.R.; Klaus, J.P.; Krementsov, D.N.; Shirley, D.J.; Ballif, B.A.; Botten, J. The lymphocytic choriomeningitis virus matrix protein ppxy late domain drives the production of defective interfering particles. *PLoS Pathog* **2016**, *12*, e1005501. [CrossRef]

41. Nishi, H.; Shaytan, A.; Panchenko, A.R. Physicochemical mechanisms of protein regulation by phosphorylation. *Front. Genet.* **2014**, *5*, 270. [CrossRef] [PubMed]

42. Keck, F.; Ataey, P.; Amaya, M.; Bailey, C.; Narayanan, A. Phosphorylation of single stranded rna virus proteins and potential for novel therapeutic strategies. *Viruses* **2015**, *7*, 5257–5273. [CrossRef] [PubMed]

43. Schwartz, D.; Church, G.M. Collection and motif-based prediction of phosphorylation sites in human viruses. *Sci. Signal.* **2010**, *3*, rs2. [CrossRef] [PubMed]

44. Bretaña, N.A.; Lu, C.-T.; Chiang, C.-Y.; Su, M.-G.; Huang, K.-Y.; Lee, T.-Y.; Weng, S.-L. Identifying protein phosphorylation sites with kinase substrate specificity on human viruses. *PLoS ONE* **2012**, *7*, e40694. [CrossRef] [PubMed]

45. Keating, J.A.; Striker, R. Phosphorylation events during viral infections provide potential therapeutic targets. *Rev. Med. Virol.* **2012**, *22*, 166–181. [CrossRef] [PubMed]

46. García, M.; Cooper, A.; Shi, W.; Bornmann, W.; Carrion, R.; Kalman, D.; Nabel, G.J. Productive replication of ebola virus is regulated by the c-abl1 tyrosine kinase. *Sci. Transl. Med.* **2012**, *4*, 123ra124. [CrossRef] [PubMed]

47. Kolesnikova, L.; Mittler, E.; Schudt, G.; Shams-Eldin, H.; Becker, S. Phosphorylation of marburg virus matrix protein vp40 triggers assembly of nucleocapsids with the viral envelope at the plasma membrane. *Cell. Microbiol.* **2012**, *14*, 182–197. [CrossRef]

48. Bajorek, M.; Caly, L.; Tran, K.C.; Maertens, G.N.; Tripp, R.A.; Bacharach, E.; Teng, M.N.; Ghildyal, R.; Jans, D.A. The thr205 phosphorylation site within respiratory syncytial virus matrix (m) protein modulates m oligomerization and virus production. *J. Virol.* **2014**. [CrossRef]

49. Pei, Z.; Harrison, M.S.; Schmitt, A.P. Parainfluenza virus 5 m protein interaction with host protein 14-3-3 negatively affects virus particle formation. *J. Virol.* **2011**, *85*, 2050–2059. [CrossRef]

50. Hemonnot, B.; Mollé, D.; Bardy, M.; Gay, B.; Laune, D.; Devaux, C.; Briant, L. Phosphorylation of the htlv-1 matrix l-domain-containing protein by virus-associated erk-2 kinase. *Virology* **2006**, *349*, 430–439. [CrossRef]

51. Ziegler, C.M.; Eisenhauer, P.; Bruce, E.A.; Beganovic, V.; King, B.R.; Weir, M.E.; Ballif, B.A.; Botten, J. A novel phosphoserine motif in the lcmv matrix protein z regulates the release of infectious virus and defective interfering particles. *J. Gen. Virol.* **2016**, *97*, 2084–2089. [CrossRef] [PubMed]

52. Volpon, L.; Osborne, M.J.; Capul, A.A.; de la Torre, J.C.; Borden, K.L.B. Structural characterization of the z ring-eif4e complex reveals a distinct mode of control for eif4e. *Proc. Natl. Acad. Sci. USA* **2010**, *107*, 5441–5446. [CrossRef] [PubMed]

53. Salvato, M.S.; Schweighofer, K.J.; Burns, J.; Shimomaye, E.M. Biochemical and immunological evidence that the 11 kda zinc-binding protein of lymphocytic choriomeningitis virus is a structural component of the virus. *Virus Res.* **1992**, *22*, 185–198. [CrossRef]

54. Salvato, M.S.; Shimomaye, E.M. The completed sequence of lymphocytic choriomeningitis virus reveals a unique rna structure and a gene for a zinc finger protein. *Virology* **1989**, *173*, 1–10. [CrossRef]

55. Hastie, K.M.; Zandonatti, M.; Liu, T.; Li, S.; Woods, V.L.; Saphire, E.O. Crystal structure of the oligomeric form of lassa virus matrix protein z. *J. Virol.* **2016**, *90*, 4556–4562. [CrossRef] [PubMed]

56. Volpon, L.; Osborne, M.J.; Borden, K.L.B. Nmr assignment of the arenaviral protein z from lassa fever virus. *Biomol. NMR Assign.* **2008**, *2*, 81–84. [CrossRef]

57. May, E.R.; Armen, R.S.; Mannan, A.M.; Brooks, C.L. The flexible c-terminal arm of the lassa arenavirus z-protein mediates interactions with multiple binding partners. *Proteins* **2010**, *78*, 2251–2264. [CrossRef]

58. Capul, A.A.; de la Torre, J.C.; Buchmeier, M.J. Conserved residues in lassa fever virus z protein modulate viral infectivity at the level of the ribonucleoprotein. *J. Virol.* **2011**, *85*, 3172–3178. [CrossRef]

59. Xing, J.; Chai, Z.; Ly, H.; Liang, Y. Differential inhibition of macrophage activation by lymphocytic choriomeningitis virus and pichinde virus is mediated by the z protein n-terminal domain. *J. Virol.* **2015**, *89*, 12513–12517. [CrossRef]

60. Li, W.; Cowley, A.; Uludag, M.; Gur, T.; McWilliam, H.; Squizzato, S.; Park, Y.M.; Buso, N.; Lopez, R. The embl-ebi bioinformatics web and programmatic tools framework. *Nucleic Acids Res.* **2015**, *43*, W580–W584. [CrossRef]

61. Manning, J.T.; Forrester, N.; Paessler, S. Lassa virus isolates from mali and the ivory coast represent an emerging fifth lineage. *Front. Microbiol.* **2015**, *6*, 1037. [CrossRef] [PubMed]

62. Bowen, M.D.; Rollin, P.E.; Ksiazek, T.G.; Hustad, H.L.; Bausch, D.G.; Demby, A.H.; Bajani, M.D.; Peters, C.J.; Nichol, S.T. Genetic diversity among lassa virus strains. *J. Virol.* **2000**, *74*, 6992–7004. [CrossRef] [PubMed]

63. Shannon, L.M.W.; Thomas, S.; Daniel, C.; Hans-Peter, D.; Kelly, F.; Ketan, P.; Shelley, M.B.; William, G.D.; John, D.K.; Pierre, E.R.; et al. New lineage of lassa virus, togo, 2016. *Emerg. Infect. Dis. J.* **2018**, *24*, 599.

64. Oloniniyi, O.K.; Unigwe, U.S.; Okada, S.; Kimura, M.; Koyano, S.; Miyazaki, Y.; Iroezindu, M.O.; Ajayi, N.A.; Chukwubike, C.M.; Chika-Igwenyi, N.M.; et al. Genetic characterization of lassa virus strains isolated from 2012 to 2016 in southeastern nigeria. *PLOS Negl. Trop. Dis.* **2018**, *12*, e0006971. [CrossRef] [PubMed]

65. Verdecia, M.A.; Bowman, M.E.; Lu, K.P.; Hunter, T.; Noel, J.P. Structural basis for phosphoserine-proline recognition by group iv ww domains. *Nat. Struct. Biol.* **2000**, *7*, 639. [CrossRef] [PubMed]

66. Smerdon, S.J.; Yaffe, M.B. Chapter 72-recognition of phospho-serine/threonine phosphorylated proteins by phospho-serine/threonine-binding domains. In *Handbook of Cell Signaling*, 2nd ed.; Bradshaw, R.A., Dennis, E.A., Eds.; Academic Press: San Diego, CA, USA, 2010; pp. 539–550.

67. Liou, Y.-C.; Zhou, X.Z.; Lu, K.P. Prolyl isomerase pin1 as a molecular switch to determine the fate of phosphoproteins. *Trends Biochem. Sci.* **2011**, *36*, 501–514. [CrossRef] [PubMed]

68. Pang, R.; Lee, T.K.W.; Poon, R.T.P.; Fan, S.T.; Wong, K.B.; Kwong, Y.L.; Tse, E. Pin1 interacts with a specific serine-proline motif of hepatitis b virus x-protein to enhance hepatocarcinogenesis. *Gastroenterology* **2007**, *132*, 1088–1103. [CrossRef]

69. Jeong, S.-J.; Ryo, A.; Yamamoto, N. The prolyl isomerase pin1 stabilizes the human t-cell leukemia virus type 1 (htlv-1) tax oncoprotein and promotes malignant transformation. *Biochem. Biophys. Res. Commun.* **2009**, *381*, 294–299. [CrossRef]

70. Peloponese, J.-M.; Yasunaga, J.; Kinjo, T.; Watashi, K.; Jeang, K.-T. Peptidylproline cis-trans-isomerase pin1 interacts with human t-cell leukemia virus type 1 tax and modulates its activation of nf-κb. *J. Virol.* **2009**, *83*, 3238–3248. [CrossRef]

71. Misumi, S.; Inoue, M.; Dochi, T.; Kishimoto, N.; Hasegawa, N.; Takamune, N.; Shoji, S. Uncoating of human immunodeficiency virus type 1 requires prolyl isomerase pin1. *J. Biol. Chem.* **2010**, *285*, 25185–25195. [CrossRef]

72. Dochi, T.; Nakano, T.; Inoue, M.; Takamune, N.; Shoji, S.; Sano, K.; Misumi, S. Phosphorylation of human immunodeficiency virus type 1 capsid protein at serine 16, required for peptidyl-prolyl isomerase-dependent uncoating, is mediated by virion-incorporated extracellular signal-regulated kinase 2. *J. Gen. Virol.* **2014**, *95*, 1156–1166. [CrossRef] [PubMed]

73. Manganaro, L.; Lusic, M.; Gutierrez, M.I.; Cereseto, A.; Del Sal, G.; Giacca, M. Concerted action of cellular jnk and pin1 restricts hiv-1 genome integration to activated cd4+ t lymphocytes. *Nat. Med.* **2010**, *16*, 329. [CrossRef] [PubMed]

74. Narita, Y.; Murata, T.; Ryo, A.; Kawashima, D.; Sugimoto, A.; Kanda, T.; Kimura, H.; Tsurumi, T. Pin1 interacts with the epstein-barr virus DNA polymerase catalytic subunit and regulates viral DNA replication. *J. Virol.* **2013**, *87*, 2120–2127. [CrossRef]

75. Guito, J.; Gavina, A.; Palmeri, D.; Lukac, D.M. The cellular peptidyl-prolyl cis/trans isomerase pin1 regulates reactivation of kaposi's sarcoma-associated herpesvirus from latency. *J. Virol.* **2014**, *88*, 547–558. [CrossRef]

76. Denu, J.M.; Tanner, K.G. Specific and reversible inactivation of protein tyrosine phosphatases by hydrogen peroxide: Evidence for a sulfenic acid intermediate and implications for redox regulation. *Biochemistry* **1998**, *37*, 5633–5642. [CrossRef] [PubMed]

77. Dephoure, N.; Gould, K.L.; Gygi, S.P.; Kellogg, D.R.; Drubin, D.G. Mapping and analysis of phosphorylation sites: A quick guide for cell biologists. *Mol. Biol. Cell* **2013**, *24*, 535–542. [CrossRef] [PubMed]

78. Huang, A.S.; Baltimore, D. Defective viral particles and viral disease processes. *Nature* **1970**, *226*, 325–327. [CrossRef]

79. Dutko, F.J.; Pfau, C.J. Arenavirus defective interfering particles mask the cell-killing potential of standard virus. *J. Gen. Virol.* **1978**, *38*, 195–208. [CrossRef]

80. Carnec, X.; Baize, S.; Reynard, S.; Diancourt, L.; Caro, V.; Tordo, N.; Bouloy, M. Lassa virus nucleoprotein mutants generated by reverse genetics induce a robust type i interferon response in human dendritic cells and macrophages. *J. Virol.* **2011**, *85*, 12093–12097. [CrossRef]

81. Popescu, M.; Schaefer, H.; Lehmann-Grube, F. Homologous interference of lymphocytic choriomeningitis virus: Detection and measurement of interference focus-forming units. *J. Virol.* **1976**, *20*, 1–8.

82. Welsh, R.M.; Pfau, C.J. Determinants of lymphocytic choriomeningitis interference. *J. Gen. Virol.* **1972**, *14*, 177–187. [CrossRef] [PubMed]

83. Chesarino, N.M.; McMichael, T.M.; Hach, J.C.; Yount, J.S. Phosphorylation of the antiviral protein interferon-inducible transmembrane protein 3 (ifitm3) dually regulates its endocytosis and ubiquitination. *J. Biol. Chem.* **2014**, *289*, 11986–11992. [CrossRef] [PubMed]

84. Sotgia, F.; Lee, H.; Bedford, M.T.; Petrucci, T.; Sudol, M.; Lisanti, M.P. Tyrosine phosphorylation of β-dystroglycan at its ww domain binding motif, ppxy, recruits sh2 domain containing proteins. *Biochemistry* **2001**, *40*, 14585–14592. [CrossRef] [PubMed]

85. Chesarino, N.M.; McMichael, T.M.; Yount, J.S. E3 ubiquitin ligase nedd4 promotes influenza virus infection by decreasing levels of the antiviral protein ifitm3. *PLOS Pathogens* **2015**, *11*, e1005095. [CrossRef] [PubMed]

86. Cornillez-Ty, C.T.; Liao, L.; Yates, J.R.; Kuhn, P.; Buchmeier, M.J. Severe acute respiratory syndrome coronavirus nonstructural protein 2 interacts with a host protein complex involved in mitochondrial biogenesis and intracellular signaling. *J. Virol.* **2009**, *83*, 10314–10318. [CrossRef] [PubMed]

87. Klaus, J.P.; Eisenhauer, P.; Russo, J.; Mason, A.B.; Do, D.; King, B.; Taatjes, D.; Cornillez-Ty, C.; Boyson, J.E.; Thali, M.; et al. The intracellular cargo receptor ergic-53 is required for the production of infectious arenavirus, coronavirus, and filovirus particles. *Cell Host Microbe* **2013**, *14*, 522–534. [CrossRef] [PubMed]

88. Ziegler, C.M.; Eisenhauer, P.; Kelly, J.A.; Dang, L.N.; Beganovic, V.; Bruce, E.A.; King, B.R.; Shirley, D.J.; Weir, M.E.; Ballif, B.A.; et al. A proteomics survey of junín virus interactions with human proteins reveals host factors required for arenavirus replication. *J. Virol.* **2018**, *92*, e01565-17. [CrossRef]

89. Degasperi, A.; Birtwistle, M.R.; Volinsky, N.; Rauch, J.; Kolch, W.; Kholodenko, B.N. Evaluating strategies to normalise biological replicates of western blot data. *PLoS ONE* **2014**, *9*, e87293. [CrossRef]

9

Clinical and Epidemiological Patterns of Scrub Typhus, an Emerging Disease

Kezang Dorji [1,2], Yoenten Phuentshok [1,3], Tandin Zangpo [1,4], Sithar Dorjee [5], Chencho Dorjee [5], Peter Jolly [1], Roger Morris [6], Nelly Marquetoux [1,*] and Joanna McKenzie [1]

[1] School of Veterinary Science, Massey University, Palmerston North 4442, New Zealand; kezangt.dorjee@gmail.com (K.D.); vetyoen@gmail.com (Y.P.); zheynuapa@gmail.com (T.Z.); P.D.Jolly@massey.ac.nz (P.J.); J.S.McKenzie@massey.ac.nz (J.M.)

[2] Samdrup Jongkhar Hospital, Ministry of Health, Samdrup Jongkhar 41001, Bhutan

[3] National Centre for Animal Health, Department of Livestock, Ministry of Agriculture and Forests, Serbithang, Thimphu 11001, Bhutan

[4] Dechencholing BHU-I, Ministry of Health, Thimphu 11001, Bhutan

[5] Faculty of Nursing and Public Health, Khesar Gyalpo University of Medical Sciences of Bhutan, Thimphu 11001, Bhutan; s.dorjee@yahoo.co.nz (S.D.); director@rihs.edu.bt (C.D.)

[6] Morvet Ltd., Consultancy Services in Health Risk Management and Food Safety Policy and Programs, Masterton 5885, New Zealand; roger.morris@morvet.co.nz

* Correspondence: nelly.marquetoux@gmail.com.

Abstract: Scrub typhus (ST) is a vector-borne rickettsial infection causing acute febrile illness. The re-emergence of ST in the Asia-Pacific region represents a serious public health threat. ST was first detected in Bhutan in 2008. However, the disease is likely to be under-diagnosed and under-reported, and the true impact is difficult to estimate. At the end of 2014, the SD Bioline Tsutsugamushi Test™ rapid diagnostic test (RDT) kits became available in all hospitals to assist clinicians in diagnosing ST. We conducted a retrospective descriptive study, reviewing records from all hospitals of Bhutan to identify all RDT-positive clinical cases of ST in Bhutan in 2015. The aim was to evaluate the burden of ST in Bhutan, describe the demographic, spatial and temporal patterns of disease, and identify the typical clinical presentations. The annual incidence of RDT-positive cases of ST reporting to Bhutanese hospitals in 2015 was estimated to be 62 per 100,000 population at risk. The incidence of disease was highest in the southern districts with a subtropical climate and a high level of agricultural production. The highest proportion of cases (87%) was rural residents, with farmers being the main occupational category. The disease was strongly seasonal, with 97% of cases occurring between June and November, coinciding with the monsoon and agricultural production seasons. Common ST symptoms were not specific, and an eschar was noted by clinicians in only 7.4% of cases, which is likely to contribute to an under-diagnosis of ST. ST represents an important and neglected burden, especially in rural communities in Bhutan. The outcomes of this study will inform public health measures such as timely-awareness programmes for clinicians and the public in high-risk areas, to improve the diagnosis, treatment and clinical outcomes of this disease.

Keywords: scrub typhus; One Health; incidence; clinical pattern; descriptive epidemiology; vector-borne disease; emerging disease

1. Introduction

Scrub typhus (ST) or tsutsugamushi disease is a vector-borne rickettsial disease that is caused by the obligate intracellular bacterium *Orientia tsutsugamushi*. The primary reservoir is a trombiculid mite of the genus *Leptotrombidium*, which maintains the infection within populations through both transovarial and transtadial means of transmission [1]. Transmission to humans and other mammals occurs when the larval stage of infected mites feed on a human host [1]. A high risk of exposure to ST is associated with outdoor activities, agricultural work in particular, or living near grasslands or fields [2,3]. Humans are dead-end hosts, with no evidence of horizontal transmission of *O. tsutsugamushi* between people.

The geographic distribution of endemic ST is associated with the distribution of the reservoir mite in an area known as the 'tsutsugamushi triangle', centered on South-East and Pacific Asia [4]. ST has been described in this region for over a century [1,5]. The recent resurgence and re-emergence of ST in the endemic area has been associated with global climate change, influencing the distribution of infected mites [1]. Other putative factors are changes in agricultural practices and human behaviour, as well as improvements in diagnostic capabilities [5,6].

ST clinically presents as an acute non-specific febrile illness, which is difficult to diagnose [7]. Other common symptoms include nausea, vomiting, headache, myalgia and respiratory signs [8,9]. An eschar at the site of the bite, occurring before the onset of other symptoms, is pathognomonic [8,10]. However, the presence of an eschar, usually on the front of the body [11], is variably reported in 1–97% of ST patients, depending on the region of the world [1]. While ST is readily treated with antibiotics such as tetracycline, doxycycline, azithromycin and rifampicin [12], the nonspecific flu-like symptoms lead to the under-diagnosis and the under-treatment of this disease in many countries. Untreated ST can cause major complications and ultimately death. The median case fatality rate in untreated patients was estimated to be between 6 and 10% [1,13], but fatalities of up to 70% have been reported [1]. The duration of illness before effective antibiotic treatment is positively associated with progression to severe disease [14]. Hospital-based studies in South India reported a case fatality of 8–9% in ST patients reporting to the hospital, with multi-organ dysfunction observed in 34% of these patients [9,15]. Prompt clinical diagnosis and timely appropriate treatment are thus critical for improving the clinical outcome in individual patients [8,15], and for decreasing the public health impact of this disease [1].

In Bhutan, located within the tsutsugamushi triangle, ST was first identified as a cluster of pyrexia cases of unknown origin reporting to the Gedu hospital in the summer of 2008 [16]. A second outbreak occurred in Gedu in July 2009, of which 70% of cases were confirmed as ST by the Armed Forces Research Institute of Medical Sciences in Bangkok [17]. The disease was made notifiable in Bhutan in 2010. Notifications began to increase, particularly from the southern subtropical regions, which remain hot and humid for most of the year, and are exposed to the Indian summer monsoon [18]. However, given the non-specific presentation of ST, the disease was likely to be under-reported with only 22 to 67 cases being notified annually between 2012 and 2014. Misdiagnosis by clinicians and a lack of awareness amongst the public will respectively result in inappropriate case management, and delays in seeking treatment for febrile illness, in turn increasing the impact of ST in Bhutan.

In 2014, the Ministry of Health of Bhutan initiated a national sero-surveillance programme to gather more information on the incidence of ST, and to raise awareness among clinicians. In Bhutan, 19 of the 20 districts have a government district hospital, in which doctors provide in-patient and out-patient clinical services for the general public. The Gasa district in the far-north Himalayan area only has a Basic Healthcare Unit—Grade 1 (BHU-I) which functions as a district hospital. The country has two regional referral hospitals: in Gelephu, servicing southern Bhutan, and in Monggar, servicing eastern Bhutan. A national referral hospital is located in the capital city, Thimphu. There are no private medical services in Bhutan. As part of the sero-surveillance programme, the Ministry of Health approved the use of a commercial point-of-care rapid diagnostic test (RDT), the SD Bioline Tsutsugamushi Test^{TM}, in all hospitals and the BHU-I in Gasa, to support clinicians with the differential diagnosis and timely treatment of ST. The test has the advantage of low cost, rapidity, a single test result and simple interpretation [19]. The SD Bioline Tsutsugamushi Test^{TM} is an immunochromatographic test that is designed for use in clinical settings. It detects IgM, IgG and IgA antibodies against *O. tsutsugamushi*, which increases the sensitivity of the test in patients that may seek treatment once past the acute phase, and those which have been re-infected with *O tsutsugamushi* and have an elevated IgG titre [20].

Under the national sero-surveillance programme, clinicians were encouraged to send samples from patients positive to the RDT to the Royal Centre for Disease Control (RCDC), which functions as the national public health laboratory in Thimphu, for confirmatory testing using the Scrub Typhus Detect TM IgM Enzyme-Linked Immunosorbent Assay (ELISA) test (Inbios International, Inc., Seattle, WA, USA). Cut-off values for the ELISA were calculated for samples collected from Bhutan with the assistance of a laboratory in Pune, India.

Before 2015, no population-wide information on ST was available in Bhutan. With new diagnostic capabilities becoming widely available in hospitals in 2015, a rise in diagnosed ST in Bhutan was expected, irrespective of the level of notification to the Ministry of Health. The aim of this descriptive epidemiology study was therefore to compile the first year of data that was generated by the improved diagnostic capability in hospitals and the national sero-surveillance programme, to gain insight into the epidemiological patterns of ST and the likely impact of ST in Bhutan.

The objectives of our study were to: (1) obtain a more accurate estimate of the incidence of clinical ST, (2) describe the clinical patterns of ST, and (3) describe the demographic, spatial and temporal epidemiological characteristics of clinical ST in Bhutan. The outcomes of this study would contribute to more accurate estimates of the national burden of disease, and support the development and implementation of public health measures to reduce the impact of ST.

2. Materials and Methods

We conducted a national descriptive study of laboratory-confirmed ST cases that were identified in hospitals in Bhutan in 2015. The case definition was clinically suspected ST cases that were confirmed by the Rapid Diagnostic Test (RDT; SD Bioline Tsutsugamushi Test[TM]) during routine practice in hospitals in Bhutan during 2015.

2.1. Data Collection

ST cases were identified retrospectively by examining the clinical records of all district and referral hospitals and the BHU-I in Gasa district in early 2016. RDT-positive cases that were identified during a hospital-based case control study conducted from October to December 2015 in 11 districts with a higher incidence of ST were included. RDT-positive samples from this case-control study were sent to the RCDC for confirmatory IgM ELISA testing.

Data were obtained from RCDC on IgM ELISA-positive cases tested under the national sero-surveillance programme and the case control study.

For cases that were eligible for the case control study, demographic, clinical and epidemiological information were collected by interview during the study. For other patients, the clinical data were retrieved from the hospital records, and the demographic data was retrieved directly from the patient using their recorded contact details, where necessary.

The national census data issued by the Ministry of Health, Bhutan's Statistical Bureau, was used as the denominator to calculate national and district-level incidence, and age-based incidence rates of RDT-positive ST cases. The district population, as well as the rural versus urban population data was derived from 2015 statistics and age demographic data from 2017 statistics.

2.2. Analysis

We used descriptive methods to analyse the clinical and epidemiological characteristics of ST cases, including demographic, temporal and spatial distributions. Temporal patterns were based on the date of consultation in local hospitals. Spatial distribution was based on the address of the patient at the time of consultation. We mapped the district-level incidence of the RDT+ ST cases with and without the cases identified during the case control study, to identify a potential confounding of the case control study on the spatial distribution of ST. The age distribution between male and female patients was compared by using a two-sample Kolmogorov-Smirnov (KS) test. The proportion of patients experiencing each group of symptoms was compared between males and females using the Pearson's Chi-squared test. The proportion of rural versus urban cases was compared to that in the general population, using a test of equal proportions between samples.

Incidence rates were expressed as the cumulative number of ST cases per 100,000 persons at risk in 2015.

All analyses were performed using R [21].

2.3. Ethical Considerations

The ethical clearance was approved by the Research Ethics Board of Health (REBH), Ministry of Health, Royal Government of Bhutan, Thimphu via letter number REBH/PO/2015/042 on the 25 November 2015.

3. Results

A total of 470 RDT-positive clinical cases of ST was identified in this study, representing an observed annual incidence of 62 cases per 100,000 persons at risk in Bhutan in 2015. Among the 470 cases, 160 samples were sent to the RCDC for IgM ELISA testing, as part of the national sero-surveillance programme, of which 85 (53%) were ELISA-positive. A further subset of the 470 cases included 125 RDT-positive samples identified through the case control study which were tested with the IgM ELISA at RCDC, of which 79 (63%) were ELISA-positive.

There was a similar proportion of females (51.3%) and males (48.7%) among the cases. The median age of ST patients was 30 years old, with the highest percentage of cases within the 20–40-year-old period (Figure 1). The age distribution of ST in males and females was very similar (Figure 1) and statistically not different (KS p-value = 0.65). While the highest number of ST cases occurred in the 20–40-year old age group, the age-specific incidence was highest in age groups between 40 and 70 years old (Figure 2).

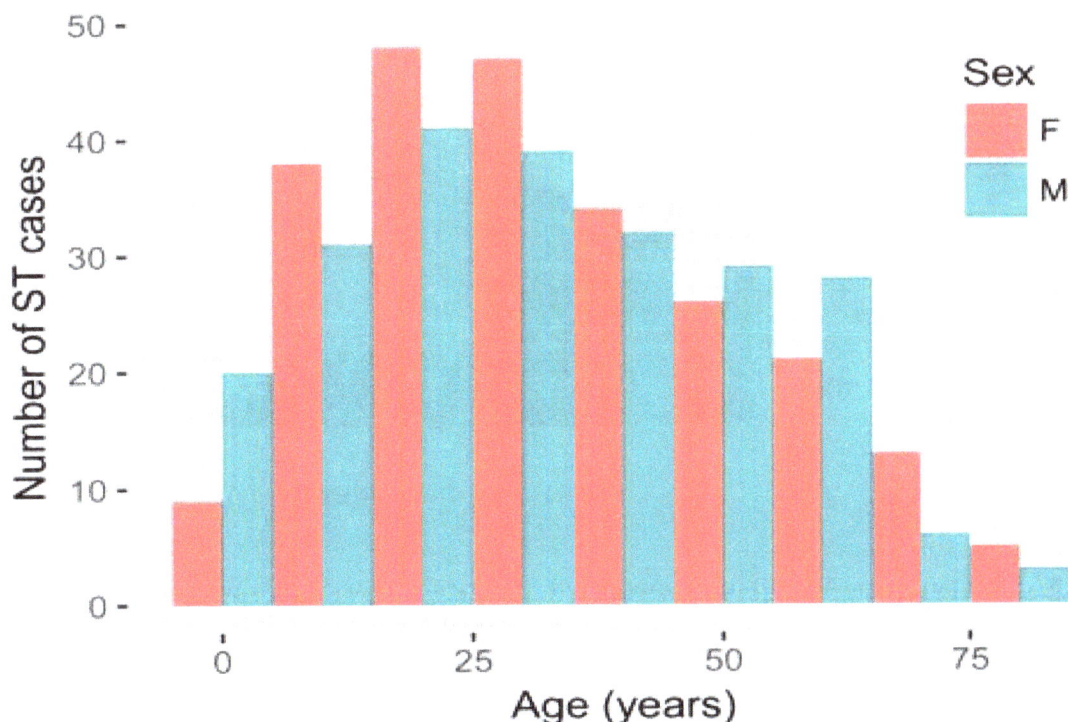

Figure 1. Age distribution of 470 clinically suspected scrub typhus (ST) cases that were positive to the SD Bioline Tsutsugamushi test in Bhutan in 2015.

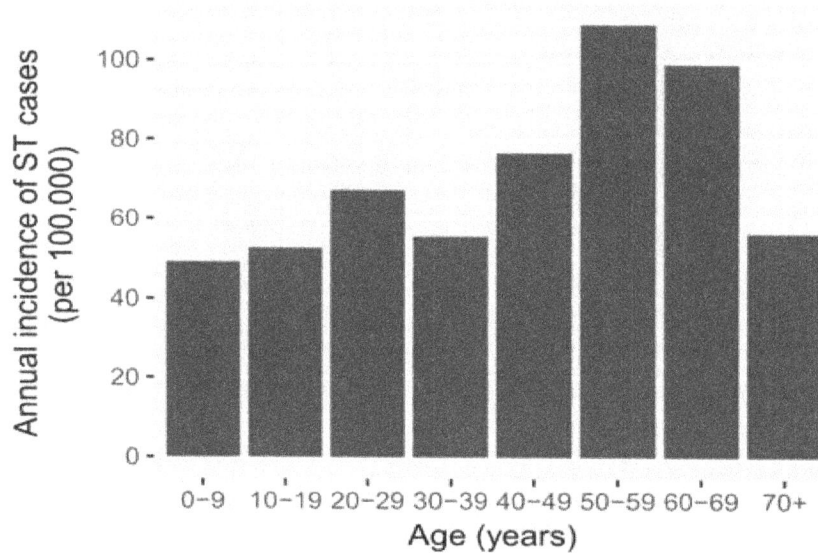

Figure 2. Age-specific incidences of 470 clinically suspected ST cases that were positive to the SD Bioline Tsutsugamushi test in Bhutan in 2015.

Farmers represented the main line of occupation among ST patients (45%), followed by students (22%) and housewives (17%) (Figure 3). The vast majority of patients were from rural areas (88%, $n =$ 412) compared to 62% in the general population. Rural cases were overrepresented in the RDT-positive population, compared to the general population ($p < 0.0001$).

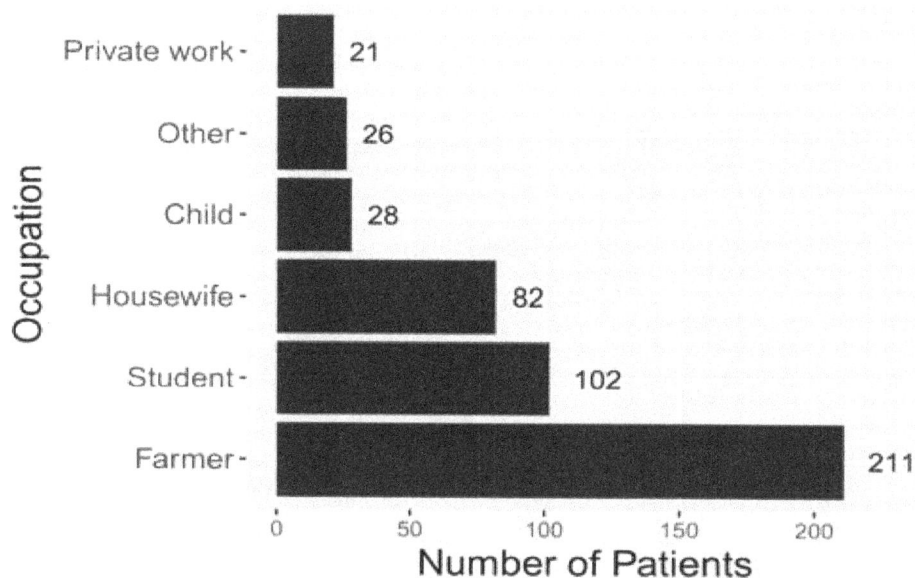

Figure 3. Occupation of 470 clinically suspected ST cases that were positive to the SD Bioline Tsutsugamushi test in Bhutan in 2015 (the "Other" category encompasses gomchen (lay priests), patients from India, military personnel, monks and civil servants).

The highest annual incidence of RDT-positive ST cases was observed in sub-tropical districts in the south of Bhutan (Figure 4). This spatial pattern was consistent with and without the cases identified through the case control study, which was conducted in the southern districts (Figure 4). Cases were observed in all districts except Gasa, which is located in the higher Himalayas.

a. Excluding 125 RDT–positive ST cases identified during the case–control study
conducted in 11 southern districts between October and December 2015

b. Including all 470 RDT–positive ST cases identified during 2015

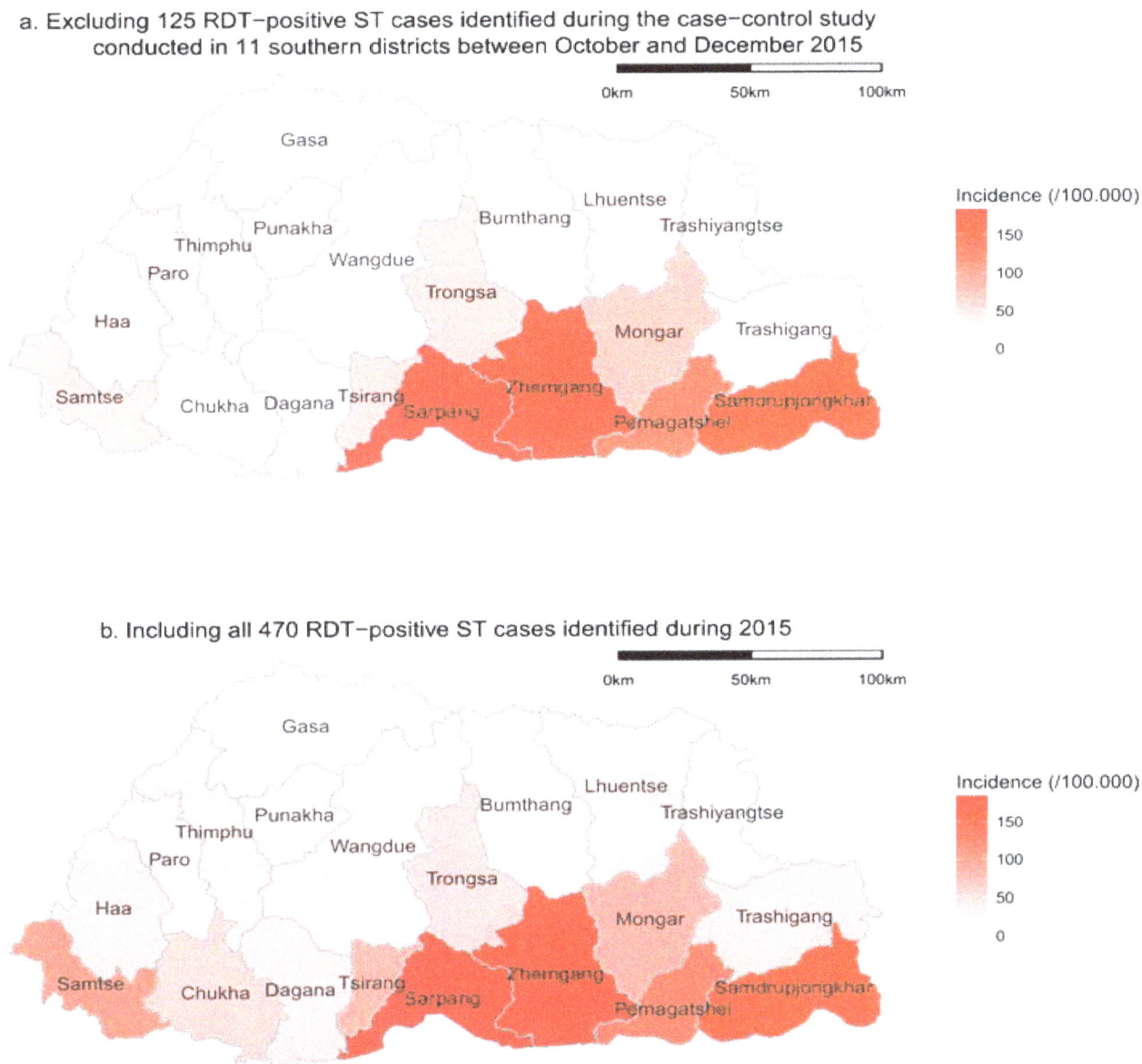

Figure 4. Spatial distribution of the incidences of clinically suspected scrub typhus cases that tested positive to the SD Bioline Tsutsugamushi test in Bhutan in 2015 ((a) excluding 125 RDT-positive ST cases that were identified during the case-control study conducted in 11 southern districts between October and December 2015, (b) including all 470 RDT-positive ST cases that were identified during 2015).

The temporal distribution of ST cases showed a strong trend of seasonality that was associated with the monsoon season. There were virtually no cases between December and June, followed by a sharp increase in July with a peak of incidence in September, and a sudden drop from October onwards (Figure 5).

Most RDT-positive ST cases presented with nonspecific flu-like symptoms. Fever was present in all patients, since this was generally the criterion for clinicians to perform the RDT, headache in 87%, myalgia and poly-arthralgia, respectively, in 56% and 40% of patients, and diarrhea or vomiting in 22% (Table 1). The presence of a pathognomonic eschar was only observed in 7.4% of the patients, twice as commonly in males (10%) as females (5%) ($p = 0.06$). Males and females mostly presented with a similar pattern of symptoms. However, respiratory and vascular symptoms were significantly 1.7 ($p = 0.01$) and 1.9 ($p = 0.04$) times more frequent in males.

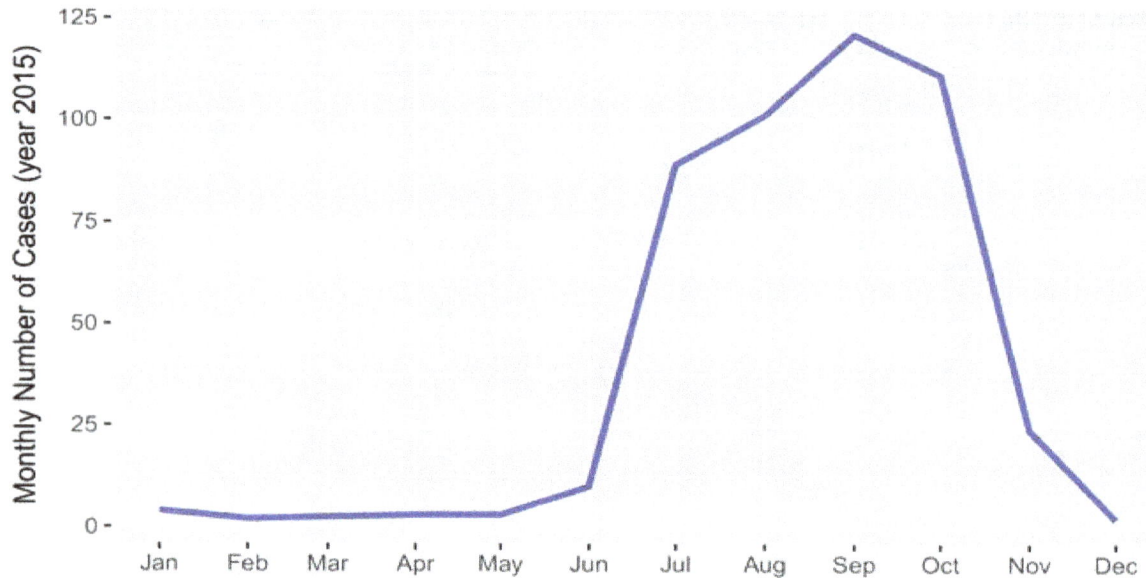

Figure 5. Temporal distribution of 470 clinically suspected scrub typhus cases that tested positive to the SD Bioline Tsutsugamushi test in Bhutan in 2015.

Table 1. Comparison of the clinical manifestations of 470 clinically suspected ST cases that tested positive to the SD Bioline Tsustugamushi test in males (241) and females (229) in Bhutan in 2015.

	Positive	n	Proportion (Overall)	Proportion (Males)	Proportion (Females)	p-Value
Fever	470	470	100%	100%	100%	NA
Headache	407	470	86.6%	83.8%	89.2%	0.12
Myalgia	265	470	56.4%	55.9%	56.8%	0.91
Malaise	216	468	46.2%	48.7%	43.8%	0.33
Polyarthralgia	189	470	40.2%	41.5%	39%	0.65
Other Digestive Symptoms	179	470	38.1%	37.1%	39%	0.74
Chills	130	469	27.7%	28.1%	27.4%	0.95
Diarrhoea/Vomiting	102	470	21.7%	21%	22.4%	0.79
Giddiness	95	467	20.3%	16.8%	23.7%	0.09
Respiratory Symptoms	91	470	19.4%	24.5%	14.5%	0.01
Rashes	88	469	18.8%	18.8%	18.8%	1
Vascular Symptoms	45	470	9.6%	12.7%	6.6%	0.04
Eschar	35	470	7.4%	10%	5%	0.06
Restlessness	31	470	6.6%	7%	6.2%	0.88
Lymphadenopathy	9	470	1.9%	2.2%	1.7%	0.94
Jaundice	3	470	0.6%	0.4%	0.8%	1

4. Discussion

The emergence of reported ST cases in Bhutan between 2010 and 2014 indicated the potential for ST to be a significant health issue in Bhutan. However, most healthcare workers as well as the public were not aware of the disease at that time. This is the first national study of ST in Bhutan, providing more accurate evidence for the overall incidence and the spatial, temporal and demographic distributions of ST in Bhutan's population in 2015.

The identification of 470 cases of RDT-positive ST in Bhutan in 2015, representing an observed annual incidence of 62 RDT-confirmed clinical ST cases/100,000 persons at risk, is a much higher incidence of ST than that reflected through the national sero-surveillance data from previous years. These results suggest that ST is a common cause of febrile illness in Bhutan. However, there are many challenges that are associated with serological testing for ST that make it difficult to interpret the extent to which this result reflects the true incidence of clinical ST in the Bhutanese population. Given the SD Bioline Tsutsugamushi test measures IgM, IgG and IgA antibodies it is likely to overestimate the incidence of clinical ST infections that occurred during 2015, given the test also captures antibodies that are associated with historical exposure in an unknown proportion of febrile cases [20]. This is supported by the IgM ELISA test results being positive in only 53% and 63% of the subset of RDT+ cases that were tested with the ELISA, respectively, in the sero-surveillance programme and the case control study. The IgM test results are likely to reflect the proportions of RDT+ cases that have current infections. The InBios Scrub Typhus Detect IgM ELISA was reported to have a sensitivity and specificity of 93% and 91% respectively, when measured against patients with typhus-like illness that fulfilled robust scrub typhus criteria in Thailand [22]. On the other hand, reinfection with *O. tsutsugamushi* is not uncommon in endemic areas, and such cases can be expected to have a rising IgG titre, which would not be captured in the IgM ELISA test results [20]. Furthermore, a proportion of cases who sought treatment after only a few days of fever may not have developed IgM antibodies, and this would have been missed by both serological tests [20]. In general, the RDT-positive incidence is more likely to reflect the overall exposure to *O. tsutsugamushi* amongst febrile patients, including recent and historical exposure, while the IgM ELISA incidence is more likely to reflect clinical disease that is associated with recent exposure. Both tests are likely to underestimate the true incidence of clinical ST in the study populations. Due to ST's non-specific flu-like symptoms, it is likely that not all cases would have sought treatment at the hospitals; milder or self-limiting cases of ST might not be seen in the hospital. The disease is also likely to be under-diagnosed, due to a lack of awareness of clinicians and non-specific clinical presentation. Moreover, anecdotal reports indicate that clinicians may have faced a shortage in the supply of RDT kits in some district hospitals in 2015, especially in high-incidence areas, and an unknown number of clinical ST cases may not have been tested.

There is considerable variation in the information on sensitivity and specificity of the SD Bioline Tsutsugamushi test. While the company selling the test claims a sensitivity and specificity of 99% and 96% respectively, one study evaluating this test against the immunofluorescence assay (IFA) in Thailand found a sensitivity of only 20.9% (95% CI: 10.0–36.0) in acute samples that are collected from patients who had a fever for a mean of 2–3 days. A higher sensitivity of 76.7% (95% CI: 61.4–88.2) was found in convalescent samples that were collected from the same patients at a median interval of 14 days (range 11–30 days). The specificity was similar in acute (74.4%; 95% CI: 58.8–86.5) and convalescent (76.7%; 95% CI: 61.4–88.2) samples [23]. Other studies have found that the same test had a sensitivity of 66.7% (95% CI 57.1–75.1%) and 72.6% in acute samples from febrile patients in Thailand and Korea, respectively, when assessed against the IFA [20,24]. Specificity was estimated to be 98.4% (95% CI: 91.5–99.7) in the Thai study [20]. Furthermore, there are acknowledged problems with evaluating the test accuracy by using the IFA as a gold standard, which may result in underestimates of sensitivity and specificity in the tests being evaluated [22]. The authors recommend the widespread use of the IgM ELISA, with optical density cut-offs, calibrated for an individual country, as a gold standard for the acute diagnosis of ST infections. The accuracy of serological tests may also be influenced by the variation in the circulating strains of *O. tsutsugamushi* [22,24]. The authors acknowledge the need for ST diagnostic tests to be validated within the country in which they are to be used, to provide more accurate results. The SD Bioline Tsutsugamushi test has not been validated for Bhutan, which further complicates the interpretation of how well the results represent the true ST situation in the country.

While there are challenges in interpreting how well the results of the RDT testing of clinically suspected ST cases reflect the true incidence of clinical ST in the national Bhutanese population, the results are reasonably comparable between sub-groups within the tested population, given that the same test was used throughout the country. It was previously thought that ST was endemic only in the southern part of the country. However, this study has shown that while the highest incidence of RDT-positive clinical ST cases occurred in the subtropical southern districts of Bhutan, cases occurred throughout Bhutan in all but one district, Gasa, which is located in the higher Himalaya area (Figure 4). Hence, ST is a vector-borne zoonotic disease of national importance. The higher incidence in subtropical areas is likely to be associated with the climate favouring the survival of chigger mites, together with higher levels of exposure to the vector through the more intensive farming activities undertaken in the favourable growing climate in this region. The lack of cases in the mountainous Gasa district may be due to an unsuitable environment for the reservoir's sustenance. However, it may also be influenced by the district not having a district-level hospital, which may have led to potential ST cases not being diagnosed and/or tested. Furthermore, the local population may experience difficulty in accessing medical services in this mountainous area, which could further contribute to an underestimation of the incidence of ST in this district.

There was a very strong temporal pattern in the occurrence of RDT-positive clinical ST cases, with 97% of cases observed between June and November, peaking in September (Figure 5). A similar pattern was found in a study in West Bengal, India [25]. This time of the year coincides with the monsoon and the cropping season, which might favour both the density of the chiggers and people's exposure to the vector through agricultural work.

The observed seasonal and spatial patterns of RDT-positive clinical ST cases could be affected by clinicians in high-risk areas having greater awareness of ST during the high-risk season. Data on the total number of clinically suspected ST cases and the number of cases tested with the RDT in hospitals were not available. Hence, we cannot assess the consistency with which the RDT was applied across the clinically suspected ST cases in all hospitals, nor the variation in the proportion of RDT-tested cases that were positive. However, it is unlikely that clinicians' prior knowledge of ST biased the results in this study. While clinicians in the southern areas of Bhutan are generally aware of a higher incidence of febrile disease during the monsoon season, they were mostly unaware of ST and its epidemiology at the time of the study, hence variable awareness of ST is unlikely to have had a significant effect on the clinical suspicion of ST, or the application of the RDT.

The case control study on clinical ST cases diagnosed from October to December 2015 in 11 districts in the south of Bhutan is likely to influence the observed spatial and temporal patterns, as clinicians would have had a greater awareness of ST during the study. Given the study did not begin until October 2015, it would not have influenced the increased incidence showing from July until the peak in September. Furthermore, it would provide more confidence that the incidence declined significantly in November and December. Mapping the RDT-positive ST cases without those from the case control study showed the same spatial pattern with a higher incidence in the southern districts of Bhutan. This gives confidence that there is a higher risk of ST in the subtropical southern districts of Bhutan. A possible source of bias in the spatial and temporal distribution of diagnosed ST may have arisen from a shortage of kits in some hospitals. There is no data available on the timing of diagnostic kit supply to district hospitals during 2015. However, anecdotal reports indicate that some hospitals experienced a temporary shortage of diagnostic kits, particularly hospitals in the high-incidence areas during the high-incidence time of year. This might have influenced the observed distribution of diagnosed cases.

ST predominantly affected people living in rural areas (87%), primarily farmers (45%) (Figure 3). This is consistent with previous observations throughout South-East Asia [25–28]. Students were the second-highest group with clinical ST. This is consistent with results from previous studies, highlighting the importance of ST in the differential diagnosis of children with pyrexia of unknown origin [29].

The highest age-specific incidence of clinical ST occurred in 40–70 year olds. The national statistics [30] show that a larger proportion of people aged 40 years and over live in rural areas (72%) compared with urban areas (28%). Hence, this age-related result is likely to be confounded with a higher risk of exposure of older people to rural environments and agricultural activities. It may also reflect the cumulative exposure of the at-risk population to *O. tsutsugamushi*, which is captured by the RDT measuring IgG and IgA, as well as IgM antibodies. Further studies that include multi-variable analyses would provide more accurate indications of the risk factors for ST.

Cases of ST in Bhutan presented as a nonspecific febrile illness, with signs of myalgia or poly-arthralgia in half the patients, consistent with reports in the literature [13,31]. Respiratory and vascular symptoms were significantly more frequent in males compared to females (respectively

1.7 and 1.9 times). Such a difference has not been reported in other studies, and it is difficult to propose an explanation for these differences. It may be confounded by variable distribution of these conditions between males and females in the over 40 year old age group. The presence of an eschar at the site of the chigger bite is described as pathognomonic [9], and it can thus be a precious diagnostic clue for clinicians. In Japan, 87% of patients presented with an eschar [27]. In contrast, this lesion was noted by the clinician in only 7.4% of patients (10% in males and 5% in females) in the present study. It is possible that clinicians did not thoroughly investigate patients for this lesion, especially female patients. The low detection rate of eschars may also be influenced by the inclusion of febrile patients with historical exposure to ST in the RDT-positive population, given the test measures of IgG and IgA, as well as IgM antibodies.

Among the 470 RDT-positive cases identified in hospitals, samples from only 160 cases were submitted from only four hospitals to the RCDC under the national sero-surveillance programme. The hospitals were: the national referral hospital in Thimphu, the regional referral hospitals in Sarpang and Mongar, and the secondary referral hospital in Paro. District hospitals in the rest of the country did not contribute samples, due to the perceived difficulty of transporting the samples to Thimphu, and a general lack of awareness about the sero-surveillance programme. As a result, the data generated through the national sero-surveillance programme significantly under-represents the true incidence of clinical ST in Bhutan. Raising clinicians' awareness of the sero-surveillance programme and ensuring facilities are available to transport samples from district hospitals to the RCDC in Thimphu would improve the representativeness of the sero-surveillance data. This would improve the ability of the Ministry of Health to monitor trends and to determine if clinical ST continues to emerge over time and over geographic areas in Bhutan. It would also indicate hospitals that may be under-diagnosing ST, which would enable targeted measures to be implemented to improve treatment-seeking behaviours of the public, and/or the diagnosis and treatment of ST in such areas where there is a difference between the expected and actual reported cases.

Despite the limitations of the SD Bioline Tsutsugamushi test, such commercial point of care tests are considered to be useful in clinical settings in limited resource environments to guide the differential diagnosis of ST [32], with the advantages of affordability, rapidity, single test results and ease of interpretation [19]. However, the tests need to be used with appropriate clinical discernment. It is important for clinicians to rule out other causes of acute febrile illness and the possibility of co-infection of patients with other infections that are associated with similar exposures, such as dengue and other rickettsial diseases. Given the limitations in the sensitivity of the test, clinicians should be encouraged to initiate treatment in patients in which they strongly suspect ST, even if the sample tests negative to the RDT, and to send samples from such patients to RCDC for confirmatory testing with the IgM ELISA. The epidemiological information generated through this study provides supplementary information that clinicians can use to diagnose ST, even in the absence of a positive RDT. Furthermore, epidemiological information can significantly contribute to the formulation and timely implementation of public health measures to reduce the burden of ST in Bhutan. Communication programmes can be implemented in all areas, to raise the awareness of the public to seek treatment if they are suffering flu-like symptoms. Likewise, providing clinicians with guidelines and professional training in risk factors for ST, such as the times of year, geographic areas, occupations and types of exposure to potential chigger habitat could increase the probability of considering ST in the differential diagnosis for patients presenting with nonspecific febrile illness. The timely supply of test kits and therapeutic drugs to hospitals, especially in high-risk areas, may contribute to the improved diagnosis and treatment of ST cases.

This study represents an important step towards understanding the incidence and associated risk factors for ST in Bhutan, which can inform both public health measures and the design of future studies. It would be valuable to validate the SD Bioline Tsutsugamushi test in Bhutan. Furthermore, studies to identify the antigenic variants of *O. tsutsugamushi* in Bhutan and in neighbouring areas of northern India could help with the development of more sensitive serological tests. Given the complex nature of this vector-borne zoonotic disease, One Health studies, involving collaboration between multiple sectors and disciplines, are required to explore the roles of the environmental and anthropologic factors, and the ecology of the reservoir and vector population, to understand the drivers of the spatial, temporal and demographic distributions of ST in Bhutan.

Author Contributions: Conceptualisation, K.D., Y.P., T.Z., S.D., N.M. and J.M.; Data curation, K.D., Y.P., T.Z. and N.M.; Formal analysis, N.M.; Funding acquisition, P.J. and R.M.; Investigation, K.D., Y.P. and T.Z.; Methodology, K.D., S.D., N.M. and J.M.; Project administration, K.D., S.D., C.D. and J.M.; Resources, C.D., P.J., R.M. and J.M.; Supervision, S.D., P.J., R.M. and J.M.; Validation, K.D., Y.P., T.Z. and N.M.; Visualization, N.M.; Writing—original draft, K.D., Y.P., T.Z. and S.D.; Writing—review & editing, P.J., N.M. and J.M.

Acknowledgments: We acknowledge the dedicated support of the district health staff who were instrumental in this study. The program was implemented by Massey University, in collaboration with Khesar Gyalpo University of Medical Sciences, and the Royal University of Bhutan.

References

1. Xu, G.; Walker, D.H.; Jupiter, D.; Melby, P.C.; Arcari, C.M. A review of the global epidemiology of scrub typhus. *PLoS Negl. Trop. Dis.* **2017**, *11*, e0006062. [CrossRef] [PubMed]

2. Lyu, Y.; Tian, L.; Zhang, L.; Dou, X.; Wang, X.; Li, W.; Zhang, X.; Sun, Y.; Guan, Z.; Li, X.; et al. A Case-Control Study of Risk Factors Associated with Scrub Typhus Infection in Beijing, China. *PLoS ONE* **2013**, *8*, e63668. [CrossRef]

3. Newton, P.N.; Day, N.P. 63—Scrub Typhus. In *Hunter's Tropical Medicine and Emerging Infectious Disease*, 9th ed.; Magill, A.J., Hill, D.R., Solomon, T., Ryan, E.T., Eds.; W.B. Saunders: London, UK, 2013; pp. 542–545.

4. Yang, H.-H.; Huang, I.-T.; Lin, C.-H.; Chen, T.-Y.; Chen, L.-K. New Genotypes of *Orientia tsutsugamushi* Isolated from Humans in Eastern Taiwan. *PLoS ONE* **2012**, *7*, e46997. [CrossRef] [PubMed]

5. Chakraborty, S.; Sarma, N. Scrub Typhus: An Emerging Threat. *Indian J. Dermatol.* **2017**, *62*, 478–485. [PubMed]

6. Wei, Y.; Huang, Y.; Li, X.; Ma, Y.; Tao, X.; Wu, X.; Yang, Z. Climate variability, animal reservoir and transmission of scrub typhus in Southern China. *PLoS Negl. Trop. Dis.* **2017**, *11*, e0005447. [CrossRef]

7. Chang, K.; Lee, N.-Y.; Ko, W.-C.; Tsai, J.-J.; Lin, W.-R.; Chen, T.-C.; Lu, P.-L.; Chen, Y.-H. Identification of factors for physicians to facilitate early differential diagnosis of scrub typhus, murine typhus, and Q fever from dengue fever in Taiwan. *J. Microbiol. Immunol. Infect.* **2017**, *50*, 104–111. [CrossRef]

8. Rajapakse, S.; Rodrigo, C.; Fernando, D. Scrub typhus: Pathophysiology, clinical manifestations and prognosis. *Asian Pac. J. Trop. Med.* **2012**, *5*, 261–264. [CrossRef]

9. Varghese, G.M.; Trowbridge, P.; Janardhanan, J.; Thomas, K.; Peter, J.V.; Mathews, P.; Abraham, O.C.; Kavitha, M. Clinical profile and improving mortality trend of scrub typhus in South India. *Int. J. Infect. Dis.* **2014**, *23*, 39–43. [CrossRef]

10. Jeong, Y.J.; Kim, S.; Wook, Y.D.; Lee, J.W.; Kim, K.-I.; Lee, S.H. Scrub Typhus: Clinical, Pathologic, and Imaging Findings1. *Radio Graph.* **2007**, *27*, 161–172. [CrossRef]

11. Kim, D.-M.; Shin, H.; Lee, S.-H.; Song, H.-J.; Park, C.Y.; Lee, J.H.; Kim, H.S.; Kim, H.K.; Won, K.J.; Yang, T.Y.; et al. Distribution of eschars on the body of scrub typhus patients: A prospective study. *Am. J. Trop. Med. Hyg.* **2007**, *76*, 806–809. [CrossRef]

12. El Sayed, I.; Liu, Q.; Wee, I.; Hine, P. Antibiotics for treating scrub typhus. *Cochrane Database Syst. Rev.* **2018**. [CrossRef] [PubMed]

13. Paris, D.H.; Shelite, T.R.; Day, N.P.; Walker, D.H. Unresolved Problems Related to Scrub Typhus: A Seriously Neglected Life-Threatening Disease. *Am. J. Trop. Med. Hyg.* **2013**, *89*, 301–307. [CrossRef]

14. Zhang, L.; Zhao, Z.; Bi, Z.; Kou, Z.; Zhang, M.; Yang, L.; Zheng, L. Risk factors associated with severe scrub typhus in Shandong, northern China. *Int. J. Infect. Dis.* **2014**, *29*, 203–207. [CrossRef]

15. Varghese, G.M.; Janardhanan, J.; Trowbridge, P.; Peter, J.V.; Prakash, J.A.; Sathyendra, S.; Thomas, K.; David, T.S.; Kavitha, M.; Abraham, O.C.; et al. Scrub typhus in South India: Clinical and laboratory manifestations, genetic variability, and outcome. *Int. J. Infectious Dis.* **2013**, *17*, e981–e987. [CrossRef] [PubMed]

16. Dorji, T.; Wangchuk, S.; Lhazeen, K. Clinical Characteristics of Scrub Typhus in Gedu and Mongar (Bhutan). 2010. Available online: http://www.rcdc.gov.bt/web/clinical-characteristics-of-scrub-typhus-in-gedu-and-mongarbhutan/ (accessed on 4 April 2018).

17. Tshokey, T.; Choden, T.; Sharma, R. Scrub typhus in Bhutan: A synthesis of data from 2009 to 2014. *WHO South East Asia J. Public Health* **2016**, *5*, 117. [CrossRef]

18. Banerjee, A.; Bandopadhyay, R. Biodiversity Hotspot of Bhutan and its Sustainability. *Curr. Sci.* **2016**, *110*, 521. [CrossRef]

19. Shivalli, S. Diagnostic evaluation of rapid tests for scrub typhus in the Indian population is needed. *Infect. Dis. Poverty* **2016**, *5*, 894. [CrossRef] [PubMed]

20. Silpasakorn, S.; Waywa, D.; Hoontrakul, S.; Suttinont, C.; Losuwanaluk, K.; Suputtamongkol, Y. Performance of SD Bioline Tsutsugamushi assays for the diagnosis of scrub typhus in Thailand. *J. Med. Assoc. Thai* **2012**, *95*, 5.

21. R Development Core Team. *R: A Language and Environment for Statistical Computing*; R Foundation for Statistical Computing: Vienna, Austria, 2014.

22. Blacksell, S.D.; Tanganuchitcharnchai, A.; Nawtaisong, P.; Kantipong, P.; Laongnualpanich, A.; Day, N.P.J.; Paris, D.H. Diagnostic Accuracy of the InBios Scrub Typhus Detect Enzyme-Linked Immunoassay for the Detection of IgM Antibodies in Northern Thailand. *Clin. Vaccine Immunol.* **2016**, *23*, 148–154. [CrossRef] [PubMed]

23. Watthanaworawit, W.; Hanboonkunupakarn, B.; Nosten, F.; Tanganuchitcharnchai, A.; Jintaworn, S.; Blacksell, S.D.; Turner, P.; Turner, C.; Richards, A.L.; Day, N.P.J. Diagnostic Accuracy Assessment of Immunochromatographic Tests for the Rapid Detection of Antibodies against *Orientia tsutsugamushi* Using Paired Acute and Convalescent Specimens. *Am. J. Trop. Med. Hyg.* **2015**, *93*, 1168–1171. [CrossRef]

24. Lee, K.-D.; Moon, C.; Oh, W.S.; Sohn, K.M.; Kim, B.-N. Diagnosis of scrub typhus: Introduction of the immunochromatographic test in Korea. *Korean J. Intern. Med.* **2014**, *29*, 253–255. [CrossRef] [PubMed]

25. Sharma, P.K.; Ramakrishnan, R.; Hutin, Y.; Barui, A.; Manickam, P.; Kakkar, M.; Mittal, V.; Gupte, M. Scrub typhus in Darjeeling, India: Opportunities for simple, practical prevention measures. *Trans. R. Soc. Trop. Med. Hyg.* **2009**, *103*, 1153–1158. [CrossRef]

26. Lee, Y.-S.; Wang, P.-H.; Tseng, S.-J.; Ko, C.-F.; Teng, H.-J. Epidemiology of scrub typhus in eastern Taiwan, 2000–2004. *Jpn. J. Infect. Dis.* **2006**, *59*, 235–238. [PubMed]

27. Ogawa, M.; Hagiwara, T.; Kishimoto, T.; Shiga, S.; Yoshida, Y.; Furuya, Y.; Kaiho, I.; Ito, T.; Nemoto, H.; Yamamoto, N.; et al. Scrub typhus in Japan: Epidemiology and clinical features of cases reported in 1998. *Am. J. Trop. Med. Hyg.* **2002**, *67*, 162–165. [CrossRef]

28. Vallée, J.; Thaojaikong, T.; Moore, C.E.; Phetsouvanh, R.; Richards, A.L.; Souris, M.; Fournet, F.; Salem, G.; Gonzalez, J.-P.J.; Newton, P.N. Contrasting Spatial Distribution and Risk Factors for Past Infection with Scrub Typhus and Murine Typhus in Vientiane City, Lao PDR. *PLOS Negl. Trop. Dis.* **2010**, *4*, e909. [CrossRef]

29. Yadav, D.; Chopra, A.; Dutta, A.K.; Kumar, S.; Kumar, V. Scrub Typhus: An Uncommon Cause of Pyrexia without Focus. *J. Nepal Paedtr. Soc.* **2013**, *33*, 234–235. [CrossRef]

30. National Statistics Bureau. *Population Projections for Bhutan 2017–2047*; Royal Government of Bhutan: Thimphu, Bhutan, 2019.

31. Rapsang, A.G.; Bhattacharyya, P. Scrub typhus. *Indian J. Anaesth.* **2013**, *57*, 127. [PubMed]

32. Chanana, L.; Atre, K.; Galwankar, S.; Kelkar, D. State of the Globe: What's the Right Test for Diagnosing Rickettseal Diseases. *J. Glob. Infect. Dis.* **2016**, *8*, 95–96. [CrossRef] [PubMed]

10

Insights into Australian Bat Lyssavirus in Insectivorous Bats of Western Australia

Diana Prada [1,*], **Victoria Boyd** [2], **Michelle Baker** [2], **Bethany Jackson** [1,†] **and Mark O'Dea** [1,†] (ID)

[1] School of Veterinary Medicine, Murdoch University, Perth, WA 6150, Australia; b.jackson@murdoch.edu.au (B.J.); m.odea@murdoch.edu.au (M.O.)

[2] Australian Animal Health Laboratory, CSIRO, Geelong, VIC 3220, Australia; vicky.boyd@csiro.au (V.B.); michelle.baker@csiro.au (M.B.)

* Correspondence: 32589004@student.murdoch.edu.au.

† These authors contributed equally.

Abstract: Australian bat lyssavirus (ABLV) is a known causative agent of neurological disease in bats, humans and horses. It has been isolated from four species of pteropid bats and a single microbat species (*Saccolaimus flaviventris*). To date, ABLV surveillance has primarily been passive, with active surveillance concentrating on eastern and northern Australian bat populations. As a result, there is scant regional ABLV information for large areas of the country. To better inform the local public health risks associated with human-bat interactions, this study describes the lyssavirus prevalence in microbat communities in the South West Botanical Province of Western Australia. We used targeted real-time PCR assays to detect viral RNA shedding in 839 oral swabs representing 12 species of microbats, which were sampled over two consecutive summers spanning 2016–2018. Additionally, we tested 649 serum samples via Luminex® assay for reactivity to lyssavirus antigens. Active lyssavirus infection was not detected in any of the samples. Lyssavirus antibodies were detected in 19 individuals across six species, with a crude prevalence of 2.9% (95% CI: 1.8–4.5%) over the two years. In addition, we present the first records of lyssavirus exposure in two *Nyctophilus* species, and *Falsistrellus mackenziei*.

Keywords: Australian bat lyssavirus; microbats; Western Australia; serology; Luminex; real-time PCR

1. Introduction

Australian bat lyssavirus (ABLV) is one of the 16 classified species of lyssaviruses within the family *Rhabdoviridae* [1]. It was first discovered in Australia in 1996 [2] and early studies distinguished two variants, the pteropid variant carried by all four species of flying fox within continental Australia [3], and the insectivorous variant detected only in the yellow-bellied sheath-tailed bat (*Saccolaimus flaviventris*) [4]. Although there is evidence of ABLV exposure in 11 genera within four microbat families [5], additional reservoir species have yet to be identified.

Both ABLV strains are associated with clinical disease in the host species [2,4]. Although spillover events are extremely rare, they have resulted in fatal neurological disease in humans and horses [6–8], making ABLV an agent of significant public health concern. Current public health policy recommends a prophylactic rabies vaccination for bat handlers, with the administration of post-exposure treatment including vaccination and rabies immunoglobulin based on vaccination history and individual immune status [9]. However, the perceived risk from exposure to microbats is potentially limited by the relative lack of media exposure these species receive compared to the larger pteropids, coupled with only a single documented microbat to human transmission of ABLV to date.

Since the discovery of ABLV, surveillance has predominantly relied on passive sampling regimes, with a single published study based on active sampling in the east and north of the country [10]. Results suggest ABLV circulates at a low prevalence (<1%) in healthy wild bat populations [5]. However, the prevalence (and therefore risk) escalates to 5%–10% where bats are injured, sick or orphaned. These are precisely the conditions which are considered to drive human exposure through rescue and rehabilitation attempts, or the protection of property, pets or children [11–13]. Interestingly, the public health research on ABLV and human-bat interactions to date does not report on community knowledge or risk perceptions of microbats versus pteropid species, generally referring to 'bats' as a broad group [11–15]. Therefore, whilst basic knowledge of ABLV in bats appears to be high in some regions [11], public awareness of the specific risks and recommended post-exposure behaviours with respect to microbats warrants further research.

In Western Australia, ABLV surveillance has also been sporadic and passive, with the only targeted study focusing on the far northern part of the state and concentrating mainly on the pteropid bats in the region [5], with sample collection occurring some 15 years ago. Active surveillance of microbats has likely been hindered by the additional time and resource demands of sampling non-cave roosting species typical of the region [16]. Therefore, there is limited current information on the ABLV status of Western Australian microbat species and the disease status is assumed by the extrapolation of information from bat populations in the eastern states. Additionally, there is no local data of ABLV status in the south west of Western Australia, an area with arguably increased human-bat interaction due to the higher population density.

In order to better inform the regional risks associated with human-bat interactions, this study aimed to establish the lyssavirus status of insectivorous bats in the South-West Botanical Province of WA over a period of two years. We used an ABLV specific and a pan-lyssavirus reverse transcription real-time PCR (RRT-PCR) assay to screen oral swabs from 12 species of microbats. Additionally, we used a bead-based Luminex® assay on serum samples to determine previous lyssavirus exposure.

2. Materials and Methods

All sampling was approved by the Department of Parks and Wildlife of Western Australia, permits 08-001359-1, and CE005517. Capture, handling and sampling procedures were approved by the Murdoch University Animal Ethics Committee (R2882/16).

Harp traps and mist nets were used to capture bats at different locations of the South-West Botanical Province (SWBP), an Australian global biodiversity hotspot. The province covers approximately 44 million hectares and comprises nine bioregions [17]. Remnant natural cover in the east and west of the region is separated by the extensive monoculture known as the Western Australian wheatbelt, which acts as a major dispersion barrier for many native species.

Sampling took place over two summers between 2016 and 2018, with sites in the east and west boundaries of the wheatbelt. The northeastern sites were within the semi-arid Avon bioregion which was predominantly sampled during the first season (2016–2017). The southwestern sites were distributed across five bioregions, the Esperance Plains, Geraldton Sandplains, Jarrah Forest, Swan Coastal Plain, and Warren (Figure 1), which were mainly sampled during the second year of the study (2017–2018). Therefore, most sampling sites were visited only once over the two years, except for locations in the Avon bioregion which were sampled during both summers.

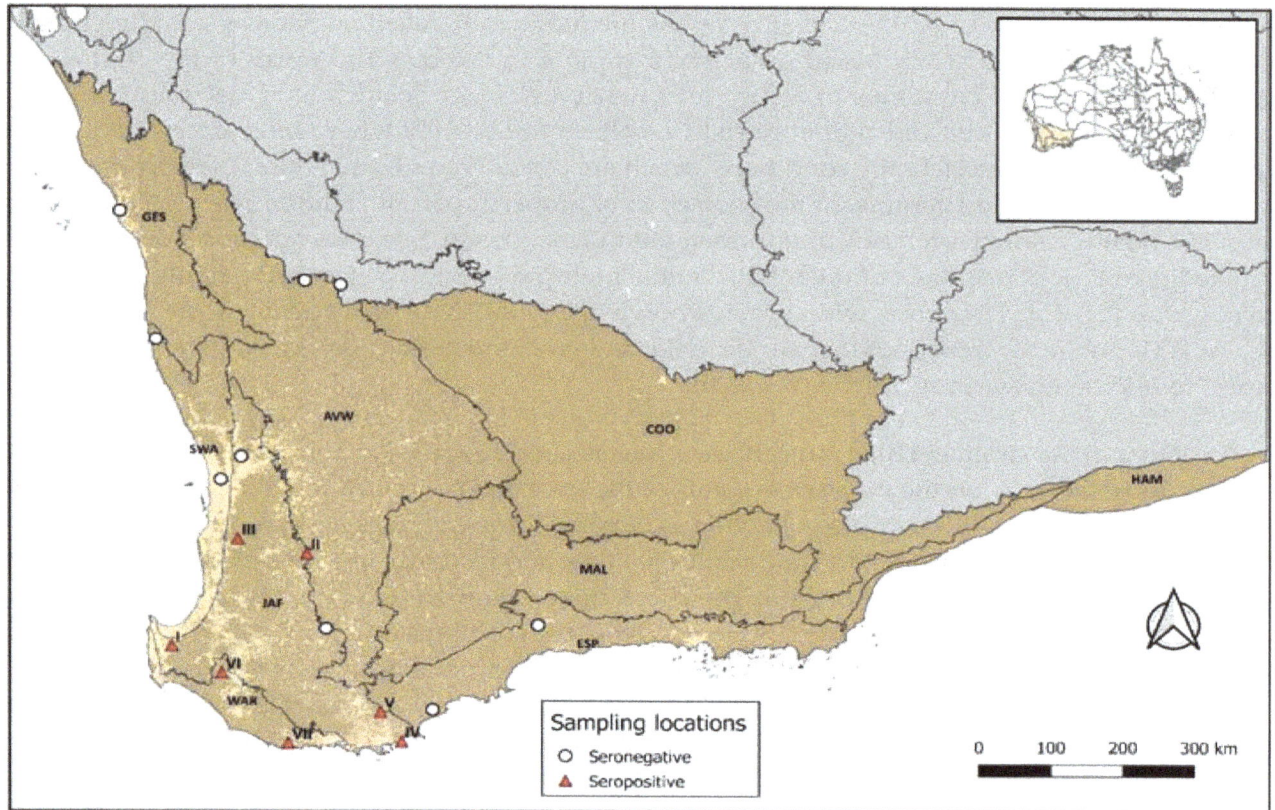

Figure 1. The South West Botanical province (SWBP) highlighted in brown. Sampling sites are shown and sites where seropositive individuals were identified are labelled I-VII. Presence (light areas) and absence (dark areas) of human populations are shown. The SWBP encompasses nine bioregions, Avon Wheatbelt (AVW), Coolgardie (COO), Esperance Plains (ESP), Geraldton Sandplains (GES), Hampton (HAM), Jarrah Forest (JAF), Mallee (MAL), Swan Coastal Plain (SWA), and Warren (WAR).

Prior to undertaking trapping, all personnel involved in handling bats underwent a complete rabies vaccination schedule. Biosecurity and biosafety protocols during handling and sampling included the use of protective gloves while manipulating bats out of traps and nets. During sample collection, double gloves were worn while restraining the animal (nitrile gloves over protective gloves), with the nitrile gloves changed between each bat. All surfaces and non-disposable equipment (e.g., calipers) were disinfected with a 10% solution of F10 (Health and Hygiene, South Africa) between each bat. Additionally, single calico bags were used for each individual and soaked in F10 before being re-used.

Following capture, bats were taxonomically identified, and a single oral swab (FLOQSwab, Copan, Brescia, Italy) was collected per individual and stored in RNAlater® (Ambion, Life Technologies, Carlsbad, CA, USA). Additionally, 10 μL of blood was taken from the brachial vein and diluted 1:10 in phosphate buffered saline (PBS).

Oral swabs were vortexed and 50 μL of the supernatant used as starting material for all extractions using a Magmax viral RNA extraction kit (Ambion, Applied Biosystems, Vilnius, Lithuania) following the manufacturer's instructions. The detection of lyssavirus RNA was performed using an Australian bat lyssavirus RRT-PCR specific for the insectivorous variant of the virus [18], and a pan-lyssavirus RRT-PCR assay [19]. Inactivated insectivorous ABLV RNA provided by the CSIRO Australian Animal Health Laboratory (AAHL, Victoria, Australia) was used as a positive control. Assays were performed on a QuantStudio 6 Flex platform (Life Technologies, Singapore). Nucleic acid extraction verification and lack of inhibitors were assessed using an endogenous 18S rRNA PCR assay (Life Technologies, Pleasanton, CA, USA).

Sera were tested for reactivity to lyssavirus antigens [20] in an indirect binding Luminex®️ assay [21], at a final working dilution of 1:50 at CSIRO AAHL. As a pilot study, samples collected during the first season were pooled one in three ($n = 246$) or one in four ($n = 24$). All samples collected during the second season were tested individually ($n = 391$). Median Fluorescence Intensity (MFI) was read using a Bio-Plex instrument (Bio-Rad Laboratories, Hercules, CA, USA). Due to the lack of known positive and known negative bat sera from the species captured in this study to validate the assay, the MFI threshold to differentiate positive and negative samples was set at 1000 MFI as per CSIRO protocols. Previous studies published by the Australian Animal Health Laboratory and elsewhere using the same Bio-Plex platform have used a threshold of at least three times the mean MFI of negative sera from other bat species with values below 250 MFI considered negative [22–25]. The same principle was used here to establish a threshold based on an MFI of 250 corresponding to a negative sample with sample MFIs above 1000 considered positive.

Prevalence estimates and 95% confidence intervals were calculated using the Wilson's Method [26] as implemented in the R package *epitools* [27].

3. Results

In total, 839 oral swabs and 661 blood samples were collected. Twelve samples did not provide a valid Luminex®️ assay result and were removed from the analysis. Therefore, the final serological dataset comprised 649 samples encompassing 12 bat species (Table 1). Captured species composition varied at each location (Figure 2) and in general *Chalinolobus gouldii* and *Vespadelus regulus* had the greatest representation in the swab and sera data sets (Table 1). A total of 270 serum samples were collected in the first year and 379 during the second year.

Table 1. Seroprevalence of Australian Bat Lyssavirus in 12 species of microbats of the South West Botanical Province of Western Australia. The total number of samples tested and positives () are shown.

Family	Species	Swabs	Sera	Seroprevalence [1]
	Chalinolobus gouldii	287(0)	262(2)	0.7 (0.2–2.7)
	Chalinolobus morio	105(0)	64(3)	4.6 (1.6–12.8)
	Falsistrellus mackenziei	14(0)	7(1)	NC [2]
	Nyctophilus geoffroyi	69(0)	48(0)	
	Nyctophilus gouldi	78(0)	66(3)	4.5 (1.5–12.5)
Vespertilionidae	*Nyctophilus major*	12(0)	5(1)	NC [2]
	Nyctophilus sp [3]	6(0)	5(0)	
	Scotorepens balstoni	13(0)	8(0)	
	Vespadelus baverstocki	6(0)	5(0)	
	Vespadelus finlaysoni	1(0)	0	
	Vespadelus regulus	227(0)	164(9)	5.5 (2.9–10.1)
	Vespadelus sp [3]	2(0)	1(0)	
Molossidae	*Austronomus australis*	13(0)	11(0)	
	Ozimops sp	6(0)	3(0)	

[1] Prevalence (%) and 95% confidence intervals (CI). [2] Prevalence estimates not calculated (NC) due to small sample size. [3] These individuals were not confidently identified to species level, however will belong to either of the listed *Nyctophilus* or *Vespadelus* species, and therefore do not count towards the total number of species sampled.

Neither the ABLV specific or the pan-lyssavirus RRT-PCR reactions yielded a positive result. No inhibition was detected in any of the samples and positive and negative controls were valid.

Serological reactivity to lyssavirus antigens was detected in 19 samples (Table 1, Table S1) resulting in an overall antibody prevalence of 2.9% (95% CI: 1.8–4.5%). Seropositive samples encompassed six species, *V. regulus* had the highest prevalence at 5.5% (95% CI: 2.9–10.1%), followed by *C. morio* (4.6%, 95% CI: 1.6–12.8), *Nyctophilus gouldi* (4.5%, 95% CI: 1.5–12.5) and *C. gouldii* (0.7%, 95% CI: 0.2–2.7%). Additionally, reactivity was also detected in a single *Falsistrellus mackenziei*, and an *N. major*. Due to their small sample sizes, prevalence values were not estimated for these two species (Table 1).

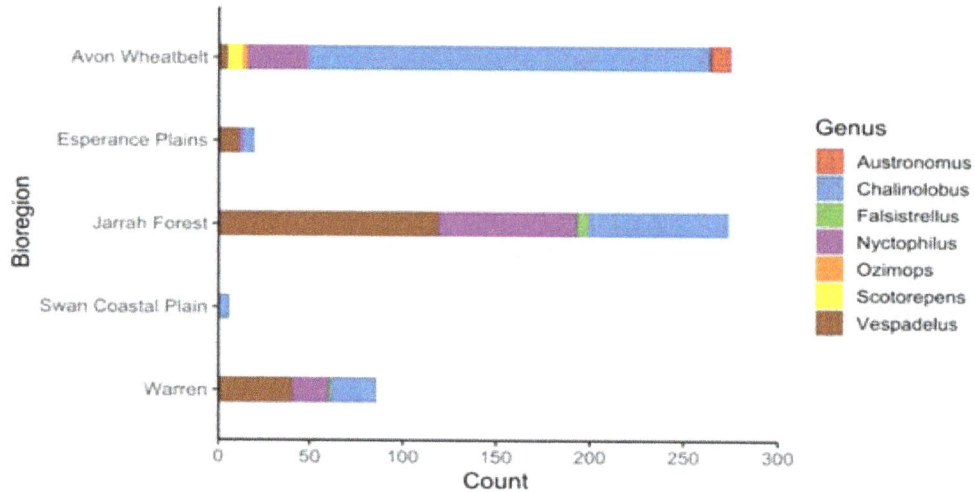

Figure 2. Number of blood samples taken by genera and bioregion. Note, no blood samples were obtained from bats in the Geraldton Sandplains bioregion.

Despite a large number of individuals being sampled during the first year ($n = 270$), none reacted on the lyssavirus serological assay, thus all seropositive bats were captured during the second year of the study, and south of the wheatbelt. Consequently, annual seroprevalence significantly increased from 0% in the first year to 5% (95% CI: 3.2–7.7%) in the second year ($p = < 0.0001$). It should be noted that the majority (78%) of captures in the first year and north of the wheatbelt were dominated by a single species, *C. gouldii*.

Seropositive individuals were captured at seven sites which were dominated by natural jarrah (*Eucalyptus marginata*) and marri (*Corymbia calophylla*) forests, and on one occasion on agricultural land transitioning to wandoo (*E. wandoo*) woodlands (Table 2). Seropositive *V. regulus* were sampled at five different locations, seropositive *N. gouldii*, and *C. morio* were captured at three and two locations, respectively, and the remaining two species were all captured at a single site. When examining the data by number of seropositive samples per location, three different species were captured at three locations, and the remaining four locations were represented by a single seropositive species.

Table 2. Distribution of seropositive individuals per bioregion and trapping location. Number of positives () per species.

Bioregion	Location	Species
Jarrah Forest	I	*Vespadelus regulus* (1)
	II	*Chalinolobus gouldii* (2)
	III	*Vespadelus regulus* (2)
		Nyctophilus major (1)
		Falsistrellus mackenziei (1)
	IV	*Nyctophilus gouldi* (1)
	V	*Vespadelus regulus* (1)
Warren	VI	*Chalinolobus morio* (2)
		Nyctophilus gouldi (1)
		Vespadelus regulus (1)
	VII	*Chalinolobus morio* (1)
		Nyctophilus gouldi (1)
		Vespadelus regulus (4)

4. Discussion

Here we report the first comprehensive study investigating the lyssavirus status of apparently healthy populations of insectivorous bats in the South West Botanical Province of WA. Significantly, this is the first active surveillance to take place in the SWBP and therefore constitutes an update to the existing limited lyssavirus data on wild microbat populations [10]. We did not detect any current ABLV infection or the presence of any other lyssavirus species circulating within the sampled populations, despite the large sample size (n = 839). The suitability of oral swabs for lyssavirus detection has previously been demonstrated in clinical studies [18,28–30], and in active lyssavirus surveillance efforts [31,32]. Nonetheless, diagnostic sensitivity in a field surveillance setting for the detection of ABLV may be limited by the combination of intermittent shedding [33], and a small window of infection [32,34] of an already low prevalence virus.

Serological results indicated previous lyssavirus exposure in 19 individuals, resulting in an overall seroprevalence of 2.9% in the study population. This result is congruent with previous sero-response estimates of wild Australian bat populations [5], albeit using a different serological assay. Antibody reactivity was detected in six Vespertilionidae species, *C. gouldii*, *C. morio*, *V. regulus*, *F. mackenziei*, *N. gouldi*, and *N. major*. The presence of lyssavirus antibodies has previously been documented for the *Chalinolobus* and *Vespadelus* genera [5], and the results here constitute the first published report of lyssavirus exposure in *Nyctophilus spp.* and *F. mackenziei*, an endemic species of the jarrah forests of the South West. It was not possible to carry out further confirmatory testing on seropositive individuals, as the volume of blood ethically permissible to be drawn from microbats was fully used in the Luminex® assay.

Seroprevalence values per species varied between 0.7% and 5.5%, with the highest values observed in *V. regulus* (5.5%), *C. morio* (4.6%) and *N. gouldi* (4.5%). Despite the existence of previously published seroprevalence figures for some Australian Vespertilionidae species [5], it is not appropriate to make direct comparisons due to previous results grouping different species by genera and being based on an alternative serological assay. Even though seropositivity for ABLV has previously been reported in *Austronomus australis* [5], we did not detect any antibody response in this species, possibly due to the small sample size (n = 11).

All seropositive individuals originated from seven locations within the Jarrah and Warren bioregions and none from the Avon bioregion, which is isolated by the Australian wheatbelt. It is unclear whether this partitioning of the data represents a geographical, temporal or a species association given these risk factors are confounded in the study population. However, temporal shedding may explain the 0% prevalence in the Avon bioregion despite the large sample size (n = 226), as this region was predominantly sampled in the first year and all the seropositive individuals occurred in the second year of the study. This hypothesis is supported by longitudinal studies elsewhere showing that inter-annual variation of seroprevalence estimates is common in wild bat populations [28,32]. Further, long term active surveillance in *Myotis myotis* has provided important insights into the infection dynamics of lyssavirus at a temporal and geographical scale [32], highlighting how similar studies would contribute to better understanding of ABLV dynamics within Australian microbat populations. It is possible that a failure to detect seropositive samples during the first year could also have been the result of decreased assay sensitivity triggered by sample pooling. However, titration studies using pools of *Pteropus alecto* sera by CSIRO AAHL have not demonstrated a loss of assay sensitivity at the pooling levels used in this study.

The detection of ABLV seropositivity in the SWBP, particularly the southern parts of the region, further supports the existence of additional lyssavirus reservoirs, as the distribution of *Pteropus spp.* and *Saccolaimus flaviventris* does not extend to the SWBP. This suggests that any hypothetical reservoir may be a member of the families Vespertilionidae or Molossidae, with serology results indicating Vespertilionidae may be a reservoir genus in the Southwest of WA. Importantly, seropositive individuals of six separate species came from a variety of areas in the south west in relatively close proximity to towns and recreational areas (<20 km).

The results from this study suggest that active infections in wild microbat populations may be even lower than previously thought. Despite this, the evidence of circulating ABLV in the region validates current recommendations for post-exposure treatment of people with bat bites and scratches, including those from microbats. We recommend public health research akin to that conducted in the eastern states [11–15] in order to evaluate knowledge, attitudes and perceptions of ABLV risks in the south west of WA specifically for microbat species. This information should be used to guide future public health campaigns in the region.

Author Contributions: M.O., B.J. and D.P. designed the study and collected the data; V.B. and M.B. carried out all the serology laboratory work; D.P. performed all the molecular laboratory work and analysed the data from the molecular and serology datasets; D.P. drafted the manuscript; M.O. and B.J. reviewed and edited the manuscript; M.O. and B.J. supervised the research.

Acknowledgments: We would like to acknowledge all the volunteers involved in the data collection. This project would not have been possible without their help and good disposition in the field. We would also like to thank Robert Bullen, Nicholas Dunlop, Terry Reardon, Andrew Grigg and Cameron Richardson from Alcoa, and members of the Department of Biodiversity, Conservation and Attractions in particular Sarah Comber, Janine Liddelow, and Peter Lacey for their assistance in identifying adequate bat trapping sites, which was fundamental to this project. We also thank the private landowners who provided access to their properties, as well as John and Lisa Lawson from the Lions Dryandra Village for facilitating our stay there. We would also like to thank the Australian Wildlife Conservancy and Bush Heritage Australia for supporting this project.

References

1. International Committee on Taxonomy of Viruses. Available online: https://talk.ictvonline.org/taxonomy/ (accessed on 14 February 2019).
2. Fraser, G.C.; Hooper, P.T.; Lunt, R.A.; Gould, A.R.; Gleeson, L.J.; Hyatt, A.D.; Russell, G.M.; Kattenbelt, J.A. Encephalitis Caused by a Lyssavirus in Fruit Bats in Australia. *Emerg. Infect. Dis.* **1996**, *2*, 327–331. [CrossRef] [PubMed]
3. Gould, A.R.; Hyatt, A.D.; Lunt, R.; Kattenbelt, J.A.; Hengstberger, S.; Blacksell, S. Characterisation of a novel lyssavirus isolated from Pteropid bats in Australia. *Virus Res.* **1998**, *54*, 165–187. [CrossRef]
4. Gould, A.R.; Kattenbelt, J.A.; Gumley, S.G.; Lunt, R.A. Characterisation of an Australian bat lyssavirus variant isolated from an insectivorous bat. *Virus Res.* **2002**, *89*, 1–28. [CrossRef]
5. Field, H.E. Evidence of Australian bat lyssavirus infection in diverse Australian bat taxa. *Zoonoses Public Health* **2018**, *65*, 742–748. [CrossRef] [PubMed]
6. Francis, J.R.; Nourse, C.; Vaska, V.L.; Calvert, S.; Northill, J.A.; McCall, B.; Mattke, A.C. Australian Bat Lyssavirus in a child: The first reported case. *Pediatrics* **2014**, *133*, e1063–e1067. [CrossRef] [PubMed]
7. Shinwari, M.W.; Annand, E.J.; Driver, L.; Warrilow, D.; Harrower, B.; Allcock, R.J.N.; Pukallus, D.; Harper, J.; Bingham, J.; Kung, N.; et al. Australian bat lyssavirus infection in two horses. *Vet. Microbiol.* **2014**, *173*, 224–231. [CrossRef] [PubMed]
8. Hanna, J.N.; Carney, I.K.; Smith, G.A.; Tannenberg, A.E.; Deverill, J.E.; Botha, J.A.; Serafin, I.L.; Harrower, B.J.; Fitzpatrick, P.F.; Searle, J.W. Australian bat lyssavirus infection: A second human case, with a long incubation period. *Med. J. Aust.* **2000**, *172*, 597–599. [PubMed]
9. Australian Technical Advisory Group on Immunisation (ATAGI). Australian Immunisation Handbook. Available online: https://immunisationhandbook.health.gov.au/ (accessed on 14 February 2019).
10. Field, H. The Ecology of Hendra Virus and Australian Bat Lyssavirus. Ph.D. Thesis, University of Queensland, Brisbane, Australia, 2004.
11. Young, M.K.; El Saadi, D.; McCall, B.J. Preventing Australian Bat Lyssavirus: Community knowledge and risk perception of bats in southeast Queensland. *Vector-Borne Zoonotic Dis.* **2014**, *14*, 284–290. [CrossRef] [PubMed]
12. Paterson, B.J.; Butler, M.T.; Eastwood, K.; Cashman, P.M.; Jones, A.; Durrheim, D.N. Cross sectional survey of human-bat interaction in Australia: Public health implications. *BMC Public Health* **2014**, *14*, 58. [CrossRef] [PubMed]
13. Quinn, E.K.; Massey, P.D.; Cox-Witton, K.; Paterson, B.J.; Eastwood, K.; Durrheim, D.N. Understanding human—Bat interactions in NSW, Australia: Improving risk communication for prevention of Australian bat lyssavirus. *BMC Vet. Res.* **2014**, *10*, 144. [CrossRef] [PubMed]
14. McCall, B.J.; Epstein, J.H.; Neill, A.S.; Heel, K.; Field, H.; Barrett, J.; Smith, G.A.; Selvey, L.A.; Rodwell, B.; Lunt, R. Potential exposure to Australian bat lyssavirus, Queensland, 1996-1999. *Emerg. Infect. Dis.* **2000**, *6*, 259–264. [CrossRef] [PubMed]

15. Francis, J.R.; McCall, B.J.; Hutchinson, P.; Powell, J.; Vaska, V.L.; Nourse, C. Australian bat lyssavirus: Implications for public health. *Med. J. Aust.* **2014**, *201*, 647–649. [CrossRef] [PubMed]

16. Churchill, S. *Australian Bats*, 2nd ed.; Allen and Unwin: French Forest, Australia, 1998.

17. Wardell-Johnson, G.; Wardell-Johnson, A.; Bradby, K.; Robinson, T.; Bateman, P.W.; Williams, K.; Keesing, A.; Braun, K.; Beckerling, J.; Burbridge, M. Application of a Gondwanan perspective to restore ecological integrity in the south-western Australian global biodiversity hotspot. *Restor. Ecol.* **2016**, *24*, 805–815. [CrossRef]

18. Smith, I.L.; Northill, J.A.; Harrower, B.J.; Smith, G.A. Detection of Australian bat lyssavirus using a fluorogenic probe. *J. Clin. Virol.* **2002**, *25*, 285–291. [CrossRef]

19. Wadhwa, A.; Wilkins, K.; Gao, J.; Condori Condori, R.E.; Gigante, C.M.; Zhao, H.; Ma, X.; Ellison, J.A.; Greenberg, L.; Velasco-Villa, A.; et al. A Pan-*Lyssavirus* Taqman Real-Time RT-PCR assay for the detection of highly variable rabies *virus* and other lyssaviruses. *PLoS Negl. Trop. Dis.* **2017**, *11*, e0005258. [CrossRef] [PubMed]

20. Rahmadane, I.; Certoma, A.F.; Peck, G.R.; Fitria, Y.; Payne, J.; Colling, A.; Shiell, B.J.; Beddome, G.; Wilson, S.; Yu, M.; et al. Development and validation of an immunoperoxidase antigen detection test for improved diagnosis of rabies in Indonesia. *PLoS Negl. Trop. Dis.* **2017**, *11*, e0006079. [CrossRef] [PubMed]

21. Bossart, K.N.; McEachern, J.A.; Hickey, A.C.; Choudhry, V.; Dimitrov, D.S.; Eaton, B.T.; Wang, L.-F. Neutralization assays for differential henipavirus serology using Bio-Plex Protein Array Systems. *J. Virol. Methods* **2007**, *142*, 29–40. [CrossRef] [PubMed]

22. Hayman, D.T.S.; Suu-Ire, R.; Breed, A.C.; McEachern, J.A.; Wang, L.; Wood, J.L.N.; Cunningham, A.A. Evidence of Henipavirus infection in West African fruit bats. *PLoS ONE* **2008**, *3*, e2739. [CrossRef] [PubMed]

23. Hayman, D.T.S.; Wang, L.-F.; Barr, J.; Baker, K.S.; Suu-Ire, R.; Broder, C.C.; Cunningham, A.A.; Wood, J.L.N. Antibodies to henipavirus or henipa-like viruses in domestic pigs in Ghana, West Africa. *PLoS ONE* **2011**, *6*, e25256. [CrossRef] [PubMed]

24. Plowright, R.K.; Field, H.E.; Smith, C.; Divljan, A.; Palmer, C.; Tabor, G.; Daszak, P.; Foley, J.E. Reproduction and nutritional stress are risk factors for Hendra virus infection in little red flying foxes (*Pteropus scapulatus*). *Proc. R. Soc. B Biol. Sci.* **2008**, *275*, 861–869. [CrossRef] [PubMed]

25. Breed, A.C.; Yu, M.; Barr, J.A.; Crameri, G.; Thalmann, C.M.; Wang, L.F. Prevalence of henipavirus and rubulavirus antibodies in pteropid bats, Papua New Guinea. *Emerg. Infect. Dis.* **2010**, *16*, 1997–1999. [CrossRef] [PubMed]

26. Brown, L.D.; Cai, T.T.; Dasgupta, A. Interval estimation for a binomial proportion. *Stat. Sci.* **2001**, *16*, 101–133. [CrossRef]

27. Aragon, T. *epitools: Epidemiology Tools*, R Package Version 0.5-10; Published 26 October 2017; Available online: https://CRAN.R-project.org/package=epitools (accessed on 21 February 2019).

28. Hammarin, A.L.; Berndtsson, L.T.; Falk, K.; Nedinge, M.; Olsson, G.; Lundkvist, Å. Lyssavirus-reactive antibodies in Swedish bats. *Infect. Ecol. Epidemiol.* **2016**, *6*, 31262. [CrossRef] [PubMed]

29. Wakeley, P.R.; Johnson, N.; McElhinney, L.M.; Marston, D.; Sawyer, J.; Fooks, A.R. Development of a real-time, TaqMan reverse transcription-PCR assay for detection and differentiation of lyssavirus genotypes 1, 5, and 6. *J. Clin. Microbiol.* **2005**, *43*, 2786–2792. [CrossRef] [PubMed]

30. Deubelbeiss, A.; Zahno, M.-L.; Zanoni, M.; Bruegger, D.; Zanoni, R. Real-Time RT-PCR for the detection of lyssavirus species. *J. Vet. Med.* **2014**, *2014*, 476091. [CrossRef] [PubMed]

31. Echevarría, J.E.; Avellón, A.; Juste, J.; Vera, M.; Ibáñez, C. Screening of active lyssavirus infection in wild bat populations by viral RNA detection on oropharyngeal swabs. *J. Clin. Microbiol.* **2001**, *39*, 3678–3683. [CrossRef] [PubMed]

32. Amengual, B.; Bourhy, H.; López-Roig, M.; Serra-Cobo, J. Temporal dynamics of European bat lyssavirus type 1 and survival of Myotis myotis bats in natural colonies. *PLoS ONE* **2007**, *2*, e566. [CrossRef] [PubMed]

33. Franka, R.; Johnson, N.; Muller, T.; Vos, A.; Neubert, L.; Freuling, C.; Rupprecht, C.E.; Fooks, A.R. Susceptibility of North American big brown bats (*Eptesicus fuscus*) to infection with European bat lyssavirus type 1. *J. Gen. Virol.* **2008**, *89*, 1998–2010. [CrossRef] [PubMed]

34. Shankar, V.; Bowen, R.A.; Davis, A.D.; Rupprecht, C.E.; O'Shea, T.J. Rabies in a captive colony of big brown bats (*Eptesicus fuscus*). *J. Wildl. Dis.* **2004**, *40*, 403–413. [CrossRef] [PubMed]

11

Animal Models of Lassa Fever

Rachel A. Sattler [1], Slobodan Paessler [1], Hinh Ly [2] and Cheng Huang [1,*

[1]   Department of Pathology, University of Texas Medical Branch, 301 University Blvd., Galveston,
     TX 77555-0609, USA; rasattle@utmb.edu (R.A.S.); slpaessl@utmb.edu (S.P.)
[2]   Department of Veterinary Biomedical Sciences, University of Minnesota, Twin Cities, 1988 Fitch Ave.,
     295H Animal Science Veterinary Medicine Bldg., Saint Paul, MN 55108, USA; hly@umn.edu
*   Correspondence: chhuang@utmb.edu.

Abstract: Lassa virus (LASV), the causative agent of Lassa fever, is estimated to be responsible for up to 300,000 new infections and 5000 deaths each year across Western Africa. The most recent 2018 and 2019 Nigerian outbreaks featured alarmingly high fatality rates of up to 25.4%. In addition to the severity and high fatality of the disease, a significant population of survivors suffer from long-term sequelae, such as sensorineural hearing loss, resulting in a huge socioeconomic burden in endemic regions. There are no Food and Drug Administration (FDA)-approved vaccines, and therapeutics remain extremely limited for Lassa fever. Development of countermeasures depends on relevant animal models that can develop a disease strongly mimicking the pathogenic features of Lassa fever in humans. The objective of this review is to evaluate the currently available animal models for LASV infection with an emphasis on their pathogenic and histologic characteristics as well as recent advances in the development of a suitable rodent model. This information may facilitate the development of an improved animal model for understanding disease pathogenesis of Lassa fever and for vaccine or antiviral testing.

Keywords: arenaviruses; Lassa virus; viral hemorrhagic fevers; Lassa fever; animal models

1. Introduction

Lassa virus (LASV) is the causative agent of Lassa fever (LF). The virus was first isolated from two missionary nurses who died from LF in Nigeria in 1969 [1–3]. A third nurse was infected and brought to the United States; her plasma was used to treat a fourth patient who was exposed by handling infected blood samples [1]. LASV is a mammarenavirus from the *Arenaviridae* family and has a single-stranded, negative-sense, bisegmented RNA genome. LASV is endemic throughout Western Africa, especially in Nigeria, Liberia, Guinea, and Sierra Leone, where it is transmitted by the Natal mastomys (*Mastomys natalensis*) rodent, although recent work suggests viral presence in the reddish-white mastomys (*Mastomys erythroleucus*) and the "African wood mouse" (*Hylomyscus pamfi*) rodents as well [2,4]. LASV isolates of different geographic and host origins are highly diverse in genomic sequences and phylogenetically classified into up to seven lineages, with each lineage predominately localized in specific countries (refer to Table 1 for the LASV isolates covered in this review) [5–9]. A recent deep sequencing analysis revealed that the sequence variations could be as high as 25% and 32% in the viral genomic small (S) and large (L) segments, respectively, among different strains [5]. LASV causes zoonotic infections in humans, typically through the ingestion of contaminated food and/or water or inhalation of tainted aerosols from infected rodents; person-to-person transmission occurs via contact with bodily fluids [2]. Estimates from the Centers for Disease Control and Prevention (CDC) place the number of new LASV infections each year as high as 300,000 with around 5000 deaths from LF [2,10]. The average case fatality rate is approximately 1%, which can dramatically elevate to 15–20% for hospitalized cases [2]. However, a more recent report indicated only 633 confirmed cases and 171 deaths in Nigeria in 2018, with a 27% case fatality rate [11]. In the recent 2018–2019 Nigerian LF outbreaks, approximately 25% of patients died from the infection [12–14]. Therefore, it is necessary to re-evaluate the annual incidence of LASV infections and deaths.

There are no FDA-approved vaccines against LASV. Current clinical treatments are limited to an off-label use of ribavirin [2,14]. However, ribavirin treatment is expensive and only effective if administered within the first six days after the onset of symptoms [15]. When considering the high rate of misdiagnosis of LF for other endemic infections, such as typhoid or falciparum malaria [1,2,16,17], this time frame for effective LF treatment is extremely challenging [16]. Moreover, ribavirin has a high rate of side effects that often require further medical intervention, such as hemolysis [15]. Development of countermeasures against LF requires relevant animal models that can recapitulate disease and pathogenic features of LF in humans. The objective of this review is to survey the current Lassa fever animal models, including their pathologic and histologic characteristics as well as new advances in small rodent models, in order to inform the development of new animal models.

Table 1. Information for Lassa virus (LASV) strains examined in animal models *.

Strain	Lineage	Lethal/Fatal	Host	Isolation Country	Isolation Year	Reference
Josiah	IV	Yes	Human	Sierra Leone	1976	[6]
AV	V	Yes	Human	Ghana/Ivory Coast	2000	[6]
Ba366	IV	No	*Mastomys natalensis*	Guinea	2003	[6]
LF2384	IV	Yes	Human	Sierra Leone	2012	[6,8]
LF2450	IV	No	Human	Sierra Leone	2012	[6,8]
Soromba-R	V	No	*Mastomys natalensis*	Soromba, Mali	2009	[6]
Pinneo	I	No	Human	Lassa, Nigeria	1969	[6]
NJ2015	IV	Yes	Human	Liberia	2015	[9]

* Only strains mentioned in this review that have known isolation information are listed in this table.

2. Lassa Fever Symptoms and Pathogenesis

LF symptoms typically appear 1–3 weeks post-infection [2]. Eighty percent of cases are asymptomatic or present with mild, non-specific febrile symptoms such as fever, sore throat, headache, and general malaise, that may be misdiagnosed as typhoid, malaria, or appendicitis [1,2,16,17]. The other 20% of cases progress to much more severe symptomology [2]. These clinical manifestations include diarrhea, hemorrhage, disorientation, respiratory distress, abdominal pain, vomiting, facial edema, and severe pharyngitis [1,2]. Neurological signs such as hearing loss, encephalitis, and tremors also occur [2]. Of note, this hearing loss manifests as sudden-onset sensorineural hearing loss (SNHL) in approximately one-third of patients and is irreversible in two-thirds of those cases [10,18,19]. Infections during pregnancy have a greater risk of death as well as spontaneous abortion [20]. Death will typically occur due to multiorgan failure approximately two weeks post-onset of symptoms [2]. The long-term sequelae, such as SNHL, are generating a huge socioeconomic burden across Western Africa, where stigmatization and isolation lead to increased rates of depression and unemployment [21]. Aid programs in Nigeria alone can cost upwards of $43 million each year [18].

Clinical laboratory findings include thrombocytopenia, leucopenia with lymphopenia, elevated blood urea and proteinuria [22]. The aspartate aminotransferase (AST), alanine aminotransferase (ALT), amylase, and creatine phosphokinase (CPK) concentrations are also elevated in patient's serum [17], often with a higher AST level than ALT level, suggesting that the transaminases in serum are not solely derived from damaged liver, but may also be from other tissues [23]. High viral titers are measured in the spleen, lung, liver, kidney, heart, mammary gland, and placenta [17]. The level of viremia has been correlated with the severity of disease outcome.

Current knowledge on the pathology of Lassa fever is still limited due to civil unrest and social taboos and customs when dealing with the deceased in endemic areas [22]. Available pathologic analysis of clinical cases indicates lesions in the spleen, liver, and adrenal glands [17]. Histologic analysis of the liver indicates significant eosinophilic necrosis and parenchymal cell necrosis with an infiltration of eosinophils in the sinusoids [1,17,24]. Spleen samples indicate a presence of eosinophilic necrosis, lymphoid depletion, atrophied white pulp, and fibrin deposits with an infiltration of lymphocytes and mononuclear cells [1,17,24]. Adrenal gland samples indicate multifocal adrenocortical cellular necrosis, often associated with inflammation [17]. Less frequent findings include petechiae of the gastrointestinal tract, interstitial nephritis, renal tubular injury, lymph node sinus histiocytosis, mild interstitial pneumonia, renal edema and hemorrhage, as well as mild interstitial mononuclear myocarditis [1,17,24]. No alterations are detected in placental, mammary, uterine, ovarian, pancreatic, central nervous system (CNS), or brain samples [17]. These observations were made from a study performed in 1982. Our knowledge on pathology of LF in humans still lack. Studies with non-human primates have provided valuable information regarding the pathogenesis of LASV infection. As there is a limitation in study with non-human primates (NHPs), a small animal model that can resemble pathological changes in LF patients is desired.

3. Murine Models

3.1. Natal Mastomys (Mastomys Natalensis) Mice

Natal mastomys mice are the natural host of LASV. The exact subspecies that acts as a LASV reservoir remains unclear, due to multiple subspecies coexisting in endemic regions and their high genetic diversity [25,26]. There are very few studies on laboratory infections of Natal mastomys due to lack of laboratory clone of these mice. One early study reported that LASV caused a chronic asymptomatic infection despite the high virus titers detected in organs at 74 days post-infection (dpi) [25] (Table 2). Affected tissues included the lung, spleen, liver, kidney, brain, bladder, and lymph nodes [25]. Virus was also detected in the blood and urine. As the Natal mastomys mice did not develop LF signs, its use in viral pathogenesis or vaccine studies is limited. However, this model may prove useful for basic transmission studies as well as studies developing methods for limiting transmission of the virus between rodent populations or from rodents to humans.

Table 2. Mouse models of LASV infection.

Mouse	Virus Strain	Max. Dose	Route	Lethality	Signs of Disease	Affected Organs	Reference
Natal mastomys	Unknown	Not provided	IP [d]	No	asymptomatic, persistent infection, virus shed in saliva and urine	lung, spleen, liver, kidney, brain, bladder, lymph nodes	[25]
IFNAR$^{-/-}$	Josiah, AV, BA366, Nig04-10	10^5 PFU	IV [e]	No	persistent viremia, bodyweight loss, no fever and neurological signs	lung, liver, spleen brain, kidney, heart	[27–30]
Chimeric IFNAR$^{-/-B6}$	Ba366, AV, Ba289, Nig04-10, Nig-CSF	10^3 FFU	IP	100%	liver damage, vascular leakage, systemic viral dissemination, weight loss, hypothermia, elevated AST/ALT ratio	liver, lung, spleen, kidney, heart, brain	[29,31]
IFNαβ/γR$^{-/-}$	Josiah, LF2384 [a] LF2450 [b]	10^5 PFU	IP	No	minor and transient weight loss, clearance of virus by 25 dpi, no hearing loss	spleen, lung, liver, brain, kidney	[8,30]
STAT1$^{-/-}$	Josiah	10^4 PFU	IP	100%	weight loss, systematic infection	spleen, lung, liver, brain, kidney	[28]
	LF2384 [a] (fatal)	10^5 PFU	IP	80%	fever, high level viremia, weight loss, increased ALT level, decreased albumin, WBC, and monocyte counts, hearing loss associated with infiltration of CD3$^+$ lymphocytes	brain, liver, spleen, lung, kidney, heart	[8,28]
	LF2450 [b] (non-fatal)	10^5 PFU	IP	0–50%	hearing loss	brain, liver, spleen, lung, kidney, heart	[8]
CBA	Josiah	10^3 PFU	IC [f]	70–100%	scruffy fur, seizures, weight loss, immobility, and severe decubitus paralysis	not stated	[32]
HHD	Ba366 [C]	10^6 PFU	IV	22%	ruffled fur, lethargy, elevated AST level, high level viremia, severe pneumonitis	liver, lung, spleen, kidney	[33]

Note: [a] LF2384: clinical isolate from a lethally infected patient; [b] LF2450: clinical isolate from a survivor; [C] isolate from *Natal mastomys*; PFU, plaque forming unit; [d] IP: intraperitoneal; [e] IV: intravenous; [f] IC: intracranial.

3.2. IFNAR$^{-/-}$ Mice

Immune-competent laboratory mice are generally resistant to LASV infection [27–30]. Interferons play important roles in regulating host innate and adaptive immune responses against infections. LASV infection of the 129Sv mice lacking the receptor for interferon α and β (IFNAR$^{-/-}$) results in a non-lethal acute infection accompanied with persistent viremia [27–30] (Table 2). Infected mice lose approximately 15% body weight but did not develop febrile or neurological signs [26,29]. Other disease signs included ruffled fur and hypoactivity occurring by 11 dpi [28,30]. Peak viremia occurred approximately 8 dpi. The lung, liver, and spleen had the highest viral loads, and virus was also present in the brain, kidney, and heart at much lower titers [27]. Similar pathological changes and disease signs were found in the animals upon infection with a variety of LASV strains, including the Josiah, AV, BA366, and Nig04-10 strains isolated from endemic countries, Sierra Leone, Côte d'Ivoire, Guinea, and Nigeria, respectively [27,28].

A chimeric IFNAR$^{-/-B6}$ lethal mouse model had been established, in which the IFNAR$^{-/-}$ mice were irradiated and transplanted with bone marrow progenitor cells from wild type C57BL/6 mice. These IFNAR$^{-/-B6}$ chimeric mice uniformly succumbed to infections with a variety of LASV strains within 10 days [29,31]. LASV strains tested include Ba366, AV, Ba289, Nig04-10, and Nig-CSF, all of which were 100% lethal using 1000 focus-forming units (FFU) [29]. These mice presented with liver damage, vascular leakage, and systemic viral dissemination [29]. Virus titers were detected in the liver, lung, spleen, kidney, heart, brain, and blood [29,31]. Animals also presented with weight loss and hypothermia [31]. Moreover, this model featured an elevated AST/ALT ratio, as well as FAS and FAS-L [29,31] similarly observed in LF patients. Pathological findings included an infiltration of inflammatory leukocytes in the kidney, infiltration of granulocytes and T cell lymphocytes in the liver, and an increased presence of CD8+ T cells in both the spleen and lungs [29]. Lung and liver samples both presented with indications of significant vascular leakage as well as edema [29]. Interestingly, IFNAR[-/-B6] mice with a depletion of CD8+ T cells exhibited significantly increased survival rate (87.5%) despite persistent viremia [29]. This depletion also reduced the FAS and FAS-L concentrations, as well as the vascular leakage in the liver and lung [29]. This model implicates the role of T cells in the pathogenesis of LF. IFNAR[-/-] mice are less susceptible to disease probably as a result of lacking IFN receptors that are critical to stimulate a T cell response.

3.3. IFNαβ/γR[-/-] Mice

The 129Sv mice lacking interferon α, β and γ receptors (IFNαβ/γR[-/-]) did not develop clinical signs of disease upon LASV infection apart from a minor and transient weight loss [30] (Table 2). Neither did this model develop sudden onset sensorineural hearing loss when infected with either the LF2384 or LF2350 clinical isolates from a fatal and a non-fatal case respectively, from the 2012 Sierra Leone outbreak [8]. These two clinical isolates have been passaged only once in Vero cells. The animals presented with less severe disease upon infection with the Josiah strain as IFNAR[-/-] mice [30]. Virus was present in the serum, spleen, lung, liver, brain, and kidney, but was cleared by 25 dpi [30]. Tissue samples featured similar findings to the LASV-infected IFNAR[-/-] model in the brain and lung, but to significantly lesser extents [30]. Liver samples presented with mononuclear cell infiltration, although inflammation was rarely observed [30]. In the spleen, only the red pulp was affected; the kidneys showed mild, regional nephritis [30].

3.4. STAT1[-/-] Mice

Signal transducer and activator of transcription 1 (STAT1) is a transcription factor that is activated in response to IFN α, β, γ and IL-6. The 129Sv mice lacking STAT1 (STAT1[-/-]) were not only highly susceptible to LASV infection, including clinical isolates, but also presented with a lethal disease with clinically relevant manifestations, such as SNHL [8,28]. Thus, the STAT1[-/-] mouse model is promising for vaccine and therapeutic testing. Mice intraperitoneally infected with 10^4 plaque forming units (PFUs) of the Josiah strain of LASV lost ~18% of their body weight between 4 and 6 dpi, and either died or met humane endpoint criteria by 7 dpi [28]. This model also matched the differential clinical outcome of the patients from whom the viruses were isolated, with LF2384 infections being lethal and LF2350 infections non-lethal in these mice. Intraperitoneal (IP) injection with 10^5 PFU of the LF2384 or the LF2350 isolates led to 80% and 10–50% lethality, respectively [8]. Infection with 10^4 PFU of these viruses resulted in 80% lethality for the fatal isolate and 0% lethality for the non-fatal isolate [8]. LF2384 also caused fever and other signs of disease by 4–5 dpi, and death approximately 7 dpi [28]. Other signs of disease included weight loss, hypothermia, hunched posture, reduced activity, and ruffled fur [8]. In one study, fever was not noted, although the possibility that fever transiently occurred before turning into hypothermia was raised [8,28]. Virus was disseminated to the brain, liver, spleen, lung, kidney, and heart by 3 dpi with titers steadily increasing to their peak at 7 dpi [8,28]. Viremia appeared by 3 dpi and remained at high titers until death [28]. Increased ALT concentrations and decreased albumin, WBC, and monocyte counts were noted as early as 3 dpi; a moderate decrease in platelet counts was also observed [28]. Histologic analysis of the spleen indicated lesions with eosinophil accumulation in the red pulp, primarily focused around the periarteriolar lymphocytic sheaths as well as apoptotic and necrotic cells [28]. Samples also demonstrated significant fibrin deposits and an infiltration of macrophages filled with apoptotic nuclei [28]. Analysis of the liver indicated lesions with microvesicular steatosis and apoptosis in the hepatic sinusoids [28]. Of note, IFN signaling is not completely disrupted in this STAT1$^{-/-}$ mouse model as that in IFNαβ/γR$^{-/-}$ mice. A partial knockout of STAT1 gene leads to expression of a truncated form of STAT1, which may still be able to mediate a minimal T cell response. As T cells may contribute to LF pathogenesis, the difference in IFN signaling may explain why the STAT1$^{-/-}$ mice are more susceptible to disease than IFNαβ/γR$^{-/-}$ mice [29].

Additionally, the STAT1$^{-/-}$ model is the only available small animal model for SNHL [8]. Both LF2384 and LF2350 clinical isolates from the 2012 Sierra Leone outbreak caused deafness in survivors [8]. Infection with 10^5 PFU of virus caused permanent hearing loss in all survivors. With a lower dose of virus (10^4 PFU), hearing loss was present in only 20% of survivors. Histologic examination identified severe damage to the inner ear with significantly fewer outer hair cells; inner hair cells remained intact [8]. Auditory nerves in mice with hearing loss were also damaged, while the nearby facial nerves remained intact. There was significant vacuolization of the spiral ganglion, thinning of the stria vascularis, distention of Reissner's membrane, and an infiltration of blood cells in the scala tympani. Viral antigen was present in vascular-rich regions, where there was also a remarkable infiltration of CD3+ lymphocytes, indicating an immunopathologic mechanism underlying to the hearing loss [8].

3.5. CBA Mice

Intracranial infection of inbred CBA mice with the pathogenic Josiah strain of LASV resulted in disease manifestation, although it was unclear whether the animals were immunocompromised [32]. Infected CBA mice presented with scruffy fur, seizures, weight loss, immobility, severe decubitus paralysis, and death [32]. This route of inoculation allowed for onset of signs of disease between 5 and 7 dpi with 70–100% lethality within 7–12 days [32].

3.6. HHD Mice

C57BL/6 mice expressing a human/mouse chimeric HLA-A2.1 instead of the normal MHC class I gene products (humanized HHD mouse model) has recently been established as a novel model for LASV infection [33]. The HHD mouse was most susceptible to infection with the Ba366 strain and featured ~22% lethality and rapid deteriorating post-onset of signs of disease [33]. When infected with 10^6 PFU of the Ba366 strain, HHD mice began to show ruffled fur and lethargy, as well as elevated concentrations of serum AST, approximately 7–12 dpi [33]. High viral titers were observed in liver, lung, and spleen, whereas lower titers were seen in the kidney [33]. Histology examination indicated severe pneumonitis with signs of pleural effusion, thickening of the interlobular septum, and collapsed alveolar lumen with infiltration of monocytes and macrophages [33]. The liver contained altered cellular distribution, orientation, and shape of its monocytes and macrophages. The spleens also featured disruption of the white and red pulp regions, while monocytes and macrophages were found throughout with scarce T cells.

Depletion of CD4+ T cells, CD8+ T cells, or both resulted in substantial differences in disease manifestations in this model [33]. After infection, the serum AST concentrations remained normal in HHD mice lacking both CD4+ and CD8+ T cells, while the AST concentrations elevated in HHD mice. Additionally, depletion of either CD4+ T cells or CD8+ T cells resulted in partial elevation in AST concentrations [33]. In all groups, similarly high titers of viremia were developed, suggesting T cells had no substantial influence on viremia. C57BL6 mice lacking only CD4+ T cells were able to clear the viral infection, while those lacking only the CD8+ cells featured persistent viremia [33]. MHC-I$^{-/-}$ mice lacking CD8+ T cells confirmed these findings, presenting with no clinical manifestations of disease after infection, despite the high viremia [33]. CD4+ and CD8+ T cell-depleted mice did not demonstrate any significant histological changes in the lung and spleen after infection and also featured limited signs of disease, emphasizing the role of T cells in LASV pathogenesis [33].

In summary, immune-competent laboratory mice are generally resistant to LASV infection, and therefore are not suitable for modeling the severe and fatal LF diseases in humans. Immune-incompetent mice are susceptible to LASV infection but generally develop mild diseases and survive the infection (see Table 2). The chimeric IFNAR$^{-/-}$B6 mice are susceptible to lethal LASV infection but require irradiation of the mice and transplantation with bone marrow progenitor cells from wild type C57BL/6 mice. Recently, progress has been made using the STAT1$^{-/-}$ mice, which recapitulate the pathogenic potency of different LASV isolates and some LF disease signs including hearing loss. This STAT1$^{-/-}$ mouse model may be useful as a small rodent model for vaccine and therapeutic testing.

4. Guinea Pig Models

4.1. Strain 13 Guinea Pigs

Inbred Strain 13 domesticated guinea pigs have been used as a lethal LF rodent model for studying pathogenesis as well as antiviral, vaccine, and immunotherapy candidates. Unlike their Hartley outbred counterpart, this model does not require virus adaptation [34,35] (Table 3). However, Inbred Strain 13 guinea pigs are not readily available, limiting their use as a LF animal model. In this model at least 90% animals died when infected with at least 2 PFU of LASV (Josiah) [34,36,37]. The clinical isolate NJ2015, from a non-fatal infection, was also non-lethal in Strain 13 guinea pigs [36]. Guinea pigs infected with the Pinneo strain had a 100% survival rate, developing only a mild to moderate disease featuring 5–10% weight loss and lethargy approximately 10 dpi; all animals recovered by 22 dpi [38]. The Z-132 strain was 100% lethal and mimicked a Josiah infection, while the Soromba-R strain was 0–57% lethal with a very mild disease [38,39]. Survivors did not exhibit seroconversion and were susceptible to back challenge [34]. Neutralizing antibodies were not produced [37]. Signs of disease included weight loss, fever, ruffled fur, hunched posture, altered mentation, and conjunctivitis [34–36]. Guinea pigs typically became moribund between 10 and 15 dpi [37]. A persistent and high level viremia developed rapidly, typically approximately 5–6 dpi, and peaked at approximately 10 dpi. The highest viral load was identified in the lung, followed by the spleen, pancreas, lymph nodes, adrenal glands, kidneys, salivary glands, liver, and heart [34,35,39]. Histological findings included the presence of viral antigen typically associated with hepatitis, hepatic cell death, hair follicle epithelium cell death, and adrenal cortical necrosis [35]. Laryngitis and heterophilic tracheitis were noted in guinea pigs exposed via aerosol [35]. Interstitial pneumonia was found in all moribund animals with an increase in mononuclear cells, especially macrophages, surrounding the blood vessels and airways [34,35,37,39]. Edema and hemorrhage were also noted in the lungs with an expansion of the alveolar septae [35,39]. Liver samples exhibited a mild to moderate inflammation in portal and sinusoidal regions, vacuolar degeneration, and necrosis [35,37,39]. Half of the guinea pigs developed acute necrotizing nephritis and mild myocarditis or mild to moderate endocarditis and pancarditis [34,35,37]. It is important to note that this damage to the heart is not seen in clinical cases [25]. Adrenal glands featured minimal damage, although they were infected [34,35]. Further analysis of the spleen identified mild heterophilic splenitis [35,39]. The red pulp featured perifollicular to diffuse mononuclear cell proliferation [35]. Most infected guinea pigs developed petechial rashes approximately 12 dpi [35]. Lymphocytolysis and lymphoid depletion was noted in the white pulp of the spleen, thymus, and lymph nodes [35,37]. The pancreas featured acinar cell atrophy as well as other architectural changes [35]. Viral antigen was present in the reproductive tissues of both male and female infected guinea pigs, with males also featuring mild epididymitis [35]. Serum analysis indicated elevated ALT and heterophil concentrations with a transient decrease in platelets and a decrease in blood lymphocytes [35].

Table 3. Guinea pig models of LASV infection.

Guinea Pig	Strain	Max. Dose	Route	Lethality	Signs of Disease	Affected Organs	Refences
Strain 13 (inbred)	Josiah	>2 PFU10^4 TCID$_{50}$	SC^c IP	$>90\%$	weight loss, fever, ruffled fur, hunched posture, conjunctivitis, hepatitis, interstitial pneumonia, edema and hemorrhage in lungs	lung, spleen, pancreas, lymph nodes, adrenal and salivary glands, kidneys, liver, heart	[34,36,37]
	Z-132	10^4 TCID$_{50}$	IP	100%	Josiah-like	lung, liver, spleen	[38,39]
	Soromba-R	10^4 TCID$_{50}$	IP	0–57%	survivors only show minor weight loss	liver, lung, spleen	[28,34,35,38,39]
	Pinneo	10^4 TCID$_{50}$	IP	No	mild to moderate disease	N.A.*	[38]
	NJ2015	10^4 FFU	SC	No	weight loss, fever, red and swollen conjunctiva	eye (focus of the study)	[36]
Hartley (outbred)	Josiah	>2 PFU10^3 PFU	SCIP	30–67%	inapparent infection in survivors	N.A.*	[25,34,35,40,41]
	GPA-Josiah ^{a}	10^3 TCID$_{50}$	IP	100%	weight loss, fever, lethargy, respiratory distress, hypothermia	spleen, liver, lung	[25,34,35,40–42]
	LF2384 ^{b}	10^4 PFU	IP	100%	fever, weight loss, hypothermia, lethargy, thrombocytopenia, neutropenia, and lymphopenia	liver, kidney, spleen, lung, brain	[43]

* N.A: not available; ^{a} GPA-Josiah: guinea pig-adapted LASV Josiah strain; ^{b} LF2384: clinical isolate from a fatally infected LF patient; ^{c} SC: subcutaneous

Strain 13 guinea pigs presented with conjunctivitis upon LASV infection [36]. Clinically, LASV infections cause conjunctival edema and conjunctivitis in acute infections and transient blindness in survivors. No other animal models have been extensively studied for this aspect of disease, although viral titers have been identified in the aqueous humor of the eye of infected rhesus monkeys [36,44]. The lethal Josiah strain and the non-lethal NJ2015 clinical isolate both induced red and swollen conjunctiva with associated ocular discharge in the animals [36]. Viral antigen was detected in the eyes of all infected guinea pigs achieving humane euthanasia criteria, while none was detected in those of survivors [36]. Survivors presented with minimal to mild lymphocytic inflammation; lethal infections all presented with mild to moderate inflammation [36].

4.2. Hartley Guinea Pigs

Outbred Hartley domesticated guinea pigs are commercially available and susceptible to infection with the widely used Josiah strain of LASV (Table 3). However, the Josiah strain caused lethal infection in only 30–67% of animals regardless of the infection dose. Survivors seroconverted and were not susceptible to back challenge [34]. To achieve uniform lethality, the Josiah strain must be adapted in guinea pigs through serial passage [25,34,35,40,41]. Guinea pigs infected with the guinea pig-adapted LASV (GPA-LASV) developed a fever approximately 6–9 dpi as well as respiratory distress and hypothermia [41,42]. Weight loss was rapid and variable, ranging from 8% to over 20%, which is typical humane euthanasia criteria [40–42]. Other clinical manifestations included an unstable gait, a noticeable lack of grooming with associated rough/ruffled fur, delayed responsiveness/lethargy, recumbency, and a reddening of the footpads and ears [40,41]. Death occurred by an average of 15 dpi [41]. Viral titers were observed in the serum, spleen, liver, and lung [41,42]. Histologic analysis of the liver indicated lymphohistiocytic hepatitis and hepatocellular degeneration [41]. Spleen samples contained sinus histiocytosis and lung samples featured interstitial pneumonia [41]. The GPA-LASV/Hartley guinea pig model has been often used in development of antivirals and vaccine against LF [40–42].

Recently, new advances have been made in the development of the outbred LASV-infected Hartley guinea pig model by using the LF2384 clinical isolate. Uniform lethality could be achieved in outbred Hartley guinea pigs infected by the LF2384 clinical isolate without species-specific adaptation, at a dose as low as 100 PFU [45]. LF2384-infected guinea pigs presented with signs of disease such as fever, hypothermia before death, as well as weight loss by 10 dpi, scruffy coats by 12 dpi, and loss of appetite as well as lethargy by 13 dpi [45]. Neurological disease signs were not observed in this model [45]. Viral loads were detected in the liver, kidney, spleen, lung, and brain, but were not detectable in survivors of a low dose infection [45]. Guinea pigs succumbing to disease presented with thrombocytopenia, neutropenia, and lymphopenia [45]. Gross pathology indicated small spleens [45]. While this model requires further characterization, the advantages of this new LF model include the use of clinical isolates directly from patients without adaptation and the commercial availability of the animals. Additionally, the outbred background may allow for mimicking infections in humans with diverse genetic backgrounds. The newly developed LF2384 LASV/Hartley guinea pig model will be useful for vaccine and therapeutic development, which is demonstrated in a recent study showing that immunization with an adenovector-based LASV vaccine candidate efficaciously protected animals from lethal LASV infection [43].

5. Non-Human Primate Models

5.1. Squirrel Monkey Model

Squirrel monkeys (*Saimiri sciureus*) infected with the Bah strain of LASV developed variable disease. One out of four animals became moribund [46] (Table 4). These primates develop depression, tremors, drooling, anorexia, lassitude, and polydipsia as signs of disease. Serologic analysis indicated persistent viremia with no antibody development at 28 dpi [46]. High viral titers were detected primarily in the liver, kidney, and lymph nodes, while lower virus loads were found in the spleen, brain, liver, kidneys, adrenal gland, urine and heart [25,46]. The presence of the virus was associated with significant tissue necrosis [25]. Spleen and lymph node samples featured necrosis in the germinal centers; spleen samples and adrenal glands also contain regions of focal hemorrhage [46]. While the liver suffered from hepatitis with fatty metamorphosis and an infiltration of leukocytes and mononuclear cells, hepatocytic regeneration was noted [46]. Renal tubular necrosis and regeneration was present in the kidney, while heart samples featured severe myocarditis with vacuolar degeneration and necrosis [46]. Some animals developed neuropathology with chronic inflammation of the meninges, a significant infiltration of mononuclear cells and lymphocytes into the pancreas with acute arteritis, or minor pathologic changes in the adrenal gland, prostate, and bone marrow [46].

Table 4. Non-human primate (NHP) models of LASV infection [a].

NHP	LASV Strain	Max. Dose	Route	Lethality	Signs of Disease	Affected Organs	Reference
squirrel monkeys	Bah	$10^{6.8}$ TCID$_{50}$	IM [b]	25%	depression, tremors, drooling, anorexia, lassitude, polydipsia	liver, kidney, lymph nodes, spleen, brain, adrenal gland, heart	[46]
marmoset	Josiah	10^{6} PFU	SC	100%	low fever, rapid weight loss, depression, anorexia, elevated concentrations of AST, ALT, alkaline phosphatase, decreased concentrations of albumin and platelet	liver, spleen, lymph nodes, kidney, lung, adrenal gland	[47]
rhesus monkey	Josiah	$10^{6.1}$ PFU	SC	50–60%	severe petechial rash, hiccups, lethargy, aphagia, huddled posture, constipation, conjunctivitis, anorexia, weight loss, decreased water intake/dehydration, facial and periorbital edema, bleeding from the gums and nares, cough, fever	adrenal glands, liver, lung, pancreas, brain, bone marrow, kidney, lymph nodes, spleen, muscle, heart, thymus, testis, salivary gland, CSF, intestines	[44,48,49]
"crab-eating" cynomolgus macaques	Josiah	10^{4} PFU	IM	Up to 100%	fever, weight loss, lethargy, dull appearance, reluctance to move/hypoactivity, anorexia, rashes, facial edema, hunched posture, ruffled fur, piloerection, bleeding from puncture sites, dehydration, epistaxis, acute respiratory syndrome, neurological signs including deafness	lymph nodes, spleen, liver, reproductive organs, kidney, lung, heart, CNS	[38,39,50–53]
	Z-132	10^{4} TCID$_{50}$	IM	100%	Josiah-like	spleen, liver, lung	[38,39]
	Soromba-R	10^{4} TCID$_{50}$	IM	66%	less severe than Josiah strain infection, moderate to severe pulmonary lesions	similar to Josiah and Z-132	[39]

[a] Another NHP model, for which the literature was not available to the authors, is the hydramas baboon model; [b] IM: intramuscular.

5.2. Marmoset Model

The common marmoset (*Callithrix jacchus*) has been identified as a good model for Lassa fever (Table 4). Primates infected with the Josiah strain of LASV develop a systemic disease featuring low fever and rapid weight loss [47]. These monkeys also exhibited behavioral changes, such as depression and anorexia, as well as reduced stool production [47]. Severe morbidity occurred between 15 and 20 dpi [47]. Serum analysis indicated an elevation in AST, ALT, and alkaline phosphatase concentrations as well as a decrease in albumin and platelet concentrations [47]. High viral titers were observed in the liver, spleen, and lymph nodes [47]. Livers were enlarged with pale patches. Histologic analysis indicated multifocal hepatic necrosis with mild inflammation [47]. Spleens were also enlarged with mild to moderate lymphoid depletion [47]. Likewise, lymph nodes were enlarged with lymphocyte necrosis and an infiltration of inflammatory cells [47]. Kidneys were pale with interstitial nephritis [47]. Lung samples featured hemorrhage present in most lobes with mild to moderate multifocal interstitial pneumonitis, septal thickening, and multifocal edema [47]. These samples also had increased infiltration of lymphocytes and macrophages [47]. The adrenal cortex also featured mild to moderate inflammation and multifocal necrosis [47].

5.3. Rhesus Monkey (Rhesus Macaque) Model

Rhesus monkeys (*Rhesus macaques*) infected with the Josiah strain of LASV develop severe disease with prolonged viremia [44]. Succumbed animals developed disease signs by 7 dpi, including severe petechial rash, hiccups, lethargy, aphagia, huddled posture, constipation, conjunctivitis, anorexia, weight loss, decreased water intake/dehydration, facial and periorbital edema, bleeding from the gums and nares, cough, and a slight fever [44,48,49,54,55]. Fever persisted until death or a sudden hypothermia happened just before death approximately 10–14 dpi [44,49,54,55]. Subcutaneous inoculation with $10^{6.1}$ PFU of Josiah strain of LASV proved to be lethal in 60% of the animals [47]. Serologic analysis indicated antibody production by 10–12 dpi, although this was not correlated with viral clearance and animal recovery [44,49]. Elevated AST, ALT, and blood urea nitrogen (BUN) with a transient and moderate leukopenia was also noted [49,54,55]. Hematocrit, hemoglobin, fibronectin, and red blood cell counts decreased; platelet counts trended toward a decrease, although remained within the normal range [54,55]. Viremia appeared typically by 4–5 dpi with titers over 10^4 PFU/mL in lethally infected monkeys, significantly higher than those in survivors [49,54,55]. Viral loads were found in every organ tested including the adrenal glands, liver, lung, pancreas, brain, bone marrow, kidney, lymph nodes, spleen, muscle, heart, thymus, testis, salivary gland, urine, CSF, and intestines [44,49,55]. The highest titers were in the liver, spleen, and adrenal glands [55].

Gross pathological analysis indicated scattered petechial and visceral hemorrhage along with the presence of mild to moderate pleural effusions [44,48]. Liver and adrenal gland tissues presented with necrosis, with markers of regeneration of hepatocytes and a slight infiltration of inflammatory cells [44,48,49,55]. Interstitial pneumonia with edema, thickened alveolar septae, and pulmonary arteritis were present in the lung [44,48,49,55]. Spleen samples indicated lymphocytopenia and presence of viral antigens only in the red pulp [48,49]. Infected primates also developed mild to moderate interstitial and perivascular myocarditis and pericardial edema. Severe meningoencephalitis with significant perivascular cuffing was noted, albeit rarely [44,48]. Infiltration of erythrocytes and macrophages was noted in the small intestine. Lesions and a multifocal cortical interstitial mononuclear infiltrate were noted in the kidney [48,55]. Seventy-eight percent of infected primates developed lesions in the CNS with mild lymphocytic cuffing of the vessels of the brain, spinal cord, and meninges [48]. Twenty percent of primates suffered lymphocytic infiltration of the spiral ganglia; mild choriodoretinitis was also noted [48]. The arterial lesions, vasculitis, meningoencephalomyelitis and skeletal myositis observed in this monkey model were rarely, if at all, noted in human LF cases [44].

5.4. Cynomolgus Macaque Model

Josiah- or Z-132-infected "crab-eating" (cynomolgus) macaques developed a severe hemorrhagic disease with up to 100% of primates becoming moribund or dying between 11 and 18 dpi [38,39,50–53,56]. A study with the Soromba-R strain found two of three animals died (66% lethality) after infection and a prolonged time to euthanasia [39]. Infection with the Liberian LASV Z-132 strain was 100% lethal by 18 dpi [35]. Infection with 10^3 FFU AV strain featured only 67% lethality. All animals survived infection with 10^7 FFU of the AV strain, probably due to a high concentration of defective interfering (DI) viral particles in the higher dose [57]. Clinical signs, such as fever, weight loss, lethargy, dull appearance, reluctance to move/hypoactivity, anorexia, rashes, facial edema, hunched posture, ruffled fur, piloerection, bleeding from puncture sites, dehydration, epistaxis, acute respiratory syndrome, and mild to moderate depression appeared approximately 5-7 dpi, but might begin as early as 3 dpi [38,39,50–52,56–58]. Fever spiked between 7 and 10 dpi [39]. Viremia might start as early as 3–4 dpi, but was usually detectable 6–10 dpi, peaked 12–14 dpi, and continued to maintain high titers (up to 10^7 PFU/mL) until death or euthanasia [39,50,51,53,56,58]. Onset of fever was associated with detectable viremia. Survivors typically had a lower virus titer and cleared the virus by 28 dpi [50,57]. Survivors suffered neurological disorders such as tremors, reduced appetite, ataxia, convulsions/seizures, and unilateral or bilateral deafness [50,52,56,58]. Sixty-seven percent of the survivors developed hearing loss, which was thought to be driven by an immune-associated systemic vasculitis [50,56]. This hearing loss was present in all survivors of one study, presenting as unilateral or bilateral hearing loss [56].

Serologic analysis indicated elevated concentrations of AST, ALT, alkaline phosphatase (ALP), gamma-glutamyltransferase (GGT), total bilirubin (TBIL), and BUN as well as decreased concentrations of albumin, total protein, and amylase [38,39,50,51,58]. Transient lymphopenia, monocytopenia, neutropenia, and eosinopenia were also noticed at 4–10 dpi [38,39,50,51,58]. Platelet concentrations typically tended to decrease but remained within normal ranges, along with reduced hemoglobin, hematocrit, and creatinine concentrations [39,50,51,58]. The autoimmune markers C-reactive protein, antineutrophil cytoplasmic antibodies, and circulating immune complexes were also elevated in survivors with hearing loss [56]. Neutralizing antibodies were not detected in primates that succumbed to the infection but developed slowly in survivors approximately 14 dpi [50,56,57]. An early and strong T cell response was noticed in survivors [57]. Viral titers were detected at high levels in the spleen, lung, and liver, and at lower levels in the lymph nodes, kidney, and brain by 7 dpi [38,39,51,56–58].

Gross pathologic analysis revealed enlarged livers, spleens, adrenal glands, pancreas and lymph nodes, along with slight lung discoloration and pericardial effusion [38,39,57,58]. Lung samples featured mild to severe interstitial pneumonia with thickening of the alveolar septae [38,57,58]. Interestingly, although Soromba-R infections presented with a significantly less severe disease, the pathology of the lung was remarkable; 50–100% of lobes were reddened with lesions and extensive pulmonary infiltrations [38]. Liver samples were pale yellow and friable, featuring mild and multifocal portal hepatitis with random regions of necrosis [38,50,58]. Brain samples presented with meningoencephalitis in the frontal lobe, brainstem, and cerebellum with lesions. Neuritis was noted in the optic nerve [38,58]. Both lymph nodes and the white pulp of the spleen suffered follicular hyperplasia and mild lymphocytolysis. Spleens were also friable with fibrinous deposits in the red pulp [38,57,58]. Kidney samples appeared congested with mononuclear cell infiltrates [57,58]. Petechial hemorrhage and necrosis were noted on the bladder, while the ovaries and uterus were inflamed [57,58]. The thymus featured marked atrophy; myocarditis and necrotizing coronary arteritis were noted in the heart [58].

6. Surrogate Models of Lassa Fever

6.1. Pichindé Virus in Guinea Pigs

Pichindé virus (PICV) is a non-pathogenic, New World mammarenavirus isolated from cricetine rodents (*Oryzomys albigularis*) in Colombia, South America [59,60]. PICV infection of Strain 13 guinea pigs can cause Lassa-like disease and therefore has been used as a surrogate LASV model in BSL2 labs (Table 5) [61–63]. A minimum of four sequential passages of PICV in guinea pigs was required to result in 100% lethality [63,64]. Infected guinea pigs were hypoactive and lethargic, with ruffled fur, decreased food/water intake, rapid and shallow breathing, slobbering, and significant weight loss before becoming moribund [62,64]. Viremia appeared by 2 dpi and steadily increased until death at 16 dpi [62–64]. Infected guinea pigs featured extreme leukopenia beginning approximately 13 dpi and a transient neutrophilia [63]. Serologic findings included impaired platelet function, decreased activity of coagulation factors, and thrombocytopenia, decreased white blood cell concentrations and increased hematocrit [64]. AST concentrations were also elevated, starting from approximately 9 dpi [63]. Histologic analysis indicated pathological lesions in the liver, spleen, pancreas, lungs and gastrointestinal tract [61–64]. Scattered necrotic regions were found in lymphoid tissue and the bone marrow [64].

Table 5. Surrogate models of LASV infection.

Animal	Virus/Strain	Max. Dose	Route	Lethality	Signs of Disease	Affected Organs	Reference
Strain 13 (inbred) guinea pig	Pichindé virus	>3 PFU	SC	100%	hypoactivity, lethargy, ruffled fur, decreased appetite, rapid/shallow breathing, slobbering, weight loss, leukopenia, and transient neutrophilia	liver, spleen, pancreas, lung, gastrointestinal tract, lymphoid tissue, bone marrow	[61–64]
Hartley (outbred) guinea pig	Pichindé virus/P18	100 PFU	IP	100%	weight loss and fever	adrenal glands, lung, stomach, liver, brain, heart, spleen, pancreas, intestine, kidney, lymph node	[65,67]
	Pichindé virus/P2	10^4 PFU	IP	<100%	avirulent	none	[66]
	Pichindé virus/CoAn 4783	3000 PFU	IP	43%	weight loss and fever	cleared in survivors	[65]
LVG/Lak outbred golden hamsters	Pichindé virus	500 PFU	SC	0–100%	lethal infection up to 8 days post-birth; uncommon afterwards	spleen, liver, kidney	[68]
MHA/Lak inbred golden hamsters	Pichindé virus	3.5×10^6 PFU	IP	100%	lethal infection regardless of age	spleen, liver, kidney	[68]
Golden hamsters	Pirital virus	10^5 TCID$_{50}$	IP	>50%	hemorrhage, interstitial pneumonia, multifocal hepatic necrosis, splenic lymphoid depletion and necrosis	lung, liver, spleen	[69]
Rhesus monkeys	LCMV-WE	10^3 PFU	IV	100%	not listed	not listed	[70,71]
		10^8 PFU	IG [a]	20%	weight loss, elevated AST and ALT, thrombocytopenia, transient neutrophilia	liver	[72]

[a] IG: intragastric

Unlike Strain 13 guinea pigs, Hartley outbred guinea pigs did not uniformly succumb to infection by PICV CoAn 4763 strain [63,65]. The lethality was approximately 43% when animals were infected with 3000 PFU PICV CoAn 4763 [63]. Virus was cleared by 16 dpi in survivors [63]. When the CoAn 4763 strain passaged in Strain 13 guinea pigs for 18 passages, the resulting P18 strain was more virulent than the P2 strain, which was passaged only twice [65–67]. Infection with 100 PFU of the PICV P18 strain caused weight loss, fever and uniformly lethal infection in outbred guinea pigs [65–67]. Virus was present in almost all organs, with the highest titers in the adrenal glands, lungs, stomachs and livers [66]. Lower yet still notable titers were found in the brain [66]. P2-infected guinea pigs did not present with any detectable viral titer in any tested organs [66]. Additionally, P18 PICV-infected guinea pigs presented with a longer and more severe disease than their P2-infected counterparts [66]. The level of viremia was correlated with disease severity [66].

6.2. Pichindé Virus in Golden Hamsters

Pichindé virus infection also caused Lassa-like disease in Golden hamsters (*Mesocricetus auratus*) with various lethality depending on the virus strains (Table 5) [68]. The lethality could be 100% in new-born LVG/Lak outbred hamsters, and mortality was uncommon after 8 days post-birth. Peak viral titers in adults reached as high as 10^3 PFU/mL. MHA/Lak inbred hamsters demonstrated 100% lethality with as low as 35 PFU of virus regardless of ages [68]. Adults at 8 dpi developed viral titers over 10^8 PFU/mL. Both hamster models produced antibodies against the virus. Spleen, liver, and kidneys were the primary affected organs [68].

6.3. Pirital Virus in Golden Hamsters

Pirital virus, a non-human pathogenic New World mammarenavirus isolated from western Venezuela, causes a Lassa-like disease in Golden Hamsters [69]. These hamsters developed a severe disease and died approximately 7 dpi [69]. Interstitial pneumonia, multifocal hepatic necrosis, as well as splenic lymphoid depletion and necrosis were noted upon histologic analysis [69]. The brain, kidneys, and intestine were not significantly affected and there was no significant infiltration of inflammatory cells in the affected tissues [69]. Some of the infected hamsters presented with hemorrhagic signs from the mouth or puncture wounds. The clotting deficiency was noted in the collected blood samples, in which clotting rates were either non-existent or extremely slow [69].

6.4. Lymphocytic Choriomeningitis Virus (LCMV) in Rhesus Monkeys

The virulent WE strain of lymphocytic choriomeningitis virus (LCMV), a pathogenic Old World mammarenavirus, causes a uniformly lethal Lassa-like disease in rhesus monkeys infected intravenously (Table 5) [70]. Viremia was detected beginning at 4 dpi [70]. The liver especially was affected in this model, with significant gene expression changes noted [70,71]. However, of five primates infected intragastrically (IG), lethality only reached 20%, with only two of the monkeys becoming viremic [72]. Signs of disease included weight loss and serological analysis indicated elevated ALT and AST as well as thrombocytopenia, transient neutrophilia [72].

7. Summary

Animal models are essential for pathogenesis studies and LASV vaccine and antiviral developments. An ideal LF animal model should match the disease manifestation and progression, pathological changes, and the various pathogenicity of different strains in humans. Additionally, outbred animals with diverse genetic background have an advantage of mimicking infection in human populations. Other important factors include the immune-competency, the availability and the cost of the animals. The prototypic Josiah strain has been the most commonly used LASV strain in laboratory studies. However, the genetic diversity of LASV should also be considered when developing LF animal models.

The NHP models (Table 4), particularly "crab-eating" (cynomolgus) macaques, develop a disease very similar to clinical cases of LF and thus are excellent models for vaccine and antiviral evaluations as well as pathogenesis studies. However, the use of NHPs is extremely limited due to their relatively high cost, the difficulty of handling the animals, as well as the requirements for experienced staff and adequate space in high containment BSL4 facilities. Additionally, it is not easily feasible to perform NHP studies using large group sizes, making statistical significance difficult to ascertain.

Inbred Strain 13 guinea pigs are useful model animals, but the animals are not readily available and lack genetic diversity. Outbred Hartley guinea pigs are commercially available. However, the widely used Josiah strain must be adapted in guinea pigs in order to cause LF-like disease. PICV infection of Hartley guinea pigs can be used as a surrogate animal model of LF. Using the clinical LASV

LF2384 isolate, which was isolated from a fatal case and has experienced minimal passaging in the laboratory, uniformly lethality can be achieved in Hartley guinea pigs without species-specific adaptation. Although further characterization is required, this new model shows much potential as a relevant and relatively inexpensive rodent model that combines the advantages of diverse genetic background, immunocompetency as well as the convenience of the animal's small size and large numbers that can be used in an experiment, which can ensure the rigor and reproducibility of the studies. However, one limitation of using guinea pigs is the lack of available laboratory reagents and a collection of genetically modified animals for immunological and related studies. Nevertheless, guinea pig models could be ideal for vaccine and antiviral screening and potentially pathogenesis studies. A summary of guinea pig LF disease manifestations and pathologies can be found in Table 3.

Immune-competent laboratory mice are generally resistant to LASV infection (Table 2). The STAT1$^{-/-}$ mouse model is the only known animal model for studying LASV-associated hearing loss. This new mouse model has been used in studies on the pathogenesis and immunology of LF, which indicate an immunopathological mechanism of LF. This mouse model may be useful in initial vaccine and antiviral drug screening, as it is a lethal model of infection. However, its immune-incompetency should be considered, as deficiency in interferon signaling may have negative effects on such studies [73,74].

With the increased fatality of LF in the most recent 2018–2019 outbreaks, there is an urgent need for the rapid development of vaccines and antivirals. Development of small animal models that resemble human disease is crucial to facilitate vaccine and therapeutic testing. The best option at the current stage seems to be performing initial screening in lethal rodent models, such as the aforementioned STAT1$^{-/-}$ mouse model and the newly developed LF2384/outbred Hartley guinea pig model, followed by validation of promising candidates in NHPs. Additionally, the STAT1$^{-/-}$ model is useful as a new platform for investigating the mechanism of LF-associated hearing loss, which affects approximately one third of survivors.

Author Contributions: Review conceptualization and organization were conducted by all authors. The original manuscript was prepared by R.A.S. Manuscript editing was performed by all authors. All authors have read and agree to the published version of the manuscript.

Funding: R.A.S. was supported by the Institute for Translational Sciences at the University of Texas Medical Branch, which is supported in part and by the Clinical and Translational Science Award NRSA (TL1) Training Core (TL1TR001440) from the National Center for Advancing Translational Sciences at the National Institutes of Health. Work in the Paessler laboratory was supported in parts by Public Health Service grants RO1AI093445 and RO1AI129198 and the John. S. Dunn Distinguished Chair in Biodefense endowment. Work in the Ly lab was supported in parts by the Public Health Service grant R01AI131586 and by funds from the USDA National Institute of Food and Agriculture (USDA-NIFA) and from the Minnesota Agricultural Experiment Station. C.H. was supported by UTMB Commitment Fund P84373.

Acknowledgments: We apologize for any works that we were unable to include due to the constraints of the review. The authors would like to thank Junki Maruyama for consultation over the course of writing. C.H. would like to acknowledge the Galveston National Laboratory (supported by the Public Health Service award 5UC7AI094660) for support of his research activity.

References

1.   Günther, S.; Lenz, O. Lassa fever. *Br. Med. J.* **1972**, *4*, 253–254. Available online: https://www.ncbi.nlm.nih.gov/pmc/articles/PMC1788780/ (accessed on 14 June 2019).
2.   Centers for Disease Control and Prevention. Lassa Fever. 2019. Available online: https://www.cdc.gov/vhf/lassa/index.html (accessed on 15 June 2019).
3.   Frame, J.D.; Baldwin, J.M., Jr.; Gocke, D.J.; Troup, J.M. Lassa fever, a new virus disease of man from West Africa. I. Clinical description and pathological findings. *Am. J. Trop. Med. Hyg.* **1970**, *19*, 670–676. [CrossRef] [PubMed]
4.   Olayemi, A.; Oyeyiola, A.; Obadare, A.; Igbokwe, J.; Adesina, A.S.; Onwe, F.; Ukwaja, K.N.; Ajayi, N.A.; Rieger, T.; Gunther, S.; et al. Widespread arenavirus occurrence and seroprevalence in small mammals, Nigeria. *Parasit Vectors* **2018**, *11*, 416. [CrossRef]

5. Andersen, K.G.; Shapiro, B.J.; Matranga, C.B.; Sealfon, R.; Lin, A.E.; Moses, L.M.; Folarin, O.A.; Goba, A.; Odia, I.; Ehiane, P.E.; et al. Clinical Sequencing Uncovers Origins and Evolution of Lassa Virus. *Cell* **2015**, *162*, 738–750. [CrossRef]

6. Manning, J.T.; Forrester, N.; Paessler, S. Lassa virus isolates from Mali and the Ivory Coast represent an emerging fifth lineage. *Front. Microbiol.* **2015**, *6*, 1037. [CrossRef]

7. Ehichioya, D.U.; Dellicour, S.; Pahlmann, M.; Rieger, T.; Oestereich, L.; Becker-Ziaja, B.; Cadar, D.; Ighodalo, Y.; Olokor, T.; Omomoh, E.; et al. Phylogeography of Lassa Virus in Nigeria. *J. Virol.* **2019**, *93*. [CrossRef]

8. Yun, N.E.; Ronca, S.; Tamura, A.; Koma, T.; Seregin, A.V.; Dineley, K.T.; Miller, M.; Cook, R.; Shimizu, N.; Walker, A.G.; et al. Animal Model of Sensorineural Hearing Loss Associated with Lassa Virus Infection. *J. Virol.* **2015**, *90*, 2920–2927. [CrossRef]

9. Welch, S.R.; Scholte, F.E.M.; Albariño, C.G.; Kainulainen, M.H.; Coleman-McCray, J.D.; Guerrero, L.W.; Chakrabarti, A.K.; Klena, J.D.; Nichol, S.T.; Spengler, J.R.; et al. The S Genome Segment Is Sufficient to Maintain Pathogenicity in Intra-Clade Lassa Virus Reassortants in a Guinea Pig Model. *Front. Cell. Infect. Microbiol.* **2018**, *8*, 240. [CrossRef]

10. Ibekwe, T.S.; Okokhere, P.O.; Asogun, D.; Blackie, F.F.; Nwegbu, M.M.; Wahab, K.W.; Omilabu, S.A.; Akpede, G.O. Early-onset sensorineural hearing loss in Lassa fever. *Eur. Arch. Otorhinolaryngol.* **2011**, *268*, 197–201. [CrossRef]

11. Dan-Nwafor, C.C.; Furuse, Y.; Ilori, E.A.; Ipadeola, O.; Akabike, K.O.; Ahumibe, A.; Ukponu, W.; Bakare, L.; Okwor, T.J.; Joseph, G.; et al. Measures to control protracted large Lassa fever outbreak in Nigeria, 1 January to 28 April 2019. *Euro. Surveill.* **2019**, *24*. [CrossRef]

12. World Health Organization. On the Frontlines of the Fight against Lassa Fever in Nigeria. 2018. Available online: http://www.who.int/features/2018/lassa-fever-nigeria/en/ (accessed on 15 June 2019).

13. Nigeria Centers for Disease Control. 2018 Lassa Fever Outbreak in Nigeria. 2018. Available online: https://ncdc.gov.ng/themes/common/files/sitreps/00235292b8a3f55c01f9ea2eb15c8d3a.pdf (accessed on 15 June 2019).

14. World Health Organization. Emergencies Preparedness, Response Lassa Fever. 2019. Available online: https://www.who.int/csr/don/archive/disease/lassa_fever/en/ (accessed on 16 June 2019).

15. McCormick, J.B.; King, I.J.; Webb, P.A.; Scribner, C.L.; Craven, R.B.; Johnson, K.M.; Elliott, L.H.; Belmont-Williams, R. Lassa fever. Effective therapy with ribavirin. *N. Engl. J. Med.* **1986**, *314*, 20–26. [CrossRef]

16. Mustapha, A. Lassa fever: Unveiling the misery of the Nigerian health worker. *Ann. Nigerian. Med.* **2017**, *11*, 1–5.

17. Walker, D.H.; McCormick, J.B.; Johnson, K.M.; Webb, P.A.; Komba-Kono, G.; Elliott, L.H.; Gardner, J.J. Pathologic and virologic study of fatal Lassa fever in man. *Am. J. Pathol.* **1982**, *107*, 349–356.

18. Mateer, E.J.; Huang, C.; Shehu, N.Y.; Paessler, S. Lassa fever-induced sensorineural hearing loss: A neglected public health and social burden. *PLoS Negl. Trop. Dis.* **2018**, *12*, e0006187. [CrossRef]

19. Cummins, D.; McCormick, J.B.; Bennett, D.; Samba, J.A.; Farrar, B.; Machin, S.J.; Fisher-Hoch, S.P. Acute sensorineural deafness in Lassa fever. *JAMA* **1990**, *264*, 2093–2096. [CrossRef]

20. Price, M.E.; Fisher-Hoch, S.P.; Craven, R.B.; McCormick, J.B. A prospective study of maternal and fetal outcome in acute Lassa fever infection during pregnancy. *BMJ* **1988**, *297*, 584–587. [CrossRef]

21. Dunmade, A.D.; Segun-Busari, S.; Olajide, T.G.; Ologe, F.E. Profound bilateral sensorineural hearing loss in nigerian children: Any shift in etiology? *J. Deaf Stud. Deaf Educ.* **2007**, *12*, 112–118. [CrossRef]

22. Khan, S.H.; Goba, A.; Chu, M.; Roth, C.; Healing, T.; Marx, A.; Fair, J.; Guttieri, M.C.; Ferro, P.; Imes, T.; et al. New opportunities for field research on the pathogenesis and treatment of Lassa fever. *Antiviral. Res.* **2008**, *78*, 103–115. [CrossRef]

23. Johnson, K.M.; McCormick, J.B.; Webb, P.A.; Smith, E.S.; Elliott, L.H.; King, I.J. Clinical virology of Lassa fever in hospitalized patients. *J. Infect. Dis.* **1987**, *155*, 456–464. [CrossRef]

24. Winn, W.C., Jr.; Walker, D.H. The pathology of human Lassa fever. *Bull. World Health Organ.* **1975**, *52*, 535–545.

25. Walker, D.H.; Wulff, H.; Lange, J.V.; Murphy, F.A. Comparative pathology of Lassa virus infection in monkeys, guinea-pigs, and *Mastomys natalensis*. *Bull. World Health Organ.* **1975**, *52*, 523–534. [PubMed]

26. Granjon, L.; Duplantier, J.-M.; Catalan, J.; Britton-Davidian, J. Systematics of the genus Mastomys (Thomas, 1915) (Rodentia: Muridae): A review. *Belg. J. Zool.* **1997**, *127*, 7–18.

27. Rieger, T.; Merkler, D.; Gunther, S. Infection of type I interferon receptor-deficient mice with various old world arenaviruses: A model for studying virulence and host species barriers. *PLoS One* **2013**, *8*, e72290. [CrossRef]

28. Yun, N.E.; Seregin, A.V.; Walker, D.H.; Popov, V.L.; Walker, A.G.; Smith, J.N.; Miller, M.; de la Torre, J.C.; Smith, J.K.; Borisevich, V.; et al. Mice lacking functional STAT1 are highly susceptible to lethal infection with Lassa virus. *J. Virol.* **2013**, *87*, 10908–10911. [CrossRef]

29. Oestereich, L.; Lüdtke, A.; Ruibal, P.; Pallasch, E.; Kerber, R.; Rieger, T.; Wurr, S.; Bockholt, S.; Pérez-Girón, J.V.; Krasemann, S.; et al. Chimeric Mice with Competent Hematopoietic Immunity Reproduce Key Features of Severe Lassa Fever. *PLoS Pathog.* **2016**, *12*, e1005656. [CrossRef]

30. Yun, N.E.; Poussard, A.L.; Seregin, A.V.; Walker, A.G.; Smith, J.K.; Aronson, J.F.; Smith, J.N.; Soong, L.; Paessler, S. Functional interferon system is required for clearance of lassa virus. *J. Virol.* **2012**, *86*, 3389–3392. [CrossRef]

31. Oestereich, L.; Rieger, T.; Ludtke, A.; Ruibal, P.; Wurr, S.; Pallasch, E.; Bockholt, S.; Krasemann, S.; Muñoz-Fontela, C.; Gunther, S. Efficacy of Favipiravir Alone and in Combination With Ribavirin in a Lethal, Immunocompetent Mouse Model of Lassa Fever. *J. Infect. Dis.* **2016**, *213*, 934–938. [CrossRef]

32. Uckun, F.M.; Petkevich, A.S.; Vassilev, A.O.; Tibbles, H.E.; Titov, L. Stampidine prevents mortality in an experimental mouse model of viral hemorrhagic fever caused by lassa virus. *BMC Infect. Dis.* **2004**, *4*, 1. [CrossRef]

33. Flatz, L.; Rieger, T.; Merkler, D.; Bergthaler, A.; Regen, T.; Schedensack, M.; Bestmann, L.; Verschoor, A.; Kreutzfeldt, M.; Bruck, W.; et al. T cell-dependence of Lassa fever pathogenesis. *PLoS Pathog.* **2010**, *6*, e1000836. [CrossRef]

34. Jahrling, P.B.; Smith, S.; Hesse, R.A.; Rhoderick, J.B. Pathogenesis of Lassa virus infection in guinea pigs. *Infect. Immun.* **1982**, *37*, 771–778. [CrossRef]

35. Bell, T.M.; Shaia, C.I.; Bearss, J.J.; Mattix, M.E.; Koistinen, K.A.; Honnold, S.P.; Zeng, X.; Blancett, C.D.; Donnelly, G.C.; Shamblin, J.D.; et al. Temporal Progression of Lesions in Guinea Pigs Infected With Lassa Virus. *Vet. Pathol.* **2017**, *54*, 549–562. [CrossRef] [PubMed]

36. Gary, J.M.; Welch, S.R.; Ritter, J.M.; Coleman-McCray, J.; Huynh, T.; Kainulainen, M.H.; Bollweg, B.C.; Parihar, V.; Nichol, S.T.; Zaki, S.R.; et al. Lassa Virus Targeting of Anterior Uvea and Endothelium of Cornea and Conjunctiva in Eye of Guinea Pig Model. *Emerg. Infect. Dis.* **2019**, *25*, 865–874. [CrossRef] [PubMed]

37. Cashman, K.A.; Smith, M.A.; Twenhafel, N.A.; Larson, R.A.; Jones, K.F.; Allen, R.D., 3rd; Dai, D.; Chinsangaram, J.; Bolken, T.C.; Hruby, D.E.; et al. Evaluation of Lassa antiviral compound ST-193 in a guinea pig model. *Antiviral. Res.* **2011**, *90*, 70–79. [CrossRef] [PubMed]

38. Safronetz, D.; Mire, C.; Rosenke, K.; Feldmann, F.; Haddock, E.; Geisbert, T.; Feldmann, H. A recombinant vesicular stomatitis virus-based Lassa fever vaccine protects guinea pigs and macaques against challenge with geographically and genetically distinct Lassa viruses. *PLoS Negl. Trop. Dis.* **2015**, *9*, e0003736. [CrossRef] [PubMed]

39. Safronetz, D.; Strong, J.E.; Feldmann, F.; Haddock, E.; Sogoba, N.; Brining, D.; Geisbert, T.W.; Scott, D.P.; Feldmann, H. A recently isolated Lassa virus from Mali demonstrates atypical clinical disease manifestations and decreased virulence in cynomolgus macaques. *J. Infect. Dis.* **2013**, *207*, 1316–1327. [CrossRef] [PubMed]

40. Cross, R.W.; Mire, C.E.; Branco, L.M.; Geisbert, J.B.; Rowland, M.M.; Heinrich, M.L.; Goba, A.; Momoh, M.; Grant, D.S.; Fullah, M.; et al. Treatment of Lassa virus infection in outbred guinea pigs with first-in-class human monoclonal antibodies. *Antiviral. Res.* **2016**, *133*, 218–222. [CrossRef]

41. Safronetz, D.; Rosenke, K.; Westover, J.B.; Martellaro, C.; Okumura, A.; Furuta, Y.; Geisbert, J.; Saturday, G.; Komeno, T.; Geisbert, T.W.; et al. The broad-spectrum antiviral favipiravir protects guinea pigs from lethal Lassa virus infection post-disease onset. *Sci. Rep.* **2015**, *5*, 14775. [CrossRef]

42. Stein, D.R.; Warner, B.M.; Soule, G.; Tierney, K.; Frost, K.L.; Booth, S.; Safronetz, D. A recombinant vesicular stomatitis-based Lassa fever vaccine elicits rapid and long-term protection from lethal Lassa virus infection in guinea pigs. *NPJ Vaccines* **2019**, *4*, 8. [CrossRef]

43. Maruyama, J.; Mateer, E.J.; Manning, J.T.; Sattler, R.; Seregin, A.V.; Bukreyeva, N.; Jones, F.R.; Balint, J.P.; Gabitzsch, E.S.; Huang, C.; et al. Adenoviral vector-based vaccine is fully protective against lethal Lassa fever challenge in Hartley guinea pigs. *Vaccine* **2019**, *37*, 6824–6831. [CrossRef]

44. Walker, D.H.; Johnson, K.M.; Lange, J.V.; Gardner, J.J.; Kiley, M.P.; McCormick, J.B. Experimental infection of rhesus monkeys with Lassa virus and a closely related arenavirus, Mozambique virus. *J. Infect. Dis.* **1982**, *146*, 360–368. [CrossRef] [PubMed]

45. Maruyama, J.; Manning, J.T.; Mateer, E.J.; Sattler, R.; Bukreyeva, N.; Huang, C.; Paessler, S. Lethal Infection of Lassa Virus Isolated from a Human Clinical Sample in Outbred Guinea Pigs without Adaptation. *mSphere* **2019**, *4*. [CrossRef] [PubMed]

46. Walker, D.H.; Wulff, H.; Murphy, F.A. Experimental Lassa virus infection in the squirrel monkey. *Am. J. Pathol.* **1975**, *80*, 261–278. [PubMed]

47. Carrion, R., Jr.; Brasky, K.; Mansfield, K.; Johnson, C.; Gonzales, M.; Ticer, A.; Lukashevich, I.; Tardif, S.; Patterson, J. Lassa virus infection in experimentally infected marmosets: Liver pathology and immunophenotypic alterations in target tissues. *J. Virol.* **2007**, *81*, 6482–6490. [CrossRef] [PubMed]

48. Callis, R.T.; Jahrling, P.B.; DePaoli, A. Pathology of Lassa virus infection in the rhesus monkey. *Am. J. Trop. Med. Hyg.* **1982**, *31*, 1038–1045. [CrossRef] [PubMed]

49. Jahrling, P.B.; Hesse, R.A.; Eddy, G.A.; Johnson, K.M.; Callis, R.T.; Stephen, E.L. Lassa virus infection of rhesus monkeys: Pathogenesis and treatment with ribavirin. *J. Infect. Dis.* **1980**, *141*, 580–589. [CrossRef]

50. Cashman, K.A.; Wilkinson, E.R.; Shaia, C.I.; Facemire, P.R.; Bell, T.M.; Bearss, J.J.; Shamblin, J.D.; Wollen, S.E.; Broderick, K.E.; Sardesai, N.Y.; et al. A DNA vaccine delivered by dermal electroporation fully protects cynomolgus macaques against Lassa fever. *Hum. Vaccin. Immunother.* **2017**, *13*, 2902–2911. [CrossRef]

51. Geisbert, T.W.; Jones, S.; Fritz, E.A.; Shurtleff, A.C.; Geisbert, J.B.; Liebscher, R.; Grolla, A.; Ströher, U.; Fernando, L.; Daddario, K.M.; et al. Development of a new vaccine for the prevention of Lassa fever. *PLoS Med.* **2005**, *2*, e183. [CrossRef]

52. Jiang, J.; Banglore, P.; Cashman, K.A.; Schmaljohn, C.S.; Schultheis, K.; Pugh, H.; Nguyen, J.; Humeau, L.M.; Broderick, K.E.; Ramos, S.J. Immunogenicity of a protective intradermal DNA vaccine against lassa virus in cynomolgus macaques. *Hum. Vaccin. Immunother.* **2019**, *15*, 2066–2074. [CrossRef]

53. Mire, C.E.; Cross, R.W.; Geisbert, J.B.; Borisevich, V.; Agans, K.N.; Deer, D.J.; Heinrich, M.L.; Rowland, M.M.; Goba, A.; Momoh, M.; et al. Human-monoclonal-antibody therapy protects nonhuman primates against advanced Lassa fever. *Nat. Med.* **2017**, *23*, 1146–1149. [CrossRef]

54. Fisher-Hoch, S.P.; Mitchell, S.W.; Sasso, D.R.; Lange, J.V.; Ramsey, R.; McCormick, J.B. Physiological and immunologic disturbances associated with shock in a primate model of Lassa fever. *J. Infect. Dis.* **1987**, *155*, 465–474. [CrossRef]

55. Lange, J.V.; Mitchell, S.W.; McCormick, J.B.; Walker, D.H.; Evatt, B.L.; Ramsey, R.R. Kinetic study of platelets and fibrinogen in Lassa virus-infected monkeys and early pathologic events in Mopeia virus-infected monkeys. *Am. J. Trop. Med. Hyg.* **1985**, *34*, 999–1007. [CrossRef] [PubMed]

56. Cashman, K.A.; Wilkinson, E.R.; Zeng, X.; Cardile, A.P.; Facemire, P.R.; Bell, T.M.; Bearss, J.J.; Shaia, C.I.; Schmaljohn, C.S. Immune-Mediated Systemic Vasculitis as the Proposed Cause of Sudden-Onset Sensorineural Hearing Loss following Lassa Virus Exposure in Cynomolgus Macaques. *mBio* **2018**, *9*. [CrossRef] [PubMed]

57. Baize, S.; Marianneau, P.; Loth, P.; Reynard, S.; Journeaux, A.; Chevallier, M.; Tordo, N.; Deubel, V.; Contamin, H. Early and strong immune responses are associated with control of viral replication and recovery in lassa virus-infected cynomolgus monkeys. *J. Virol.* **2009**, *83*, 5890–5903. [CrossRef] [PubMed]

58. Hensley, L.E.; Smith, M.A.; Geisbert, J.B.; Fritz, E.A.; Daddario-DiCaprio, K.M.; Larsen, T.; Geisbert, T.W. Pathogenesis of Lassa fever in cynomolgus macaques. *Virol. J.* **2011**, *8*, 205. [CrossRef]

59. Buchmeier, M.; Adam, E.; Rawls, W.E. Serological evidence of infection by Pichindé virus among laboratory workers. *Infect. Immun.* **1974**, *9*, 821–823. [CrossRef]

60. Trapido, H.; Sanmartin, C. Pichindé virus, a new virus of the Tacaribe group from Colombia. *Am. J. Trop. Med. Hyg.* **1971**, *20*, 631–641. [CrossRef]

61. Aronson, J.F.; Herzog, N.K.; Jerrells, T.R. Pathological and virological features of arenavirus disease in guinea pigs. Comparison of two Pichindé virus strains. *Am. J. Pathol.* **1994**, *145*, 228–235.

62. Connolly, B.M.; Jenson, A.B.; Peters, C.J.; Geyer, S.J.; Barth, J.F.; McPherson, R.A. Pathogenesis of Pichindé virus infection in strain 13 guinea pigs: An immunocytochemical, virologic, and clinical chemistry study. *Am. J. Trop. Med. Hyg.* **1993**, *49*, 10–24. [CrossRef]

63. Jahrling, P.B.; Hesse, R.A.; Rhoderick, J.B.; Elwell, M.A.; Moe, J.B. Pathogenesis of a pichindé virus strain adapted to produce lethal infections in guinea pigs. *Infect. Immun.* **1981**, *32*, 872–880. [CrossRef]

64. Cosgriff, T.M.; Jahrling, P.B.; Chen, J.P.; Hodgson, L.A.; Lewis, R.M.; Green, D.E.; Smith, J.I. Studies of the coagulation system in arenaviral hemorrhagic fever: Experimental infection of strain 13 guinea pigs with Pichindé virus. *Am. J. Trop. Med. Hyg.* **1987**, *36*, 416–423. [CrossRef]

65. Zhang, L.; Marriott, K.; Aronson, J.F. Sequence analysis of the small RNA segment of guinea pig-passaged Pichindé virus variants. *Am. J. Trop. Med. Hyg.* **1999**, *61*, 220–225. [CrossRef] [PubMed]

66. Lan, S.; McLay Schelde, L.; Wang, J.; Kumar, N.; Ly, H.; Liang, Y. Development of infectious clones for virulent and avirulent pichindé viruses: A model virus to study arenavirus-induced hemorrhagic fevers. *J. Virol.* **2009**, *83*, 6357–6362. [CrossRef] [PubMed]

67. Zhang, L.; Marriott, K.A.; Harnish, D.G.; Aronson, J.F. Reassortant analysis of guinea pig virulence of pichindé virus variants. *Virology* **2001**, *290*, 30–38. [CrossRef]

68. Buchmeier, M.J.; Rawls, W.E. Variation between strains of hamsters in the lethality of Pichindé virus infections. *Infect. Immun.* **1977**, *16*, 413–421. [CrossRef] [PubMed]

69. Xiao, S.Y.; Zhang, H.; Yang, Y.; Tesh, R.B. Pirital virus (*Arenaviridae*) infection in the syrian golden hamster, Mesocricetus auratus: A new animal model for arenaviral hemorrhagic fever. *Am. J. Trop. Med. Hyg.* **2001**, *64*, 111–118. [CrossRef] [PubMed]

70. Djavani, M.M.; Crasta, O.R.; Zapata, J.C.; Fei, Z.; Folkerts, O.; Sobral, B.; Swindells, M.; Bryant, J.; Davis, H.; Pauza, C.D.; et al. Early blood profiles of virus infection in a monkey model for Lassa fever. *J. Virol.* **2007**, *81*, 7960–7973. [CrossRef] [PubMed]

71. Djavani, M.; Crasta, O.R.; Zhang, Y.; Zapata, J.C.; Sobral, B.; Lechner, M.G.; Bryant, J.; Davis, H.; Salvato, M.S. Gene expression in primate liver during viral hemorrhagic fever. *Virol. J.* **2009**, *6*, 20. [CrossRef]

72. Rodas, J.D.; Lukashevich, I.S.; Zapata, J.C.; Cairo, C.; Tikhonov, I.; Djavani, M.; Pauza, C.D.; Salvato, M.S. Mucosal arenavirus infection of primates can protect them from lethal hemorrhagic fever. *J. Med. Virol.* **2004**, *72*, 424–435. [CrossRef]

73. Clarke, E.C.; Bradfute, S.B. The use of mice lacking type I or both type I and type II interferon responses in research on hemorrhagic fever viruses. Part 1: Potential effects on adaptive immunity and response to vaccination. *Antiviral. Res.* **2020**, *174*, 104703. [CrossRef] [PubMed]

74. Zivcec, M.; Spiropoulou, C.F.; Spengler, J.R. The use of mice lacking type I or both type I and type II interferon responses in research on hemorrhagic fever viruses. Part 2: Vaccine efficacy studies. *Antiviral. Res.* **2020**, *174*, 104702. [CrossRef]

12

One Health—Its Importance in Helping to Better Control Antimicrobial Resistance

Peter J. Collignon [1,2,*] [ID] and Scott A. McEwen [3]

[1] Infectious Diseases and Microbiology, Canberra Hospital, Garran, ACT 2605, Australia
[2] Medical School, Australian National University, Acton ACT 2601, Australia
[3] Department of Population Medicine, University of Guelph, Guelph N1G 2W1, Canada;
    smcewen@uoguelph.ca
* Correspondence: peter.collignon@act.gov.au

Abstract: Approaching any issue from a One Health perspective necessitates looking at the interactions of people, domestic animals, wildlife, plants, and our environment. For antimicrobial resistance this includes antimicrobial use (and abuse) in the human, animal and environmental sectors. More importantly, the spread of resistant bacteria and resistance determinants within and between these sectors and globally must be addressed. Better managing this problem includes taking steps to preserve the continued effectiveness of existing antimicrobials such as trying to eliminate their inappropriate use, particularly where they are used in high volumes. Examples are the mass medication of animals with critically important antimicrobials for humans, such as third generation cephalosporins and fluoroquinolones, and the long term, in-feed use of antimicrobials, such colistin, tetracyclines and macrolides, for growth promotion. In people it is essential to better prevent infections, reduce over-prescribing and over-use of antimicrobials and stop resistant bacteria from spreading by improving hygiene and infection control, drinking water and sanitation. Pollution from inadequate treatment of industrial, residential and farm waste is expanding the resistome in the environment. Numerous countries and several international agencies have now included a One Health Approach within their action plans to address antimicrobial resistance. Necessary actions include improvements in antimicrobial use, better regulation and policy, as well as improved surveillance, stewardship, infection control, sanitation, animal husbandry, and finding alternatives to antimicrobials.

Keywords: One Health; antibiotics; antimicrobials; antimicrobial resistance; environment; water; infrastructure

1. Introduction

Antimicrobial resistance is a global public health problem [1,2]. Most bacteria that cause serious infections and could once be successfully treated with several different antibiotic classes, have now acquired resistance—often to many antibiotics. In some regions the increased resistance has been so extensive that resistance is present in some bacteria to nearly all of these drugs [2–4]. The threat is most acute for antibacterial antimicrobials (antibiotics—the focus of this paper) but also threatens antifungals, antiparastics and antivirals [5].

Antimicrobial overuse is occurring in multiple sectors (human, animal, agriculture) [3,6]. Microorganisms faced with antimicrobial selection pressure enhance their fitness by acquiring and expressing resistance genes, then sharing them with other bacteria and by other mechanisms, for example gene overexpression and silencing, phase variation. When bacteria are resistant they also present in much larger numbers when exposed to antimicrobials, whether in an individual, in a location and in the environment. Additionally important in driving the deteriorating resistance problem are factors that promote the spread of resistant bacteria (or "contagion") [7]. This spread involves not only bacteria themselves but the resistance genes they carry and that can be acquired by other bacteria [8]. Factors that facilitate "contagion" include poverty, poor housing, poor infection control, poor water supplies, poor sanitation, run off of waste from intensive agriculture, environmental contamination and geographical movement of infected humans and animals [9–11].

Wherever antimicrobials are used, there are often already large reservoirs of resistant bacteria and resistance genes. These include people and their local environments (both in hospitals and in the community), as well as animals, farms and aquaculture environments. Large reservoirs of resistance and residual antimicrobials occur in water, soil, wildlife and many other ecological niches, not only due to pollution by sewage, pharmaceutical industry waste and manure runoff from farms [10,12,13], but often resistant bacteria and resistance genes have already been there for millennia [14,15].

Most bacteria and their genes can move relatively easily within and between humans, animals and the environment. Microbial adaptations to antimicrobial use and other selection pressures within any one sector are reflected in other sectors [8,16]. Similarly, actions (or inactions) to contain antimicrobial resistance in one sector affect other sectors [17,18]. Antimicrobial resistance is an ecological problem that is characterized by complex interactions involving diverse microbial populations affecting the health of humans, animals and the environment. It makes sense to address the resistance problem by taking this complexity and ecological nature into account using a coordinated, multi-sectoral approach, such as One Health [5,19–23].

One Health is defined by WHO [24] and others [25] as a concept and approach to "designing and implementing programs, policies, legislation and research in which multiple sectors communicate and work together to achieve better public health outcomes. The areas of work in which a One Health approach is particularly relevant include food safety, the control of zoonoses and combatting antibiotic resistance" [24]. It needs to involve the "collaborative effort of multiple health science professions, together with their related disciplines and institutions—working locally, nationally, and globally—to attain optimal health for people, domestic animals, wildlife, plants, and our environment" [25]. The origins of One Health are centuries old and are based on the mutual inter-dependence of people and animals and a recognition that they share not only the same environment, but also many infectious diseases [23]. Our current concept of One Health however goes much further. It also embraces the health of the environment.

2. Use of Antimicrobials in Humans, Animals and Plants

The vast majority of antimicrobial classes are used both in humans and animals (including aquaculture; both farmed fish and shellfish). Only few antimicrobial classes are reserved exclusively for humans (e.g., carbapenems). There are also few classes limited to veterinary use (e.g., flavophospholipols, ionophores); mainly because of toxicity to humans [26–30].

Insects (e.g., bees) and some plants are frequently treated with antimicrobials. Tetracyclines, streptomycin and some other antimicrobials are used for treatment and prophylaxis of bacterial infections of fruit, such as apples and pears (e.g., "fire blight" caused by *Erwinia amylovora*) [31,32]. Antifungals, especially azoles, are used in huge quantities and applied to broad acre crops such as wheat [33].

There are marked differences in the ways antimicrobials are used in human compared to non-human sectors. In people, antimicrobials are mostly used for treatment of clinical infections in individual patients, with some limited prophylactic use in individuals (e.g., post-surgery) or occasionally in groups (e.g., prevention of meningococcal disease). Antimicrobial uses in companion animals (e.g., dogs, cats, pet birds, horses) are broadly similar to those in humans, with antimicrobials mostly administered on an individual basis to treat infection, and occasionally for prophylaxis, such as post-surgery [34,35].

In the food-producing animal sector, antimicrobials are also used therapeutically to treat individual clinically sick animals (e.g., dairy cows with mastitis) [26]. However, in intensive farming and aquaculture, for reasons of practicality and efficiency, antimicrobials are often administered through feed or water to entire groups (e.g., pens of pigs, flocks of broilers), either for prophylaxis (to healthy animals at risk of infection) or metaphylaxis (to healthy animals in the same group as diseased animals) [36]. Some have even succeeded in having this group level administration defined (and we believe inappropriately) in the animal health sector as "therapeutic" use. Growth promotion, prophylaxis and metaphylaxis account for by far the largest volumes of antimicrobials used in the food-producing animal sector [26,27,37].

Growth Promotion Use

Using antimicrobials for growth promotion is highly controversial because instead of treating sick animals they are administered to healthy animals, usually for prolonged periods of time, and often at sub-therapeutic doses in order to improve production. These conditions favor selection and spread of resistant bacteria within animals and to humans through food or other environmental pathways [38,39]. The period of exposure with growth promotion is usually greater than two weeks and often almost the entire life of an animal, for example in chicken for 36 days or more.

Based on studies, mostly conducted decades ago, the purported production benefits of antimicrobial growth promoters range widely (1–10%). Surveillance and animal production data however now suggests that benefits in animals reared in good conditions are probably quite small and may be non-existent. Many large poultry corporations are now marketing chicken raised without antimicrobials administered at hatchery or farm levels [40]. Expressed concerns are that antimicrobial growth promoters are used to compensate for poor hygiene and housing, and as replacement for proper animal health management [18,41,42]. For these reasons, the World Health Organization (WHO) advocates the termination of antimicrobial use for growth promotion [5,41]. This practice has now been banned in Europe and elsewhere and is being phased out in some other countries [43–45]. However there are still many countries where they continue to be used [46], including drugs categorized by WHO as critically important to humans, for example colistin, fluoroquinolones and macrolides [47].

Comprehensive global quantitative data on use of antimicrobial agents in humans, animals and plants is generally lacking. Table 1 shows the varying levels of antibiotic usage in people around the world, associated resistance levels, plus some social and infrastructure parameters—the latter of which can facilitate the spread of resistant bacteria (e.g., poor sanitation). Figure 1 shows antibiotic use in different regions globally in people and the lack of correlation with increased resistance levels in bacteria and human antibiotic usage. These data strongly suggest that there are other very important factors influencing antimicrobial resistance over and above simply antibiotic usage.

Table 1. Levels of antibiotic usage in people, resistance levels and other parameters globally. (All data taken from reference 7).

Country	Antibiotic Usage (Standard units per 1000 pop - CCDEP)	E. coli % Resistance 3rd gen ceph (WHO)	E. coli % Resistance Fluoroquinolones (WHO)	Staphylococcus Aureus (MRSA Rates - WHO)	2015 Corruption Index	GNP per capita 2015 (Purchasing Power Parity in 2011 Dollars)	% with Adequate Sanitation 2015	Improved Water Source (% of Population with Access)
Algeria	15.4	17	2	44.8	36	$13,795	88	87.7
Argentina	6.2	5.1	7.8	54	32	$19,102	96	98.9
Australia	11	7.7	10.6	30	79	$43,631	100	100
Austria	7.2	9.1	22.3	7.4	76	$44,048	100	100
Bahrain		55	62	10	51	$43,754	99	100
Bangladesh	4.3	57.4	89	46	25	$3,137	61	86.2
Belgium	12.6	6	21.5	17.4	77	$41,826	100	100
Bhutan		19.4	35.5	10	65	$7,861	50	100
Bosnia and Herzegovina	7.5	1.5	7.8		38	$10,119	95	99.9
Brazil	5.9	30	40	29.5	38	$14,533	83	98.1
Brunei Darussalam		6.5	12		55	$73,605	100	100
Bulgaria	9.4	22.9	30.2	22.4	41	$17,000	86	99.6
Burkina Faso		36	52.8		38	$1,593	20	82.1
Burundi		7.2	16	13	21	$683	48	75.8
Cambodia		45	71.8		21	$3,278	42	73.4
Canada	7.2	8	26.9	21	83	$42,983	100	99.8
Central African Republic		30	53		24	$581	22	68.4
Chile	4.3	23.8		90	70	$22,197	99	99
China	3	51.9	55.1	38.3	70	$13,572	77	94.8
Colombia	2.9	11.7	59	7.2	37	$12,988	81	91.3
Croatia	10.6	6	14	13	51	$20,664	97	99.6
Cuba		42.9	56		47	$21,017	93	94.6
Cyprus		36.2	47.4	41.6	61	$30,383	100	100
Czech Republic	7.5	11.4	23.5	14.5	56	$30,381	99	100
Denmark	6.7	8.5	14.1	1.2	91	$45,484	100	100
Dominican Republic	2.4	33	49	30	33	$13,372	84	86.5
Ecuador	6.7	15.1	43.8	29	32	$10,777	85	86.9
Egypt	9.1	44.4	34.9	46	36	$10,250	95	99.2
Estonia	4.4		9.9	1.7	70	$27,345	97	99.6

Table 1. *Cont.*

Country	Antibiotic Usage (Standard units per 1000 pop - CCDEP)	E. coli % Resistance 3rd gen ceph (WHO)	E. coli % Resistance Fluoroquinolones (WHO)	Staphylococcus Aureus (MRSA Rates - WHO)	2015 Corruption Index	GNP per capita 2015 (Purchasing Power Parity in 2011 Dollars)	% with Adequate Sanitation 2015	Improved Water Source (% of Population with Access)
Ethiopia		62	71	31.6	33	$1,530	28	55.4
Finland	7.2	5.1	10.8	2.8	90	$38,994	98	100
France	12.9	8.2	17.9	20.1	70	$37,775	99	100
Germany	7.1	8	23.7	16.2	81	$43,788	99	100
Greece	14.6	14.9	26.6	39.2	46	$24,095	99	100
Guatemala		39.8	41.8	52	28	$7,253	64	92.7
Honduras		36.7	43.1	30	31	$4,785	83	90.6
Hong Kong	7.5				75	$53,463	96	100
Hungary	7.3	15.1	31.2	26.2	51	$24,831	98	100
Iceland		6.2	14		79	$42,704	99	100
India	5	51.4	52.3	42.7	38	$5,733	40	94.1
Indonesia	3.6				36	$10,385	61	86.8
Iran		41	54	53	27	$16,507	90	96.2
Ireland	11.4	9	22.9	23.7	75	$61,378	91	97.9
Israel		2.6	17.9	46.7	61	$31,971	100	100
Italy	11.5	19.8	40.5	38.2	44	$34,220	100	100
Japan	5.3	16.6	34.3	53	75	$37,872	100	100
Jordan	6.3	22.5	14.5		53	$10,240	99	96.9
Kazakhstan	7.5				28	$23,522	98	93.5
Kenya		87.2	91.4	20	25	$2,901	30	63.1
Kuwait	6.3	20.1		32	49	$70,107	100	99
Latvia	5.2	15.9	16.8	9.9	55	$23,080	88	99.3
Lebanon	9.3	27.7	47	20	28	$13,089	81	99
Lesotho		2	14		44	$2,770	30	81.6
Lithuania	7.6	7	12.9	5.8	61	$26,971	92	96.6
Luxembourg	11	8.2	24.1	20.5	81	$93,900	98	100
Malaysia	4.3	17.4	23	17.3	50	$25,312	96	98.2
Malta		12.8	32	49.2	56	$32,720	100	100
Mexico	2.4	42.1	46.3	29.9	35	$16,490	85	96.1

Table 1. *Cont.*

Country	Antibiotic Usage (Standard units per 1000 pop - CCDEP)	E. coli % Resistance 3rd gen ceph (WHO)	E. coli % Resistance Fluoroquinolones (WHO)	Staphylococcus Aureus (MRSA Rates - WHO)	2015 Corruption Index	GNP per capita 2015 (Purchasing Power Parity in 2011 Dollars)	% with Adequate Sanitation 2015	Improved Water Source (% of Population with Access)
Mongolia		64.1	64.7		39	$11,478	60	64.2
Morocco	6	4	23.3	19	36	$7,365	77	85.3
Myanmar		68	55	26	22	$4,931	80	80.5
Nepal		37.9	64.3	44.9	27	$2,312	46	90.7
Netherlands	4.1	5.7	14.3	1.4	87	$46,354	98	100
New Zealand	10.9	3	6.5	10.4	88	$35,159	100	100
Nicaragua		48.1	42.9		27	$4,884	68	86.9
Nigeria		6.7	36.5	47.1	26	$5,639	29	67.6
Norway	5.9	3.6	9	0.3	87	$63,650	98	100
Pakistan	7.1	36.2	35.3	37.6	30	$4,706	64	91.3
Panama		9.2	23.3	21.1	39	$20,885	75	94.4
Papua New Guinea		24.1	13.3	43.9	25	$2,723	19	40
Paraguay		1.4	22.1	27	27	$8,639	89	96.6
Peru	3.4	44.1	62.8	65.9	36	$11,768	76	86.3
Philippines	2.2	26.7	40.9	54.9	35	$6,938	74	91.5
Poland	9.3	11.7	27.3	24.3	62	$25,323	97	98.3
Portugal	9.3	11.3	27.2	54.6	63	$26,549	100	100
Puerto Rico	9.1						99	
Republic of Moldova		28	15.3	50.3	33	$4,742	76	88.4
Russian Federation	6.2	18	25.7	29.3	29	$24,124	72	96.9
Rwanda		21.4			54	$1,655	62	75.5
Serbia	10.6	21.3	16	44.5	40	$13,278	96	99.3
Singapore	5.7	20	37.8		85	$80,192	100	100
Slovakia	9.2	31	41.9	25.9	51	$28,254	99	100
Slovenia	6.3	8.8	20.7	7.1	60	$29,097	99	99.6
South Africa	8.7	8.2	16.1	52	44	$12,393	66	92.8
South Korea	10.9	24.4	40.9	65.3	56	$34,387	100	97.6
Spain	14.3	12	34.5	22.5	55	$32,219	100	100
Sri Lanka	3.9	58.9	58.8		37	$11,048	95	95.6

Table 1. *Cont.*

Country	Antibiotic Usage (Standard units per 1000 pop - CCDEP)	E. coli % Resistance 3rd gen ceph (WHO)	E. coli % Resistance Fluoroquinolones (WHO)	Staphylococcus Aureus (MRSA Rates - WHO)	2015 Corruption Index	GNP per capita 2015 (Purchasing Power Parity in 2011 Dollars)	% with Adequate Sanitation 2015	Improved Water Source (% of Population with Access)
Sudan		49.5	56.8		12	$4,121	24	58.5
Saudi Arabia	11.1	15.9	40.9	41.9	52	$50,284	100	97
Sweden	4.8	3	7.9	0.8	89	$45,488	99	100
Switzerland	5.2	8.2	20.2	10.2	86	$56,517	100	100
Syrian Arab Republic		49.8			18	$-	96	90.1
Taiwan	8.7				62			
Thailand	7	37.9	52.5	22.4	38	$15,347	93	97.8
Tunisia	18	20.6	9.4	55.8	38	$10,770	92	97.7
Turkey	18.5	43.3	46.3	31.5	42	$19,460	95	100
United Arab Emirates	10.5	23	32.5	33.4	70	$65,717	98	99.7
United Kingdom	9	9.6	17.5	13.6	81	$38,509	99	100
United States of America	10.3	14.6	33.3	51.3	76	$52,704	100	99.2
Uruguay	6.6	0	15	40	74	$19,952	96	99.6
Venezuela	8.1	12.5	37.2	31	17	$16,769	94	93.1
Vietnam	9.4		0.2		31	$5,667	78	96.4
Zambia		37.4	50.5	32	38	$3,602	44	64.6

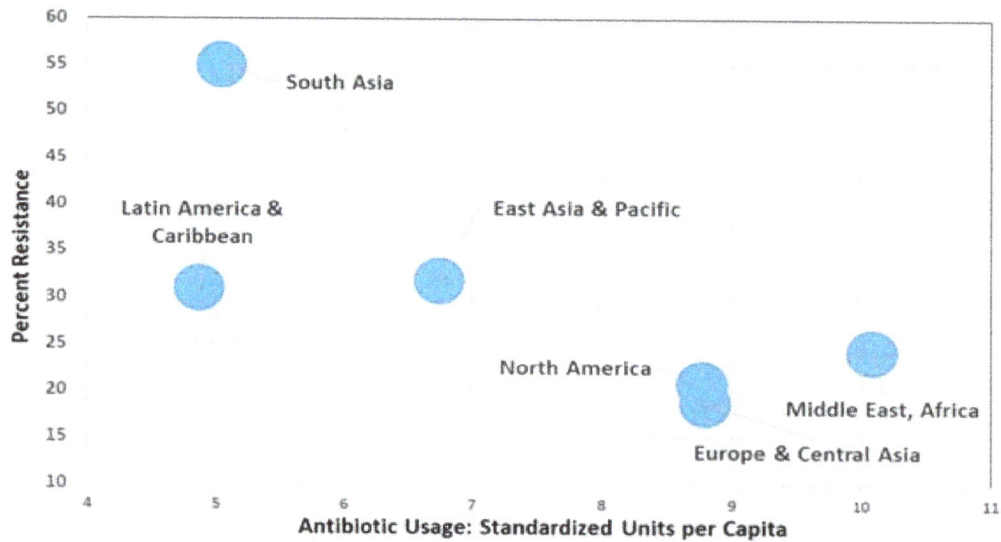

Figure 1. Global aggregated regions: antimicrobial resistance *E. coli* to third generation cephalosporins and fluoroquinolones versus antibiotic usage.

Aggregating countries into regional groupings shows a pattern where there is an inverse aggregate relationship between antimicrobial resistance and usage. These data help confirm that there are other very important factors influencing antimicrobial resistance over and above simply antibiotic usage. (Figures assembled from data taken from reference 7)

The World Organization for Animal Health has developed a global database on the use of antimicrobial agents in animals [46]. Figure 2 shows reported quantities of antimicrobials used in animals in 2014, summarized by OIE Region and expressed as total quantities (tons) and adjusted for animal biomass. Additionally, included is the per cent of countries authorizing the use of antimicrobials for growth promotion. Tetracyclines accounted for the largest proportion of overall antimicrobial use globally (37.1% of total), followed by polypeptides (15.7%), penicillins (9.8%), macrolides (8.9%) and aminoglycosides (7.8%) [46].

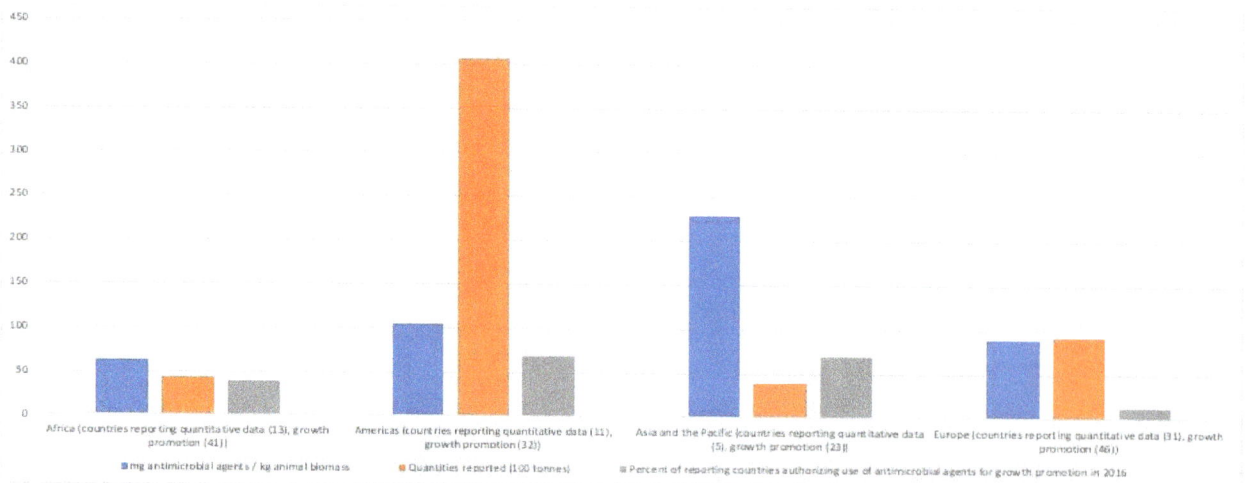

Figure 2. Reported use of antimicrobial agents in animals in 2014 by World Organisation for Animal Health (OIE) Region (adapted from [46]).

3. One Health Antimicrobial Resistance Case Studies

The following examples illustrate antimicrobial resistance problems that arise when the same classes of antimicrobials are used in humans and animals, and the challenges that arise from competing interests and imbalances of risk and benefit in various sectors.

3.1. Third Generation Cephalosporins

Third generation cephalosporins are broad spectrum beta-lactam antimicrobials that are widely used in humans and animals. In people, cefotaxime, ceftriaxone and several other members of the class are used for a wide variety of frequently serious infections, particularly in hospital settings, for example bloodstream infections due to *Escherichia coli* and other bacteria, but also in community settings, for example *Neisseria gonorrhea* [47]. Third generation cephalosporins are classified as "critically important" for human health [47].

Ceftiofur is the principal third generation cephalosporin for veterinary use; others include cefpodoxime, cefoperazone and cefovecin. Ceftiofur is injected and used in animals as therapy to treat pneumonia, arthritis, septicemia and other conditions [48,49]. However ceftiofur is also used in mass therapy (metaphylaxis or prophylaxis), either under an approved label claim (e.g., injection of feedlot cattle for control of bovine respiratory disease), or off-label (e.g., injection of hatching eggs or day-old chicks for prevention of *E. coli* infections). Factors that encourage overuse of ceftiofur are its broad spectrum activity, zero withdrawal time for milk from dairy animals (due to its high maximum residual level; MRL), and availability of a long-acting preparation [48,49].

In Europe, approximately 14 tons of third and fourth generation cephalosporins were used in 2014 for use in animals [28]. Similar volumes are used in the US [50]. In many countries, cephalosporins are commonly used in humans but with wide variations. Overall, 101 tons of third generation cephalosporins were used in people Europe in 2012 [29] and in the US, approximately 82 tons in 2011 [51].

Resistance to the third generation cephalosporins is mainly mediated by extended-spectrum beta-lactamases (ESBLs) and AmpC beta-lactamases [47]. ESBL genes are highly mobile and transmitted on plasmids, transposons and other genetic elements. AmpC beta-lactamases were originally reported to be chromosomal but have also been identified on plasmids and to have spread horizontally among *Enterobacteriaceae* [47]. Unfortunately, in many countries resistance to third generation cephalosporins is now common among *E. coli* and *K. pneumonia* [52,53]. Resistance genes are frequently co-located with genes encoding resistance to other classes of antimicrobials, including tetracyclines, aminoglycosides and sulfonamides. As a consequence, the use of other antimicrobials in animals, for example tetracyclines administered in feed, can select for ESBL strains of bacteria [54].

Ceftiofur can be administered to eggs or day-old chicks in hatcheries, using automated equipment that injects small quantities of the drug into the many thousands of hatching eggs or chicks intended for treated flocks as prophylaxis against *E. coli* infections [55,56]. This practice selected for cephalosporin resistance in *Salmonella* Heidelberg, an important cause of human illness and associated with consumption of poultry products [57]. Surveillance detected a high degree of time-related correlations in trends of resistance to ceftiofur (and ceftriaxone, a drug of choice for treatment of severe cases of salmonellosis in children and pregnant women) among *Salmonella* Heidelberg from clinical infections in humans, from poultry samples collected at retail, and in *E. coli* from retail poultry samples [55]. Voluntary termination of ceftiofur use in hatcheries in Quebec was followed by a precipitous drop in the prevalence of resistance to ceftiofur. Subsequent re-introduction of its use, was followed by a return to higher prevalence of resistance [56]. In recognition of the resultant human health risks, in 2014, the Canadian poultry industry placed a voluntary ban on the use of ceftiofur and other critically important antimicrobials for disease prophylaxis [58].

In Japan, voluntary withdrawal of the off-label use of ceftiofur in hatcheries in 2012 was also followed by a significant decrease in broad-spectrum cephalosporin resistance in *E. coli* from broilers [59]. Some other countries (e.g., Denmark and Australia) have also placed voluntary restrictions in its use [60]. The label claim for day-old injection of poultry flocks was withdrawn in Europe, while some countries banned off-label use of third generation cephalosporins (e.g., U.S.) [48,61], and in other countries there is a requirement that use is restricted to situations where no other effective approved drugs are available for treatment [62].

3.2. Colistin

Colistin is in the polymyxin class of antimicrobials, and has been used in both people and animals for over 50 years [63]. Polymyxins, when administered systemically, frequently cause nephrotoxicity and neurotoxicity in people [64]. Thus, until recently its use was mainly limited to topical use and the treatment of infections in cystic fibrosis patients by inhalation (with a colistimethate sodium).

Colistin however is now used much more frequently, as a drug of last resort by injection, for treatment of multi-resistant gram-negative infections including carbapenem-resistant *Pseudomonas aeruginosa* and *E. coli* [65–67]. Where approved for use in food animals (e.g., Brazil, Europe, China), most colistin is administered orally to groups of pigs, poultry and in some cases calves, for treatment and prophylaxis of diarrhea due to gram-negative infections or for growth promotion [63,67,68]. In countries where data are available, the quantities consumed for animal production vastly exceed those used in humans and is very variable between countries [69]. In 2013 total animal consumption in Europe was 495 tons; 99.7% in oral form (e.g., for oral solution, medicated feed premix and oral powder) [63]. In China, the world's largest producer of pigs and poultry, an estimated 12,000 tons of colistin was used in food animals [68].

Until recently, limited data on colistin resistance were available, partly because of technical difficulties in phenotypic susceptibility testing [63,70]. In Europe in 2016, resistance was found in 1.9% of indicator *E. coli* from broilers, 3.9% from broiler meat, 6.1% from turkeys and 10.1% from turkey meat [71]. Colistin resistance was thought limited to chromosomal mutation and was essentially non-transferable [63], however in 2015 the transferable plasmid-mediated colistin resistance gene, mcr-1, was found in *E. coli* isolates obtained from animals, food and human bloodstream infections from China [68]. Spread of the gene by conjugation has been shown in *Klebsiella pneumoniae, Enterobacter aerogenes, Enterobacter spp.* and *P. aeruginosa* [68]. Retrospective analyses have demonstrated the mcr-1 gene in several bacterial species isolated from humans, animals and environmental samples in numerous countries [72–76], and the gene was found in about 5% of healthy travelers [77]. The earliest identification of the gene thus far was in *E. coli* from poultry collected in the 1980s in China [78]. The mcr-1 gene has also been detected in isolates obtained from wildlife and surface water samples, demonstrating environmental contamination [79]. Recently, other plasmid-mediated colistin resistance genes has been reported for example mcr-2 in *E. coli* from pigs in Belgium [80].

Colistin illustrates some important One Health dimensions of antimicrobial resistance that differ from those of third generation cephalosporins. The toxicity with systemic use and the availability of other safer and more effective antimicrobials, meant for many years colistin was mainly used topically in people. However with the emergence of multi-drug resistance in many Gram-negative bacteria, there has been increasing need for this drug to systemically treat severe, life-threatening infections in humans in many countries. The colistin case demonstrates (once again) that using large quantities antimicrobials for group treatments or growth promotion in animals can lead to significant antimicrobial resistance problems for human health, even if the drug class is initially believed to be of lesser importance, because the relative importance of antimicrobials to human health can change. This is the same problem that arose from using avoparcin as a growth promoter until it was banned; it selected for resistance to another glycopeptide, vancomycin, which is used for the treatment of life-threatening MRSA (methicillin resistant *Staphylococcus aureus*) and for treating serious enterococcal infections (the latter especially in penicillin allergic patients) [81,82].

4. Risks to Public Health and Animal Health

Antimicrobial resistance is harmful to health because it reduces the effectiveness of antimicrobial therapy and tends to increase the severity, incidence and costs of infection [3,83]. There is now considerable evidence that antimicrobial use in animals is an important contributor to antimicrobial resistance among some pathogens of humans, in particular, common enteric pathogens such as *Salmonella spp., Campylobacter spp., Enterococcus spp.* and *E. coli* [6,18,26,38,41].

Non-typhoidal *Salmonella* (NTS) are among the most common bacteria isolated from foodborne infections of humans. Globally, there are approximately 94 million cases, including 155,000 deaths each year [1]. Animals are the most important reservoirs of NTS for humans [38,84–86]. Fecal shedding by carrier animals is an important source of antimicrobial resistant *Salmonella* contamination of meat and poultry products [38], and may also be responsible for fruit and vegetable contamination through fecal contamination of the environment [87]. *Salmonella* resistance to any medically important antimicrobial is of concern, but particularly to those critically important to human health, such as cephalosporins and fluoroquinolones [38,41,56]. Therapy in some groups (e.g., children and pregnant women) can be very restricted and beta-lactams such as third generation cephalosporins often may be the only therapy available to treat serious infections.

From the One Health antimicrobial resistance perspective, the third generation cephalosporins are good examples of antimicrobials that are considered critically important for both human and animal health. The main concern regarding selection and spread of resistance from animals to humans is their use as mass medications in large numbers of animals, either for therapy or prophylaxis. There are parallels with fluoroquinolones, another class of critically important antimicrobials, to which resistance among *Campylobacter jejuni* emerged following mass medication of poultry flocks [88–90]. In Australia where fluoroquinolones were never approved in food animals, fluoroquinolone resistant strains in food animals remain very rare [91].

Fluoroquinolone use in food animals is also linked to quinolone resistance in *Salmonella* [41,92–94]. Surveillance data compiled by WHO indicate that rates of fluoroquinolone resistance in non-typhoidal *Salmonella* vary widely by geographical region. For example, rates are relatively low in Europe (2–3%), higher in the Eastern Mediterranean region (up to 40–50%) and wide ranging in the Americas (0–96%) (1). Many *Salmonella* are also resistant to antimicrobials that have long been used as growth promoters in many countries (e.g., Canada, USA) including tetracyclines, penicillins and sulfonamides [41,84]. Antimicrobial resistance in some of the more virulent *Salmonella* serovars (e.g., Heidelberg, Newport, Typhimurium) has been associated with more severe infections in humans [38,83,86,95]. Resistance to other critically important antimicrobials continues to emerge in *Salmonella*, for example, a carbapenem resistant strain of *Salmonella* was identified on a pig farm that routinely administered prophylactic cephalosporin (ceftiofur) to piglets [96].

Escherichia coli are important pathogens of both humans and animals. In humans, *E. coli* are a common cause of serious bacterial infections, including enteritis, urinary tract infection and bloodstream infections [97–99]. Currently in England the rate for blood stream infections is about 64 cases per 100,000 per year and rising. A large and increasing proportion involves antimicrobial resistance, including fluoroquinolone resistance [100]. These higher rates are also being seen in countries with good surveillance systems in place, for example Denmark [60].

Many *E. coli* appear to behave as commensals of the gut of animals and humans, but may be opportunistic pathogens as well as donors of resistance genetic elements for pathogenic *E. coli* or other species of bacteria [101,102]. Although antimicrobial resistance is a rapidly increasing problem in *E. coli* infections of both animals and humans, the problem is better documented for isolates from human infections, where resistance is extensive, particularly in developing countries [1,103]. Humans are regularly exposed to antimicrobial resistant *E. coli* through foods and inadequately treated drinking water [104,105].

Travelers from developed countries are at risk of acquiring multi-resistance *E. coli* from other people or contaminated food and/or water [97,105,106]. There are now serious problems with extended spectrum beta lactamase (ESBL) *E. coli* in both developing and developed countries and foods from animals, in particular poultry, have been implicated as sources for humans [99,107,108], although the magnitude of the contribution from food animals is uncertain [102–104].

Given the critical importance of third and fourth generation cephalosporins and fluoroquinolones to human medicine and the clear evidence that treatment of entire groups of animals selects for resistance in important pathogens that spread from animals to humans [56,90], these drugs should be used rarely, if at all in animals, and only when supporting laboratory data demonstrate that no suitable alternatives of lesser human health importance are available. Their use as mass medications should be restricted.

Serious staphylococcal infections in people are common, including with Methicillin-resistant *Staphylococcus aureus* (MRSA) in both community and hospital settings, causing skin, wound, bloodstream and other types of infection [1,109–111]. *Staphylococcus aureus* and other staphylococci are also recognized pathogens of animals, for example they are responsible for cases of mastitis in cattle, and skin infections in pigs and companion animals [112,113]. MRSA were until recently relatively rare in animals but strains pathogenic to humans have emerged in several animal species [113–116]. Transmission to humans is thought currently to be mainly through contact with carrier animals [116]. The predominant strain isolated from animals is sequence type (ST) 398, and while pathogenic to humans, it is not considered a major epidemic strain [112,113]. Antimicrobial use in livestock, as well as lapses in biosecurity within and between farms, and international trade in animals, food or other products, are factors contributing to the spread of this pathogen in animals [113,117].

5. One Health Considerations from the Environment

One Health includes consideration of the environment as well as human and animal health [23,111]. The ecological nature of antimicrobial resistance is a reflection and consequence of the interconnectedness and diversity of life on the planet [22]. Many pathogenic bacteria, the antimicrobials that we use to treat them, and genes that confer resistance, have environmental origins (e.g., soil) [8,14,20]. Some important resistance genes, such as beta lactamases, are millions of years old [14,15]. Soil and other environmental matrices are rich sources of highly diverse populations of bacteria and their genes [14,118]. Antimicrobial resistance to a wide variety of drugs has been demonstrated in environmental bacteria isolated from the pre-antibiotic era, as well as from various sites (e.g., caves) free of other sources of exposure to modern antimicrobials [8,15,111,119]. Despite having ancient origins, there is abundant evidence that human activity has an impact on the resistome, which is the totality of resistance genes in the wider environment [13,14,118,119]. Hundreds of thousands of tons of antimicrobials are produced annually and find their way into the environment [18,27]. Waste from treatment plants and pharmaceutical industry, particularly if inadequately treated, can release high concentrations of antimicrobials into surface water [18,19,120,121]. Residues of antimicrobials are constituents of human sewage, livestock manure, and aquaculture, along with fecal bacteria and resistance genes [118,122–125]. Sewage treatment and composting of manure reduce concentrations of some but not all antimicrobials and microorganisms, which are introduced to soil upon land application of human and animal bio-solids [126].

Various environmental pathways are important routes of human exposure to resistant bacteria and their genes from animal and plant reservoirs [18,96,127] and provide opportunities for better regulations to control antimicrobial resistance. In developed countries with good quality sewage and drinking water treatment, and where most people have little to no direct contact with food-producing animals, transmission of bacteria and resistance genes from agricultural sources is largely foodborne, either from direct contamination of meat and poultry during slaughter and processing, or indirectly from fruit and vegetables contaminated by manure or irrigation water [38,87,90].

In countries with poor sewage and water treatment, drinking water is likely to be very important in transmission of resistant bacteria and/or genes from animals [11,97,111,120]). Poor sanitation also facilitates indirect person–person waterborne transmission of enteric bacteria among residents as well as international travelers who then return home colonized with resistant bacteria acquired locally [103,128]. Through these and other means, including globalized trade in animals and food, and long-distance migratory patterns of wildlife, antimicrobial resistant bacteria are globally disseminated.

General measures to address antimicrobial resistance in the wider environment include improved controls on pollution from industrial, residential and agricultural sources. Improved research as well as environmental monitoring and risk assessment is required to better understand the role of the environment in selection and spread of antimicrobial resistance, and to identify more specific measures to address resistance in this sector [12,14,18,100,103,129].

6. One Health Strategies to Address Antimicrobial Resistance

WHO and other international agencies (e.g., Food and Agriculture Organization (FAO), World Organization for Animal Health (OIE)), along with many individual countries, have developed comprehensive action plans to address the antimicrobial resistance crisis [5,130–136]. The WHO Global Action Plan seeks to address five major objectives that comprise the subtitles of the following sections. The WHO Plan embraces a One Health approach to address antimicrobial resistance, and it calls on member countries to do the same when developing their own action plans (6). There are five main pillars to the WHO Global Plan:

1. Improve Awareness and Understanding of Antimicrobial Resistance through Effective Communication, Education and Training
2. Strengthen the Knowledge and Evidence Base through Surveillance and Research
3. Reduce the Incidence of Infection through Effective Sanitation, Hygiene and Infection Prevention Measures
4. Optimize the Use of Antimicrobial Medicines in Human and Animal Health
5. Develop the Economic Case tor Sustainable Investment that Takes Account of the Needs of All Countries, and Increase Investment in New Medicines, Diagnostic Tools, Vaccines and Other Interventions

The One Health approach laid out in the WHO Global Action Plan is appropriate and consistent with statements made in action plans from other international and national organizations. There is however, a long way to go before a fully integrated One Health approach to antimicrobial resistance is implemented at country and global levels. Among the numerous barriers to overcome include the competing interests among multiple sectors (involving animals, humans, and environment) and organizations, agreement on priorities for action, and gaps in antimicrobial resistance surveillance, antimicrobial use policy, and infection control in many parts of the world.

7. Conclusions

History has shown that it is not feasible to neatly separate antimicrobial classes into those exclusively for use in human or non-human sectors, with the exception of new antimicrobial classes. These should probably be reserved for use in humans as long as there are few or no alternatives available. The majority of classes, however, will be available for use in both sectors and the challenge for One Health is to ensure that use of these drugs is optimal overall. This is likely to be achieved when antimicrobials used in both sectors are used for therapy, only rarely for prophylaxis and never for growth promotion, and when we better control the types and amounts of antimicrobials plus the numbers of resistant bacteria we allow to be placed into the environment. What is vitally important is that we do more to stop the spread of resistant bacteria—not only from person to person but between and within the human and agriculture sectors and the environment, giving particular emphasis to controls of contaminated water.

References

1. World Health Organization (WHO). *Antimicrobial Resistance: Global Report on Surveillance*; WHO: Geneva, Switzerland, 2014.

2. Centers for Disease Control (CDC). *Antibiotic Resistance Threats in the United States*; CDC: Atlanta, GA, USA, 2013.

3. O'Neill, J. Tackling Drug-Resistant Infections Globally: Final Report and Recommendations the Review On Antimicrobial Resistance. 2016. Available online: https://amr-review.org/sites/default/files/160525_Finalpaper_withcover.pdf (accessed on 15 January 2019).

4. Laxminarayan, R.; Duse, A.; Wattal, C.; Zaidi, A.K.M.; Wertheim, H.F.L.; Sumpradit, N.; Vlieghe, E.; Hara, G.L.; Gould, I.M.; Goossens, H.; et al. Antibiotic Resistance—The Need for Global Solutions. *Lancet Infect. Dis.* **2013**, *13*, 1057–1098. [CrossRef]

5. World Health Organization (WHO). *Global Action Plan on Antimicrobial Resistance*; WHO: Geneva, Switzerland, 2015. Available online: http://www.wpro.who.int/entity/drug_resistance/resources/global_action_plan_eng.pdf (accessed on 15 January 2019).

6. Aarestrup, F.M.; Wegener, H.C.; Collignon, P. Resistance in Bacteria of The Food Chain: Epidemiology and Control Strategies. *Expert Rev. Anti-Infect. Ther.* **2008**, *6*, 733–750. [CrossRef]

7. Collignon, P.; Beggs, J.J.; Walsh, T.R.; Gandra, S.; Laxminarayan, R. Anthropological and Socioeconomic Factors Contributing to Global Antimicrobial Resistance: A Univariate and Multivariable Analysis. *Lancet Planet Heal.* **2018**, *2*, e398–e405. [CrossRef]

8. Holmes, A.H.; Moore, L.S.P.; Sundsfjord, A.; Steinbakk, M.; Regmi, S.; Karkey, A.; Guerin, P.J.; Piddock, L.J. Understanding the Mechanisms and Drivers of Antimicrobial Resistance. *Lancet* **2016**, *387*, 176–187. [CrossRef]

9. Burow, E.; Käsbohrer, A. Risk Factors for Antimicrobial Resistance in *Escherichia coli* in Pigs Receiving Oral Antimicrobial Treatment: A Systematic Review. *Microb. Drug Resist.* **2017**, *23*, 194–205. [CrossRef] [PubMed]

10. Marti, E.; Variatza, E.; Balcazar, J.L. The Role of Aquatic Ecosystems as Reservoirs of Antibiotic Resistance. *Trends Microbiol.* **2014**, *22*, 36–41. [CrossRef]

11. Bürgmann, H.; Frigon, D.; Gaze, W.H.; Manaia, C.M.; Pruden, A.; Singer, A.C.; Smets, B.F.; Zhang, T. Water and Sanitation: An Essential Battlefront in the War on Antimicrobial Resistance. *FEMS Microbiol. Ecol.* **2018**, *94*, fiy101. [CrossRef]

12. Huijbers, P.M.C.; Blaak, H.; de Jong, M.C.M.; Graat, E.A.M.; Vandenbroucke-Grauls, C.M.J.E.; de Roda Husman, A.M. Role of the Environment in the Transmission of Antimicrobial Resistance to Humans: A Review. *Environ. Sci. Technol.* **2015**, *49*, 11993–12004. [CrossRef]

13. Anonymous. Initiatives for Addressing Antimicrobial Resistance in the Environment: Current Situation and Challenges. 2018. Available online: https://wellcome.ac.uk/sites/default/files/antimicrobial-resistance-environment-report.pdf (accessed on 15 January 2019).

14. Gaze, W.H.; Krone, S.M.; Larsson, D.G.J.; Li, X.-Z.; Robinson, J.A.; Simonet, P.; Smalla, K.; Timinouni, M.; Topp, E.; Wellington, E.M.; et al. Influence of Humans on Evolution and Mobilization of Environmental Antibiotic Resistome. *Emerg. Infect. Dis.* **2013**, *19*, e120871. [CrossRef]

15. Perry, J.A.; Wright, G.D. Forces Shaping the Antibiotic Resistome. *BioEssays* **2014**, *36*, 1179–1184. [CrossRef]

16. Woolhouse, M.E.J.; Ward, M.J. Sources of Antimicrobial Resistance. *Science* **2013**, *341*, 1460–1461. [CrossRef]

17. Heuer, O.E.; Kruse, H.; Grave, K.; Collignon, P.; Karunasagar, I.; Angulo, F.J. Human Health Consequences of Use of Antimicrobial Agents in Aquaculture. *Clin. Infect. Dis.* **2009**, *49*, 1248–1253. [CrossRef]

18. O'Neill, J. Antimicrobials in Agriculture and the Environment: Reducing Unnecessary Use and Waste. The Review on Antimicrobial Resistance. 2015. Available online: https://amr-review.org/sites/default/files/Antimicrobialsinagricultureandtheenvironment---Reducingunnecessaryuseandwaste.pdf (accessed on 15 January 2019).

19. So, A.D.; Shah, T.A.; Roach, S.; Ling Chee, Y.; Nachman, K.E. An Integrated Systems Approach is Needed to Ensure the Sustainability of Antibiotic Effectiveness for Both Humans and Animals. *J. Law Med. Ethics* **2015**, *43*, 38–45. [CrossRef] [PubMed]

20. Collignon, P. The Importance of a One Health Approach to Preventing the Development and Spread of Antibiotic Resistance. In *One Health: The Human-Animal-Environment Interfaces in Emerging Infectious Diseases: Food Safety and Security, and International and National Plans for Implementation of One Health Activities*; Mackenzie, J.S., Jeggo, M., Daszak, P., Richt, J.A., Eds.; Springer: Berlin/Heidelberg, Germany, 2013; pp. 19–36.

21. Torren-Edo, J.; Grave, K.; Mackay, D. "One Health": The Regulation and Consumption of Antimicrobials for Animal Use in the EU. *IHAJ* **2015**, *2*, 14–16.

22. Robinson, T.P.; Bu, D.P.; Carrique-Mas, J.; Fèvre, E.M.; Gilbert, M.; Grace, D.; Hay, S.I.; Jiwakanon, J.; Kakkar, M.; Kariuki, S.; et al. Antibiotic Resistance is the Quintessential One Health Issue. *Trans. R. Soc. Trop. Med. Hyg.* **2016**, *110*, 377–380. [CrossRef] [PubMed]

23. Zinsstag, J.; Meisser, A.; Schelling, E.; Bonfoh, B.; Tanner, M. From 'Two Medicines' to 'One Health' and Beyond. *Onderstepoort J. Vet. Res.* **2012**, *79*, a492. [CrossRef]

24. World Health Organization. One Health. 2017. Available online: https://www.who.int/features/qa/one-health/en/ (accessed on 15 January 2019).

25. One Health Commission. What is One Health? 2018. Available online: https://www.onehealthcommission.org/en/why_one_health/what_is_one_health/ (accessed on 15 January 2019).

26. McEwen, S.A.; Fedorka-Cray, P.J. Antimicrobial Use and Resistance in Animals. *Clin. Infect. Dis.* **2002**, *34*, S93–S106. [CrossRef]

27. Van Boeckel, T.P.; Brower, C.; Gilbert, M.; Grenfell, B.T.; Levin, S.A.; Robinson, T.P.; Teillant, A.; Laxminarayan, R. Global Trends in Antimicrobial Use in Food Animals. *Proc. Natl. Acad. Sci. USA* **2015**, *112*, 5649–5654. [CrossRef]

28. European Medicines Agency (EMA). *Sales of Veterinary Antimicrobial Agents in 29 European Countries in 2014*; EMA: London, UK, 2016.

29. ECDC (European Centre for Disease Prevention and Control); EFSA (European Food Safety Authority); EMA (European Medicines Agency). ECDC/EFSA/EMA First Joint Report on The Integrated Analysis of The Consumption of Antimicrobial Agents and Occurrence of Antimicrobial Resistance in Bacteria from Humans and Food-Producing Animals. *EFSA J.* **2015**, *13*, 4006. [CrossRef]

30. Food and Agriculture Organization (FAO). Drivers, Dynamics and Epidemiology of Antimicrobial Resistance in Animal Oroduction. 2016. Available online: http://www.fao.org/3/a-i6209e.pdf (accessed on 15 January 2019).

31. Vidaver, A.K. Uses of Antimicrobials in Plant Agriculture. *Clin. Infect. Dis.* **2002**, *34*, S107–S110. [CrossRef]

32. Sundin, G.W.; Wang, N. Antibiotic Resistance in Plant-Pathogenic Bacteria. *Annu. Rev. Phytopathol.* **2018**, *56*, 161–180. [CrossRef] [PubMed]

33. Collignon, P. Use of Critically Important Antimicrobials in Food Production. In *Kucers' The Use of Antibiotics: A Clinical Review of Antibacterial, Antifungal, Antiparasitic and Antiviral Drugs*, 7th ed.; Grayson, L., Ed.; American Society for Microbiology and CRC Press: Boca Raton, FL, USA, 2018; pp. 9–18.

34. Sykes, J.E. Antimicrobial Drug Use in Dogs and Cats. In *Antimicrobial Therapy in Veterinary Medicine*, 5th ed.; Giguère, S., Prescott, J.F., Dowling, P.M., Eds.; John Wiley & Sons, Inc.: Hoboken, NJ, USA, 2013; pp. 473–494.

35. Giguère, S.; Abrams-Ogg, A.C.G.; Kruth, S.A. Prophylactic Use of Antimicrobial Agents, and Antimicrobial Chemotherapy for the Neutropenic Patient. In *Antimicrobial Therapy in Veterinary Medicine*, 5th ed.; Giguère, S., Prescott, J.F., Dowling, P.M., Eds.; John Wiley & Sons, Inc.: Hoboken, NJ, USA, 2013; pp. 357–378.

36. National Research Council. *The Use of Drugs in Food Animals: Benefits and Risks*; The National Academies Press: Washington, DC, USA, 1999.

37. Murphy, D.; Ricci, A.; Auce, Z.; Beechinor, J.G.; Bergendahl, H.; Breathnach, R.; Bures, J.; Pedro, J.; da Silva, D.; Hederová, J.; et al. EMA and EFSA Joint Scientific Opinion on Measures to Reduce the Need to Use Antimicrobial Agents in Animal Husbandry in the European Union, and the Resulting Impacts on Food Safety (RONAFA). *EFSA J.* **2017**, *15*, 4666.

38. Food and Agriculture Organization (FAO); World Organisation for Animal Health (OIE); World Health Organization (WHO) (FAO/OIE/WHO). *Joint FAO/OIE/WHO Expert Workshop on Non-Human Antimicrobial Usage and Antimicrobial Resistance: Scientific Assessment*; WHO: Geneva, Switzerland, 2003.

39. Food and Agriculture Organization (FAO); World Health Organization (WHO). *FAO/WHO Expert Meeting on Foodborne Antimicrobial Resistance: Role of Environment, Crops and Biocides. Summary Report*; FAO: Rome, Italy, 2018.

40. Zuraw, L. Perdue Announces Dramatic Reduction in Antibiotic Use in its Chickens. Food Safety News. 2014. Available online: http://www.foodsafetynews.com/2014/09/perdue-dramatically-reduces-antibiotic-use-in-chickens/#.WjLZulQ-dTZ (accessed on 15 January 2019).

41. World Health Organization (WHO). *Impacts of Antimicrobial Growth Promoter Termination in Denmark. The WHO International Review Panel's Evaluation of the Termination of the Use of Antimicrobial Growth Promoters in Denmark*; WHO: Foulum, Denmark, 2003.

42. World Health Organization (WHO). *The Medical Impact of the Use of Antimicrobials in Food Animals*; WHO: Berlin, Germany, 1997.

43. European Union (EU). Guidelines for the Prudent Use of Antimicrobials in Veterinary Medicine (2015/C 299/04). *Off. J. Eur. Union* **2015**, *C299*, C299:7–C299:26.

44. Food and Drug Administration (FDA). *Guidance for Industry #213. New Animal Drugs and New Animal Drug Combination Products Administered in or on Medicated Feed or Drinking Water of Food-Producing Animals: Recommendations for Drug Sponsors for Voluntarily Aligning Product Use Conditions with GFI #209*; FDA: Rockville, MD, USA, 2013.

45. Mehrotra, M.; Li, X.-Z.; Ireland, M.J. Enhancing Antimicrobial Stewardship by Strengthening the Veterinary Drug Regulatory Framework. *Can. Commun. Dis. Rep.* **2017**, *43*, 220–223. [CrossRef]

46. World Organisation for Animal Health (OIE). *OIE Annual Report on Antimicrobial Agents Intended for Use in Animals. Second Report*; OIE: Paris, France, 2018. Available online: http://www.oie.int/fileadmin/Home/eng/Our_scientific_expertise/docs/pdf/AMR/Annual_Report_AMR_2.pdf (accessed on 15 January 2019).

47. WHO Advisory Group on Integrated Surveillance of Antimicrobial Resistance (AGISAR). *Critically Important Antimicrobials for Human Medicine*; 4th revision 2013; World Health Organization: Geneva, Switzerland, 2016.

48. European Medicines Agency (EMA). *Revised Reflection Paper on the Use of 3rd and 4th Generation Cephalosporins in Food Producing Animals in the European Union: Development of Resistance and Impact on Human and Animal Health*; EMA: London, UK, 2009.

49. Prescott, J.F. Beta-lactam Antibiotics. In *Antimicrobial Therapy in Veterinary Medicine*, 5th ed.; Giguère, S., Prescott, J.F., Dowling, P.M., Eds.; John Wiley & Sons, Inc.: Hoboken, NJ, USA, 2013; pp. 153–173.

50. Food and Drug Administration (FDA). *2017 Summary Report on Antimicrobials Sold or Distributed for Use in Food-Producing Animals*; FDA: Washington, DC, USA, 2018.

51. Food and Drug Administration (FDA). *Drug Use Review. Food and Drug Administration, Department of Health and Human Services*; FDA: Washington, DC, USA, 2012. Available online: http://www.fda.gov/downloads/Drugs/DrugSafety/InformationbyDrugClass/UCM319435.pdf (accessed on 15 January 2019).

52. de Kraker, M.E.A.; Wolkewitz, M.; Davey, P.G.; Koller, W.; Berger, J.; Nagler, J.; Icket, C.; Kalenic, S.; Horvatic, J.; Seifert, H.; et al. Burden of Antimicrobial Resistance in European Hospitals: Excess Mortality and Length of Hospital Stay Associated with Bloodstream Infections due to *Escherichia coli* Resistant to Third-Generation Cephalosporins. *J. Antimicrob. Chemother.* **2011**, *66*, 398–407. [CrossRef]

53. Park, S.H. Third-Generation Cephalosporin Resistance in Gram-Negative Bacteria in the Community: A Growing Public Health Concern. *Korean J. Intern. Med.* **2014**, *29*, 27–30. [CrossRef] [PubMed]

54. Kanwar, N.; Scott, H.M.; Norby, B.; Loneragan, G.H.; Vinasco, J.; McGowan, M.; Cottell, J.L.; Chengappa, M.M.; Bai, J.; Boerlin, P. Effects of Ceftiofur and Chlortetracycline Treatment Strategies on Antimicrobial Susceptibility and on tet(A), tet(B), and blaCMY-2 Resistance Genes among *E. coli* Isolated from the Feces of Feedlot Cattle. *PLoS ONE* **2013**, *8*, e80575. [CrossRef]

55. Canadian Integrated Program for Antimicrobial Resistance (CIPARS). *Salmonella* Heidelberg—Ceftiofur-Related Resistance in Human and Retail Chicken Isolates. 2009. Available online: http://www.phac-aspc.gc.ca/cipars-picra/heidelberg/pdf/heidelberg_e.pdf (accessed on 15 January 2019).

56. Dutil, L.; Irwin, R.; Finley, R.; Ng, L.K.; Avery, B.; Boerlin, P.; Bourgault, A.M.; Cole, L.; Daignault, D.; Desruisseau, A.; et al. Ceftiofur Resistance in *Salmonella enterica* Serovar Heidelberg From Chicken Meat and Humans, Canada. *Emerg. Infect. Dis.* **2010**, *16*, 48–54. [CrossRef] [PubMed]

57. Smith, K.E.; Medus, C.; Meyer, S.D.; Boxrud, D.J.; Leano, F.; Hedberg, C.W.; Elfering, K.; Braymen, C.; Bender, J.B.; Danila, R.N. Outbreaks of Salmonellosis in Minnesota (1998 through 2006) Associated with Frozen, Microwaveable, Breaded, Stuffed Chicken Products. Vol. 71. *J. Food Prot.* **2008**, *71*, 2153–2160. [CrossRef] [PubMed]

58. Chicken Farmers of Canada. Antibiotics. 2018. Available online: https://www.chickenfarmers.ca/antibiotics/ (accessed on 15 January 2019).

59. Hiki, M.; Kawanishi, M.; Abo, H.; Kojima, A.; Koike, R.; Hamamoto, S.; Asai, T. Decreased Resistance to Broad-Spectrum Cephalosporin in *Escherichia coli* from Healthy Broilers at Farms in Japan After Voluntary Withdrawal of Ceftiofur. *Foodborne Pathog. Dis.* **2015**, *12*, 639–643. [CrossRef]

60. DANMAP 2014. Use of Antimicrobial Agents and Occurrence of Antimicrobial Resistance in Bacteria from Food Animals, Food and Humans in Denmark. Statens Serum Institut, National Veterinary Institute, Technical University of Denmark, National Food Institute, Technical University of Denmark, 2015. Available online: https://www.danmap.org/downloads/reports.aspx (accessed on 15 January 2019).

61. Department of Health and Human Services, Food and Drug Administration. 2012, 21 CFR Part 530 [Docket No. FDA–2008–N–0326] New Animal Drugs; Cephalosporin Drugs; Extra Label Animal Drug Use; Order of Prohibition. *Fed. Regist.* **2012**, *77*, 735–745.

62. European Medicines Agency (EMA). Answers to the Request for Scientific Advice on the Impact on Public Health and Animal Health of the Use of Antibiotics in Animals. 2014. Available online: http://www.ema.europa.eu/docs/en_GB/document_library/Other/2014/07/WC500170253.pdf (accessed on 15 January 2019).

63. European Medicines Agency (EMA). Updated Advice on the Use of Colistin Products in Animals Within the European Union: Development of Resistance and Possible Impact on Human and Animal Health. In *Committee for Medicinal Products for Veterinary use (CVMP), Committee for Medicinal Products*; EMA: London, UK, 2016.

64. Falagas, M.E.; Kasiakou, S.K. Toxicity of Polymyxins: A Systematic Review of the Evidence from Old and Recent Studies. *Crit. Care* **2006**, *10*, R27. [CrossRef] [PubMed]

65. Falagas, M.E.; Kasiakou, S.K.; Saravolatz, L.D. Colistin: The Revival of Polymyxins for the Management of Multidrug-Resistant Gram-Negative Bacterial Infections. *Clin. Infect. Dis.* **2005**, *40*, 1333–1341. [CrossRef] [PubMed]

66. Linden, P.K.; Kusne, S.; Coley, K.; Fontes, P.; Kramer, D.J.; Paterson, D. Use of Parenteral Colistin for the Treatment of Serious Infection Due to Antimicrobial-Resistant *Pseudomonas aeruginosa*. *Clin. Infect. Dis.* **2003**, *37*, e154–e160. [CrossRef]

67. Fernandes, M.R.; Moura, Q.; Sartori, L.; Silva, K.C.; Cunha, M.P.V.; Esposito, F.; Lopes, R.; Otutumi, L.K.; Gonçalves, D.D.; Dropa, M.; et al. Silent Dissemination of Colistin-Resistant *Escherichia coli* in South America Could Contribute to the Global Spread of the mcr-1 Gene. *Eurosurveillance* **2016**, *21*. [CrossRef]

68. Liu, Y.-Y.; Wang, Y.; Walsh, T.R.; Yi, L.-X.; Zhang, R.; Spencer, J.; Doi, Y.; Tian, G.; Dong, B.; Huang, X.; et al. Emergence of Plasmid-Mediated Colistin Rresistance Mechanism MCR-1 in Animals and Human Beings in China: A Microbiological and Molecular Biological Study. *Lancet Infect. Dis.* **2016**, *16*, 161–168. [CrossRef]

69. European Centers for Disease Control and Prevention (ECDC). *Summary of the Latest Data on Antibiotic Consumption in the European Union. Antibiotic Consumption in Europe*; ECDC: Stockholm, Sweden, 2015.

70. Landman, D.; Georgescu, C.; Martin, D.A.; Quale, J. Polymyxins Revisited. *Clin. Microbiol. Rev.* **2008**, *21*, 449–465. [CrossRef]

71. European Food Safety Authority (EFSA), European Centre for Disease Prevention and Control (ECDC). The European Union Summary Report on Antimicrobial Resistance in Zoonotic and Indicator Bacteria from Humans, Animals and Food in 2016. *EFSA J.* **2018**, *16*, e05182.

72. Catry, B.; Cavaleri, M.; Baptiste, K.; Grave, K.; Grein, K.; Holm, A.; Jukes, H.; Liebana, E.; Navas, A.L.; Mackay, D.; et al. Use of Colistin-Containing Products Within the European Union and European Economic Area (EU/EEA): Development of Resistance in Animals and Possible Impact on Human and Animal Health. *Int. J. Antimicrob Agents* **2015**, *46*, 297–306. [CrossRef]

73. Prim, N.; Rivera, A.; Rodríguez-Navarro, J.; Español, M.; Turbau, M.; Coll, P.; Mirelis, B. Detection of mcr-1 Colistin Resistance Gene in Polyclonal *Escherichia coli* Isolates in Barcelona, Spain, 2012 to 2015. *Eurosurveillance* **2016**, *21*. [CrossRef]

74. Irrgang, A.; Roschanski, N.; Tenhagen, B.-A.; Grobbel, M.; Skladnikiewicz-Ziemer, T.; Thomas, K.; Roesler, U.; Käsbohrer, A. Prevalence of mcr-1 in *E. coli* from Livestock and Food in Germany, 2010–2015. *PLoS ONE* **2016**, *11*, e0159863. [CrossRef]

75. Hasman, H.; Hammerum, A.M.; Hansen, F.; Hendriksen, R.S.; Olesen, B.; Agersø, Y.; Zankari, E.; Leekitcharoenphon, P.; Stegger, M.; Kaas, R.S.; et al. Detection of mcr-1 Encoding Plasmid-Mediated Colistin-Resistant *Escherichia coli* Isolates from Human Bloodstream Infection and Imported Chicken Meat, Denmark 2015. *Eurosurveillance* **2015**, *20*. [CrossRef] [PubMed]

76. Wang, R.; van Dorp, L.; Shaw, L.P.; Bradley, P.; Wang, Q.; Wang, X.; Jin, L.; Zhang, Q.; Liu, Y.; Rieux, A.; et al. The Global Distribution and Spread of the Mobilized Colistin Resistance Gene mcr-1. *Nat. Commun.* **2018**, *9*, 1179. [CrossRef]

77. von Wintersdorff, C.J.H.; Wolffs, P.F.G.; van Niekerk, J.M.; Beuken, E.; van Alphen, L.B.; Stobberingh, E.E.; Oude Lashof, A.M.L.; Hoebe, C.J.P.A.; Savelkoul, P.H.M.; Penders, J. Detection of the Plasmid-Mediated Colistin-Resistance Gene mcr-1 in Faecal Metagenomes of Dutch Travellers. *J. Antimicrob Chemother.* **2016**, *71*, 3416–3419. [CrossRef]

78. Shen, Z.; Wang, Y.; Shen, Y.; Shen, J.; Wu, C. Early Emergence of mcr-1 in *Escherichia coli* from Food-Producing Animals. *Lancet Infect. Dis.* **2016**, *16*, 293. [CrossRef]

79. Zurfuh, K.; Poirel, L.; Nordmann, P.; Nüesch-Inderbinen, M.; Hächler, H.; Stephan, R. Occurrence of the Plasmid-Borne mcr-1 Colistin Resistance Gene in Extended-Spectrum-β-Lactamase-Producing Enterobacteriaceae in River Water and Imported Vegetable Samples in Switzerland. *Antimicrob. Agents Chemother.* **2016**, *60*, 2594–2595. [CrossRef] [PubMed]

80. Xavier, B.B.; Lammens, C.; Ruhal, R.; Kumar-Singh, S.; Butaye, P.; Goossens, H.; Malhotra-Kumar, S. Identification of a Novel Plasmid-Mediated Colistin-Resistance Gene, mcr-2, in *Escherichia coli*, Belgium, June 2016. *Eurosurveillance* **2016**, *21*. [CrossRef]

81. Levine, D.P. Vancomycin: A History. *Clin. Infect. Dis.* **2006**, *42*, S5–S12. [CrossRef]

82. Bager, F.; Madsen, M.; Christensen, J.; Aarestrup, F.M. Avoparcin Used as a Growth Promoter is Associated with the Occurrence of Vancomycin-Resistant *Enterococcus faecium* on Danish Poultry and Pig Farms. *Prev. Vet. Med.* **1997**, *31*, 95–112. [CrossRef]

83. Barza, M. Potential Mechanisms of Increased Disease in Humans from Antimicrobial Resistance in Food Animals. *Clin. Infect. Dis.* **2002**, *34*, S123–S125. [CrossRef]

84. Anderson, E.S. Drug Resistance in *Salmonella typhimurium* and its Implications. *Br. Med. J.* **1968**, *3*, 333–339. [CrossRef] [PubMed]

85. Swann, M.M. *The Use of Antibiotics in Animal Husbandry and Veterinary Medicine*; HMSO: London, UK, 1969.

86. Institute of Medicine. *Human Health Risks with the Subtherapeutic Use of Penicillin or Tetracyclines in Animal Feed*; The National Academies Press: Washington, DC, USA, 1989.

87. Hanning, I.B.; Nutt, J.D.; Ricke, S.C. Salmonellosis Outbreaks in the United States Due to Fresh Produce: Sources and Potential Intervention Measures. *Foodborne Pathog. Dis.* **2009**, *6*, 635–648. [CrossRef] [PubMed]

88. Endtz, H.; Ruijs, G.; van Klingeren, B.; Jansen, W.H.; Reijden, T.; Mouton, R.P. Quinolone Resistance in *Campylobacter* Isolated from Man and Poultry Following the Introduction of Fluoroquinolones in Veterinary Medicine. *J. Antimicrob Chemother.* **1991**, *27*, 199–208. [CrossRef] [PubMed]

89. McDermott, P.F.; Bodeis, S.M.; English, L.L.; White, D.G.; WalkeR, R.D.; Zhao, S.; Simjee, S.; Wagne, D.D. Ciprofloxacin Resistance in *Campylobacter jejuni* Evolves Rapidly in Chickens Treated with Fluoroquinolones. *J. Infect. Dis.* **2002**, *185*, 837–840. [CrossRef]

90. Nelson, J.M.; Chiller, T.M.; Powers, J.H.; Angulo, F.J. Fluoroquinolone-Resistant *Campylobacter Species* and the Withdrawal of Fluoroquinolones from Use in Poultry: A Public Health Success Story. *Clin. Infect. Dis.* **2007**, *44*, 977–980. [CrossRef] [PubMed]

91. Cheng, A.C.; Turnidge, J.; Collignon, P.; Looke, D.; Barton, M.; Gottlieb, T. Control of Fluoroquinolone Resistance through Successful Regulation, Australia. *Emerg. Infect. Dis.* **2012**, *18*, 1453–1460. [CrossRef]

92. World Health Organization (WHO). *Use of Quinolones in Food Animals and Potential Impact on Human Health*; WHO: Geneva, Switzerland, 1998.

93. Chiu, C.H.; Wu, T.L.; Su, L.H.; Chu, C.; Chia, J.H.; Kuo, A.J.; Chien, M.S.; Lin, T.Y. The Emergence in Taiwan of Fluoroquinolone Resistance in *Salmonella enterica* Serotype Choleraesuis. *N. Engl. J. Med.* **2002**, *346*, 413–419. [CrossRef] [PubMed]

94. European Medicines Agency (EMA). *Reflection Paper on the Use of Fluoroquinolones in Food-Producing Animals in the European Union: Development of Resistance and Impact on Human and Animal Health*; EMEA/CVMP/SAGAM/184651/2005; EMA: London, UK, 2006.

95. Helms, M.; Simonsen, J.; Mølbak, K. Quinolone Resistance Is Associated with Increased Risk of Invasive Illness or Death during Infection with *Salmonella* Serotype Typhimurium. *J. Infect. Dis.* **2004**, *190*, 1652–1654. [CrossRef] [PubMed]

96. Mollenkopf, D.F.; Stull, J.W.; Mathys, D.A.; Bowman, A.S.; Feicht, S.M.; Grooters, S.V.; Daniels, J.B.; Wittum, T.E. Carbapenemase-Producing Enterobacteriaceae Recovered from the Environment of a Swine Farrow-to-Finish Operation in the United States. *Antimicrob. Agents Chemother.* **2017**, *61*, e01298-16. [CrossRef] [PubMed]

97. Kennedy, K.; Collignon, P. Colonisation with *Escherichia coli* Resistant to "Critically Important" Antibiotics: A High Risk for International Travellers. *Eur. J. Clin. Microbiol. Infect. Dis.* **2010**, *29*, 1501–1506. [CrossRef]

98. Laupland, K.B.; Church, D.L. Population-Based Epidemiology and Microbiology of Community-Onset Bloodstream Infections. *Clin. Microbiol. Rev.* **2014**, *27*, 647–664. [CrossRef] [PubMed]

99. Lazarus, B.; Paterson, D.L.; Mollinger, J.L.; Rogers, B.A. Do Human Extraintestinal *Escherichia coli* Infections Resistant to Expanded-Spectrum Cephalosporins Originate From Food-Producing Animals? A Systematic Review. *Clin. Infect. Dis.* **2015**, *60*, 439–452. [CrossRef] [PubMed]

100. Bou-Antoun, S.; Davies, J.; Guy, R.; Johnson, A.P.; Sheridan, E.A.; Hope, R.J. Descriptive Epidemiology of *Escherichia coli* Bacteraemia in England, April 2012 to March 2014. *Eurosurveillance* **2016**, *21*. [CrossRef] [PubMed]

101. Hammerum, A.M.; Larsen, J.; Andersen, V.D.; Lester, C.H.; Skovgaard Skytte, T.S.; Hansen, F.; Olsen, S.S.; Mordhorst, H.; Skov, R.L.; Aarestrup, F.M.; et al. Characterization of Extended-Spectrum β-lactamase (ESBL)-Producing *Escherichia coli* Obtained from Danish Pigs, Pig farmers and Their Families from Farms with High or no Consumption of Third- or Fourth-Generation Cephalosporins. *J. Antimicrob Chemother.* **2014**, *69*, 2650–2657. [CrossRef] [PubMed]

102. Collignon, P. Antibiotic Resistance: Are we all Doomed? *Intern. Med. J.* **2015**, *45*, 1109–1115. [CrossRef]

103. Walsh, T.R.; Weeks, J.; Livermore, D.M.; Toleman, M.A. Dissemination of NDM-1 positive Bacteria in the New Delhi Environment and its Implications for Human Health: An Environmental Point Prevalence Study. *Lancet Infect. Dis.* **2011**, *11*, 355–362. [CrossRef]

104. Graham, D.W.; Collignon, P.; Davies, J.; Larsson, D.G.J.; Snape, J. Underappreciated Role of Regionally Poor Water Quality on Globally Increasing Antibiotic Resistance. *Environ. Sci. Technol.* **2014**, *48*, 11746–11747. [CrossRef]

105. Tängdén, T.; Cars, O.; Melhus, Å.; Löwdin, E. Foreign Travel Is a Major Risk Factor for Colonization with *Escherichia coli* Producing CTX-M-Type Extended-Spectrum β-Lactamases: A Prospective Study with Swedish Volunteers. *Antimicrob. Agents Chemother.* **2010**, *54*, 3564–3568. [CrossRef]

106. Vieira, A.R.; Collignon, P.; Aarestrup, F.M.; McEwen, S.A.; Hendriksen, R.S.; Hald, T.; Wegener, H.C. Association Between Antimicrobial Resistance in *Escherichia coli* Isolates from Food Animals and Blood Stream Isolates From Humans in Europe: An Ecological Study. *Foodborne Pathog. Dis.* **2011**, *8*, 1295–1301. [CrossRef]

107. De Been, M.; Lanza, V.F.; de Toro, M.; Scharringa, J.; Dohmen, W.; Du, Y.; Hu, J.; Lei, Y.; Li, N.; Tooming-Klunderud, A.; et al. Dissemination of Cephalosporin Resistance Genes between *Escherichia coli* Strains from Farm Animals and Humans by Specific Plasmid Lineages. *PLOS Genet.* **2014**, *10*, e1004776. [CrossRef] [PubMed]

108. Jakobsen, L.; Kurbasic, A.; Skjøt-Rasmussen, L.; Ejrnæs, K.; Porsbo, L.J.; Pedersen, K.; Jensen, L.B.; Emborg, H.-D.; Agersø, Y.; Olsen, K.E.P.; et al. *Escherichia coli* Isolates from Broiler Chicken Meat, Broiler Chickens, Pork, and Pigs Share Phylogroups and Antimicrobial Resistance with Community-Dwelling Humans and Patients with Urinary Tract Infection. *Foodborne Pathog. Dis.* **2009**, *7*, 537–547. [CrossRef] [PubMed]

109. ECDC (European Centre for Disease Prevention and Control); EFSA (European Food Safety Authority); EMA (European Medicines Agency). Joint Scientific Report of ECDC, EFSA and EMEA on Meticillin Resistant *Staphylococcus aureus* (MRSA) in Livestock, Companion Animals and Food. *EFSA J.* **2009**, *7*. [CrossRef]

110. European Centre for Disease Prevention and Control (ECDC). *Antimicrobial Resistance Surveillance in Europe 2014. Annual Report of the European Antimicrobial Resistance Surveillance Network (EARS-Net)*; ECDC: Stockholm, Sweden, 2015.

111. Finley, R.L.; Collignon, P.; Larsson, D.G.J.; McEwen, S.A.; Li, X.-Z.; Gaze, W.H.; Reid-Smith, R.; Timinouni, M.; Graham, D.W.; Topp, E. The Scourge of Antibiotic Resistance: The Important Role of the Environment. *Clin. Infect. Dis.* **2013**, *57*, 704–710. [CrossRef] [PubMed]

112. Price, L.B.; Stegger, M.; Hasman, H.; Aziz, M.; Larsen, J.; Andersen, P.S.; Pearson, T.; Waters, A.E.; Foster, J.T.; Schupp, J.; et al. *Staphylococcus aureus* CC398: Host Adaptation and Emergence of Methicillin Resistance in Livestock. *mBio* **2012**, e00305-11. [CrossRef] [PubMed]

113. Weese, J.S.; van Duijkeren, E. Methicillin-Resistant *Staphylococcus aureus* and *Staphylococcus pseudintermedius* in Veterinary Medicine. *Vet. Microbiol.* **2010**, *140*, 418–429. [CrossRef] [PubMed]

114. Boost, M.V.; O'Donoghue, M.M.; Siu, K.H.G. Characterisation of Methicillin-Resistant *Staphylococcus aureus* Isolates from Dogs and Their Owners. *Clin. Microbiol. Infect.* **2007**, *13*, 731–733. [CrossRef]

115. Lewis, H.C.; Mølbak, K.; Reese, C.; Aarestrup, F.M.; Selchau, M.; Sørum, M.; Skov, R.L. Pigs as Source of Methicillin-Resistant *Staphylococcus aureus* CC398 Infections in Humans, Denmark. *Emerg. Infect. Dis.* **2008**, *14*, 1383–1389. [CrossRef]

116. Voss, A.; Loeffen, F.; Bakker, J.; Klaassen, C.; Wulf, M. Methicillin-Resistant *Staphylococcus aureus* in Pig Farming. *Emerg. Infect. Dis. J.* **2005**, *11*, 1965. [CrossRef]

117. Dorado-Garcia, A.; Dohmen, W.; Bos, M.E.H.; Verstappen, K.M.; Houben, M.; Wagenaar, J.A.; Heederik, D.J. Dose-Response Relationship Between Antimicrobial Drugs and Livestock-Associated MRSA in Pig Farming. *Emerg. Infect. Dis.* **2015**, *21*, 950–959. [CrossRef]

118. Ruuskanen, M.; Muurinen, J.; Meierjohan, A.; Parnanen, K.; Tamminen, M.; Lyra, C.; Kronberg, L.; Virta, M. Fertilizing with Animal Manure Disseminates Antibiotic Resistance Genes to the Farm Environment. *J. Environ. Qual.* **2016**, *45*, 488–493. [CrossRef]

119. Wellington, E.M.H.; Boxall, A.B.; Cross, P.; Feil, E.J.; Gaze, W.H.; Hawkey, P.M.; Johnson-Rollings, A.S.; Jones, D.L.; Lee, N.M.; Otten, W.; et al. The Role of the Natural Environment in the Emergence of Antibiotic Resistance in Gram-Negative Bacteria. *Lancet Infect. Dis.* **2013**, *13*, 155–165. [CrossRef]

120. Aubertheau, E.; Stalder, T.; Mondamert, L.; Ploy, M.-C.; Dagot, C.; Labanowski, J. Impact of Wastewater Treatment Plant Discharge on the Contamination of River Biofilms by Pharmaceuticals and Antibiotic Resistance. *Sci. Total Environ.* **2017**, *579*, 1387–1398. [CrossRef]

121. Singer, A.C.; Shaw, H.; Rhodes, V.; Hart, A. Review of Antimicrobial Resistance in the Environment and Its Relevance to Environmental Regulators. *Front. Microbiol.* **2016**, *7*, 1728. [CrossRef] [PubMed]

122. Rizzo, L.; Manaia, C.; Merlin, C.; Schwartz, T.; Dagot, C.; Ploy, M.C.; Michael, I.; Fatta-Kassinos, D. Urban Wastewater Treatment Plants as Hotspots for Antibiotic Resistant Bacteria and Genes Spread into the Environment: A Review. *Sci. Total Environ.* **2013**, *447*, 345–360. [CrossRef]

123. Zhang, Q.-Q.; Ying, G.-G.; Pan, C.-G.; Liu, Y.-S.; Zhao, J.-L. Comprehensive Evaluation of Antibiotics Emission and Fate in the River Basins of China: Source Analysis, Multimedia Modeling, and Linkage to Bacterial Resistance. *Environ. Sci. Technol.* **2015**, *49*, 6772–6782. [CrossRef] [PubMed]

124. Cabello, F.C.; Godfrey, H.P.; Buschmann, A.H.; Dölz, H.J. Aquaculture as yet Another Environmental Gateway to the Development and Globalisation of Antimicrobial Resistance. *Lancet Infect. Dis.* **2016**, *16*, e127–e133. [CrossRef]

125. Wang, H.; Yang, J.; Yu, X.; Zhao, G.; Zhao, Q.; Wang, N.; Jiang, Y.; Jiang, F.; He, G.; Chen, Y.; et al. Exposure of Adults to Antibiotics in a Shanghai Suburban Area and Health Risk Assessment: A Biomonitoring-Based Study. *Environ. Sci. Technol.* **2018**, *52*, 13942–13950. [CrossRef]

126. Rahube, T.O.; Marti, R.; Scott, A.; Tien, Y.-C.; Murray, R.; Sabourin, L.; Duenk, P.; Lapen, D.R.; Topp, E. Persistence of antibiotic resistance and plasmid-associated genes in soil following application of sewage sludge and abundance on vegetables at harvest. *Can. J. Microbiol.* **2016**, *62*, 600–607. [CrossRef]

127. European Medicines Agency (EMA). Reflection Paper on Antimicrobial Resistance in the Environment: Considerations for Current and Future Risk Assessment of Veterinary Medicinal Products Draft. 2018. Available online: https://www.ema.europa.eu/documents/scientific-guideline/draft-reflection-paper-antimicrobial-resistance-environment-considerations-current-future-risk_en.pdf (accessed on 15 January 2019).

128. Collignon, P.; Kennedy, K.J. Long-Term Persistence of Multidrug-Resistant Enterobacteriaceae after Travel. *Clin. Infect. Dis.* **2015**, *61*, 1766–1767. [CrossRef] [PubMed]

129. Ashbolt, N.J.; Amézquita, A.; Backhaus, T.; Borriello, P.; Brandt, K.K.; Collignon, P.; Coors, A.; Finley, R.; Gaze, W.H.; Heberer, T.; et al. Human Health Risk Assessment (HHRA) for Environmental Development and Transfer of Antibiotic Resistance. *Environ. Health Perspect.* **2013**, *121*, 993–1001. [CrossRef] [PubMed]

130. World Organisation for Animal Health (OIE). *The OIE Strategy on Antimicrobial Resistance and the Prudent Use of Antimicrobials*; OIE: Paris, France, 2016.

131. Department of Health and Department for Environment Food & Rural Affairs. *UK Five-Year Antimicrobial Resistance Strategy 2013 to 2018*; Department of Health and Department for Environment Food & Rural Affairs: London, UK, 2013.

132. Public Health Agency of Canada. *Federal Action Plan on Antimicrobial Resistance and Use in Canada*; Public Health Agency of Canada: Ottawa, ON, Cananda, 2015.

133. Commonwealth of Australia. *Responding to the Threat of Antimicrobial Resistance. Australia's First National Antimicrobial Resistance Strategy 2015-2019*; Commonwealth of Australia: Canberra, Australia, 2016.

134. European Union (EU). *Communication from the Commission to the European Parliament and the Council. Action Plan against the Rising Threats from Antimicrobial Resistance*; EU: Brussels, Belgium, 2011.

135. The White House. *National Action Plan for Combating Antibiotic-Resistant Bacteria*; The White House: Washington, DC, USA, 2015.

136. Food and Agriculture Organization (FAO). *The FAO Action Plan on Antimicrobial Resistance 2016-2020*; FAO: Rome, Italy, 2016.

13

Attenuated Replication of Lassa Virus Vaccine Candidate ML29 in STAT-1$^{-/-}$ Mice

Dylan M. Johnson [1,3,*]**, Jenny D. Jokinen** [2,3] **and Igor S. Lukashevich** [2,3,*]

[1]   Department of Microbiology and Immunology, University of Louisville Health Sciences Center, Louisville, KY 40292, USA

[2]   Department of Pharmacology and Toxicology, University of Louisville Health Sciences Center, Louisville, KY 40292, USA; jenny.jokinen@louisville.edu

[3]   Center for Predictive Medicine for Biodefense and Emerging Infectious Diseases, NIH Regional Biocontainment Laboratory, Louisville, KY 40222, USA

*   Correspondence: dylan.johnson@louisville.edu (D.M.J.); igor.lukashevich@louisville.edu (I.S.L.)

Abstract: Lassa virus (LASV), a highly prevalent mammalian arenavirus endemic in West Africa, can cause Lassa fever (LF), which is responsible for thousands of deaths annually. LASV is transmitted to humans from naturally infected rodents. At present, there is not an effective vaccine nor treatment. The genetic diversity of LASV is the greatest challenge for vaccine development. The reassortant ML29 carrying the L segment from the nonpathogenic Mopeia virus (MOPV) and the S segment from LASV is a vaccine candidate under current development. ML29 demonstrated complete protection in validated animal models against a Nigerian strain from clade II, which was responsible for the worst outbreak on record in 2018. This study demonstrated that ML29 was more attenuated than MOPV in STAT1$^{-/-}$ mice, a small animal model of human LF and its sequelae. ML29 infection of these mice resulted in more than a thousand-fold reduction in viremia and viral load in tissues and strong LASV-specific adaptive T cell responses compared to MOPV-infected mice. Persistent infection of Vero cells with ML29 resulted in generation of interfering particles (IPs), which strongly interfered with the replication of LASV, MOPV and LCMV, the prototype of the Arenaviridae. ML29 IPs induced potent cell-mediated immunity and were fully attenuated in STAT1$^{-/-}$ mice. Formulation of ML29 with IPs will improve the breadth of the host's immune responses and further contribute to development of a pan-LASV vaccine with full coverage meeting the WHO requirements.

Keywords: Lassa virus vaccine; ML29 vaccine; STAT-1$^{-/-}$ mice; Lassa virus; Mopeia virus; interfering particles

1. Introduction

Lassa virus (LASV) is a highly prevalent arenavirus in West Africa, where it infects several hundred thousand individuals annually. This results in a large number of Lassa fever (LF) cases associated with high morbidity and mortality rates [1,2]. The natural LASV reservoir is the rodent *Mastomys natalensis*, which is widely distributed throughout sub-Saharan Africa. The area where LASV is endemic covers large regions of West Africa [3], putting a population of up to 200 million people at risk for infection [4]. Furthermore, there is evidence that LASV-endemic regions are expanding [5]. The high degree of LASV genetic diversity [6,7] likely contributes to underestimates of its prevalence [8]. With the exception of dengue fever, LF has the greatest estimated global burden among all viral hemorrhagic fevers (HFs) [9]. LF outbreaks are associated with mortality rates as high as 60%, as documented during the 2015–2016 outbreak in Nigeria [10]. The currently ongoing 2018 outbreak is the worst on record [11]. There is no FDA-approved LASV vaccine or therapeutic. Treatment options are limited to off-label ribavirin with varying degrees of success. In 2017–2018, the WHO included LASV on the top priority pathogens list and issued a Target Product Profile (TPP) for LASV vaccine development [12–14].

LASV belongs to the Old World (OW) group (former lymphocytic choriomeningitis virus, LCMV-LASV sero-complex) of the genus *Mammarenavirus* of the *Arenaviridae* family [15]. The LASV genome has two RNA segments that each encode two open reading frames in opposite polarities, separated by a structured intergenic region. The L-RNA encodes for a large L protein, which functions as a RNA-dependent RNA polymerase (RdRp), and a RING finger protein Z, which comprises the matrix of virions. The S-RNA encodes for a nucleoprotein (NP) which tightly associates with viral RNA and a glycoprotein precursor (GPC) that is processed into three subunits: a stable signal peptide, SSP; a receptor-binding GP1; and a transmembrane GP2, which mediates fusion with cell membranes. All three glycoprotein subunits associate to form club-shaped features on the surface of pleomorphic viral particles, which vary in the diameter from 50 to 300 nm. In addition to LASV, the OW group includes genetically related nonpathogenic viruses: Mopeia (MOPV), Morogoro (MORV), Gairo (GAIV) and Luna (LUNV) hosted by the same rodents [16–19]. The New World (NW) mammalian arenaviruses (former Tacaribe virus, TCRV, sero-complex) comprise viruses that circulate in the Americas, and include the causative agents of South American HFs [20].

Reassortant studies using genetically related mammalian arenaviruses with different pathogenic potential demonstrated that the L gene is responsible for high levels of virus replication in vivo, and is associated with acute disease in experimental animals [21,22]. Coinfection of cells with LASV and MOPV resulted in generation of MOPV/LASV reassortants [23,24]. One of the rationally selected clones, ML29, carrying the L-RNA from MOPV and the S-RNA from the Josiah strain of LASV (LASV/JOS), is a promising LASV vaccine candidate [24–26].

While MOPV L-RNA is the major driving force of ML29 attenuation, 18 mutations incorporated in the ML29 genome during in vitro selection additionally seem to contribute to the attenuation of ML29 [25,27]. Indeed, transcriptome profiling of human peripheral blood mononuclear cells (hPBMC) exposed to LASV or ML29 exhibited distinct molecular signatures that can be useful biomarkers of pathogenicity and protection [28,29]. Similar studies comparing MOPV and ML29 infected hPBMC revealed that gene expression patterns in mock and ML29 infected hPBMC clustered together and differed from the expression pattern observed in MOPV infected hPBMC [28].

Recently, recombinant ML29 (rML29) was rescued from cDNA clones and demonstrated the same features as a biological ML29 (bML29) [30]. Reverse genetics provides a powerful tool for elucidation of the individual contributions of ML29-specific mutations to attenuation. However, the absence of a reliable small animal model for LASV pathogenicity is a major obstacle for the field. LASV, as well as other mammalian arenaviruses, stimulate antiviral immunity differently in natural rodent hosts and in humans and non-human primates, NHPs [31–33]. While some pathogenic features of human LF can be observed in strain 13 guinea pigs [34–36], there is a poor correlation between clinical outcome of LF in humans and virulence of LASV in guinea pigs [37]. Results of LASV vaccination/challenge studies in strain 13 guinea pigs are not reproducible in NHPs [32,38,39]. In addition, strain 13 guinea pigs are no longer commercially available and difficult to breed.

Rodent models remain useful to study some mechanisms of LF pathogenesis and protective immune responses, and to provide valuable information during preclinical development of vaccine candidates [31,40]. Previous research has documented that mice lacking a functional STAT1 pathway are highly susceptible to LASV infection, and develop fatal disease with some pathological features that mimic human LF [41]. Notably, human LASV isolates from fatal LF cases in Sierra Leone induced clinically similar fatal disease including high viral load in blood and visceral organs of STAT-1$^{-/-}$ mice after intraperitoneal inoculation (i.p.). In contrast, LASV isolated from a non-lethal human case induced disease with moderate mortality. Surviving mice developed hearing loss that mimicked the sensorineural hearing loss (SNHL) commonly observed in LF patients during convalescence [42].

In this study, we provided additional evidence of deep ML29 attenuation by modeling the LASV infection protocol for STAT$^{-/-}$ mice as a means to assess the safety profile of ML29 (bML29 or rML29) in comparison with MOPV. We also generated ML29 stocks enriched with interfering particles (IPs) produced by ML29-persisitently infected cells. The growing body of evidence indicates that, during natural infection, IPs are critically involved in the modulation of viral load, innate immune responses, disease outcome, and contribute to the evolutionary persistence of viruses [43–45]. An accumulation of IPs with genome deletions has been documented during the production of live-attenuated polio [46], influenza [47,48] and measles [49–51] vaccines, and was associated with modulating vaccine potency and immunostimulatory properties. Here, we demonstrated that STAT$^{-/-}$ mice are a susceptible model capable of discriminating between viruses with different levels of attenuation, MOPV and ML29. ML29 IPs were completely attenuated in these mice, enhancing immunogenic features of ML29. The broad cross-protection activity of ML29 IPs and their intrinsic adjuvant features can be potentially used for rational formulation of a pan-LASV ML29-based vaccine by developing vaccine-manufacturing protocols to optimize the ratio between infectious ML29 and IPs.

2. Results

2.1. Generation of Interfering Particles (IPs) by ML29-Persisitently Infected Cells

Arenavirus IPs can be generated at high multiplicity of infection (MOI) by serial infection of fresh tissue cultures with undiluted culture medium harvested from previous passages. Alternatively, initially infected cells can be subjected to serial passages. Both methods resulted in the accumulation of IPs. Earlier studies suggested a contribution of IPs in the establishment and/or maintenance of LCMV persistent infection in vitro and in vivo, and in the inhibition of virus-induced immunopathology in mice [52–58]. The protocol previously applied for the generation of LASV IPs in cell cultures was used to establish ML29 persistent infection of Vero cells. In line with previous observations [59–61], passages of ML29-infected cells, either infected with bML29 or with rML29, resulted in the gradual decline of infectious particles released in culture medium. As seen in Figure 1, the infectious titers of ML29 released into the medium of persistently infected Vero cells (Vero/ML29) were reduced almost 100-fold after 10 passages, and was under detectable levels after 15 passages. Vero/ML29 cells strongly interfered with replication of homologous (ML29) or genetically related LASV/JOS, LCMV, and MOPV and did not generate infectious plaques after super infection of Vero/ML29 with these viruses. Meanwhile, neither the replication of TCRV, a NW arenavirus, nor the nonrelated Ebola virus, was affected in these cells. ML29 IPs released from persistently infected Vero/ML29 cells were able to suppress replication of homologous virus in a dose-dependent manner (Figure 1f).

While the replication of ML29 or LASV was not detectable in ML29/Vero cells after passage 10, viral proteins were detected in these cells by immunofocus (IF) assay (Figure 1c). In contrast to infectious "plaques", this assay detects cells expressing virus antigens stained by specific antibodies. With an increasing number of passages, ML29-infected cells lost their ability to produce plaques after homologous superinfection, but were strongly positive for ML29-specific antigens as demonstrated by quantitated analyses (Figure 1c; Appendix A, Figure A1). Differences in the morphology of IF foci between naïve and Vero/ML29 cells after infection and superinfection with ML29, respectively, seems to be related to differences in the expression of NP and GP proteins in different passages of Vero/ML29 (Appendix A, Figure A1F).

The viral RNA load in Vero/ML29 cells, as assessed by quantitative qRT-PCR targeting the NP gene, declined about tenfold during the first five passages and persisted approximately at the same levels during subsequent passages of Vero/ML29 (Figure 1b). The viral RNA load remained at a similar level through 50 passages (data not shown). Our attempts failed to detect genomic RNA deletions using RT-PCR, either in infected cells or in virions released from infected cells (not shown, see Discussion).

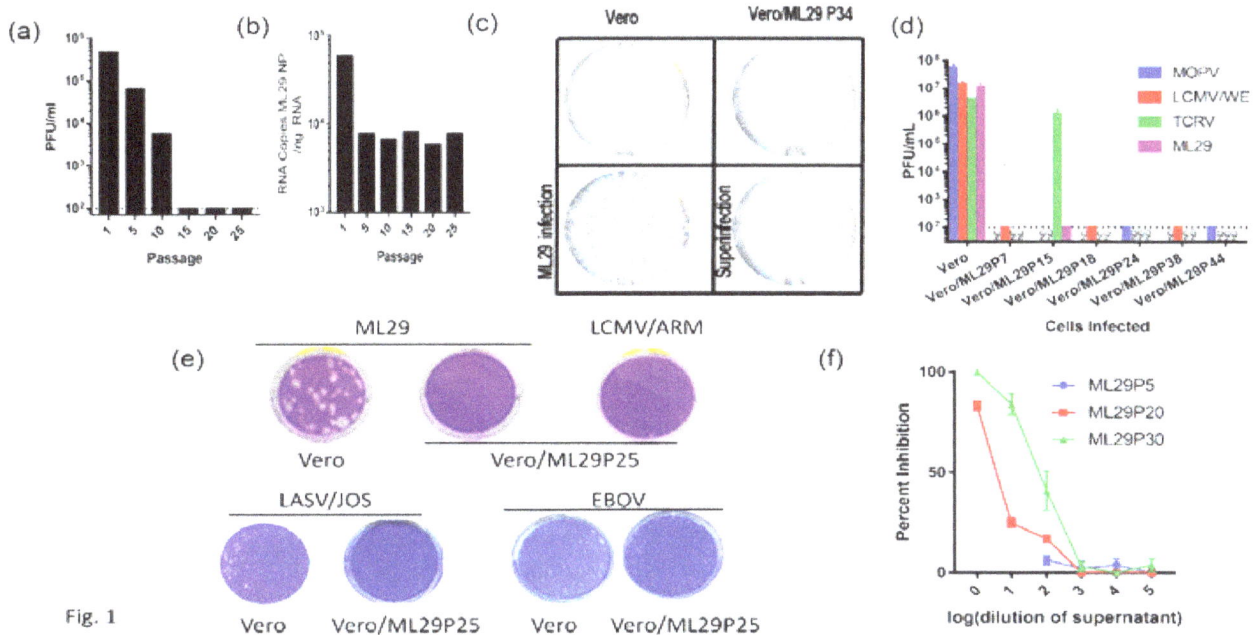

Figure 1. Vero cells persistently infected with ML29 interfere with replication of homologous and genetically related arenaviruses. (**a**) Supernatants from a Vero cell line persistently infected with ML29 (Vero/ML29) were titrated for infectious virus by plaque assay at the indicated passages. (**b**) Total RNA was isolated from a Vero/ML29 cells at the indicated passages and was assayed using qRT-PCR with a LASV/JOS nucleoprotein (NP) TaqMan probe. Copy number was determined by regression against a standard curve. (**c**) Immunofocus assay using polyclonal moneky-anti-ML29 on uninfected Vero E6 cells (top left), Vero/ML29 passage 34 cells (top right), Vero E6 cells infected with a 0.1 MOI of ML29 for 3 days (bottom left), and Vero/ML29 passage 34 cells superinfected with a 0.1 MOI of ML29 for 3 days (bottom right). (**d**) Naïve or persistently infected Vero/ML29 cells at different passages were used to titer MOPV, LCMV/WE, TCRV, ML29 by plaque assay. (**e**) Plaque-forming activity of Vero/ML29 cells. ML29 (top left and top center), LCMV/ARM (top right), LASV/JOS (bottom left and bottom left center), and EBOV (bottom right center and bottom right) were used in a plaque assay on Vero E6 cell (top left, bottom left, and bottom right center) or the 25th passage of a Vero cell line persistently infected with ML29, Vero/ML29P25 (top center, top right, bottom center left, bottom right.) (**f**) Dose-dependent effects of IPs on replication of ML29. Vero E6 cells were pre-incubated for 1 h with the indicated dilution of ML29 IPs produced by Vero/ML29 cells at passage 5, 20 or 30. The pretreated cells were then infected with standard ML29 and viral titer was determined by plaque assay. Percent inhibition is normalized to infectious titer determined on Vero E6 cells that were not pretreated.

2.2. MOPV and Attenuated Reassortant ML29 Induce Experimental Disease with Different Clinical Manifestations and Outcome in STAT-1$^{-/-}$ Mice

In STAT1$^{-/-}$ mice, LASV infection resulted in experimental disease with the outcome depending on the pathogenic potential of the LASV isolate [42]. Based on these observations, we tested the attenuation of MOPV and ML29 in these mice. Using the LASV infection protocol, three groups of mice (n = 9) were IP inoculated with MOPV, ML29 and ML29P50 (IPs produced by Vero/ML29, passage 50). MOPV infection resulted in poor grooming, lethargy and signs of dehydration starting around day 8-post-infection. These symptoms aggravated, and the mice gradually lost weight, and experienced a drop in body temperature. All animals in this group met euthanasia criteria within 11–17 days following infection (Figure 2). In ML29 infected STAT1$^{-/-}$ mice, the symptoms started to improve at the late stage of the infection. Body temperature quickly recovered after day 10 and 33% of mice survived at day 21. No clinical signs were observed in the ML29P50 group. These mice gained weight at the end of the observation period and their temperature fluctuated within a normal range.

As a control, wild-type mice with an identical genetic background were i.p. inoculated with MOPV, ML29 and ML29P50. The mice were successfully infected with these viruses as was documented by detection of viral RNA in tested tissues (Appendix A, Figure A2). However, in the wild-type mice, the replication of the viruses was well-controlled and viral RNA was barely detectable at day 21. As expected, infection did not induce clinical manifestations in any of the wild-type study groups, and these mice gained weight at the end of the 21-day observation period.

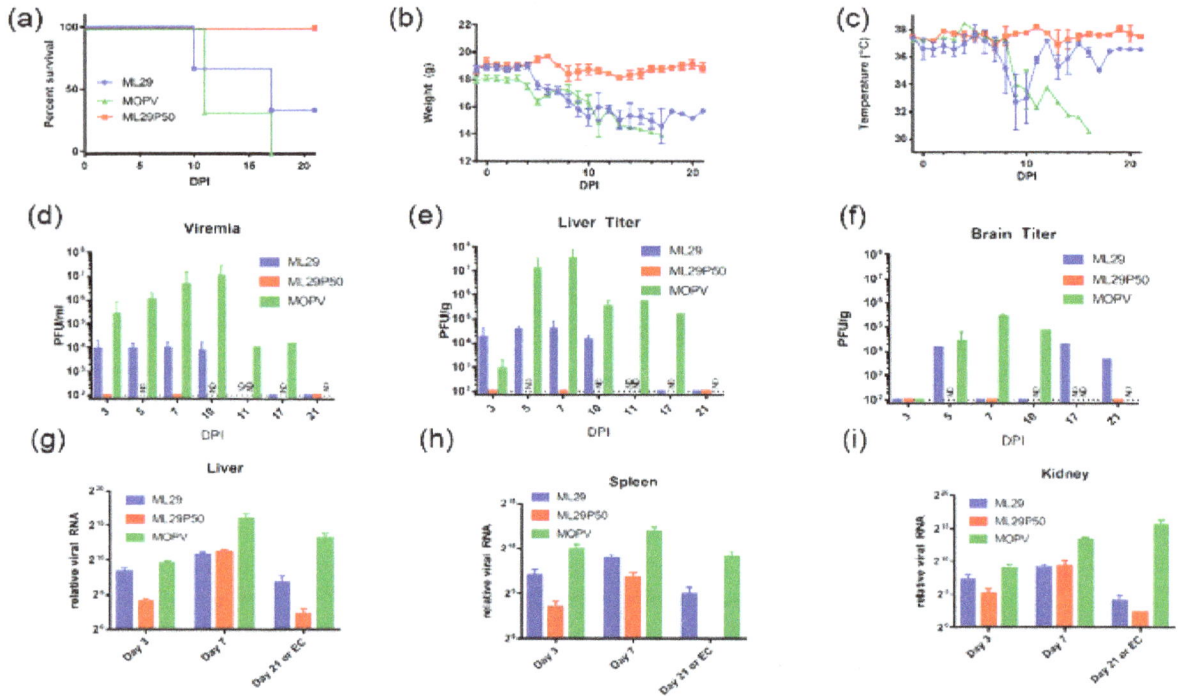

Figure 2. Clinical manifestation and outcome of MOPV and ML29 infections in STAT-1$^{-/-}$ mice. (**a**) Mice were infected (i.p.) with 1×10^3 PFU of MOPV An20410, ML29 (standard infectious virus) or with ML29P50 (IPs collected from culture medium of Vero/ML29P50 cells). ML29P50 IPs were quantified by MOPV L gene qRT-PCR and used in genome-equivalent dose, 1×10^3 PFU. (**b**) Weight and (**c**) Temperature of infected mice. (**d**) Viremia, (**e**) Infectious viral load in liver, and (**f**) brain of STAT-1$^{-/-}$ mice. (**g–i**) Viral RNA load assessed as relative expression of MOPV-L gene by qRT-PCR in the indicated tissues at the time point indicated. DPI, days post-infection. EC, endpoint criteria.

2.3. Replication of MOPV and ML29 in Tissues of STAT-$^{-/-}$ Mice: No Viremia and Infectious Virus in Tissues of ML29P50-Infected Mice

High viremia, infectious titers, and viral RNA loads were associated with replication of MOPV in tissues of STAT-1$^{-/-}$ mice as assessed by infectious plaque assay and qRT-PCR (Figure 2). At the peak of clinical manifestation, days 7–10, viremia and viral load in the liver reached more than 1×10^7 PFU/mL or PFU/g, respectively. RNAscope in situ hybridization confirmed extensive liver infection with strong signals associated with hepatocytes and endothelial cells (Figure 3, arrowed). In contrast, replication of ML29 was more attenuated in STAT-1$^{-/-}$ mice. Viremia and viral load in the liver was 3-logs lower in these mice compared with MOPV infection, and only a few weakly positive hepatocytes were seen in ML29-infected liver samples. In brain tissue, replication of infectious ML29 was transiently detected at early and late stages of infection. Replication of infectious ML29P50 in STAT-1$^{-/-}$ mice was below detectable levels in blood, liver and brain. However, replication of ML29P50 was detected in tissues by viral RNA-based assays, qRT-PCR, and RNAscope in situ hybridization. As seen in Figure 2g–i, at early stage of the infection, relative levels of ML29P50 viral RNA in tissues were lower than MOPV and ML29 viral RNAs. ML29P50 was barely detectable in the tissues at late stage of the infection.

This indicates that ML29P50 was well-controlled, an observation that is in line with the absence of clinical manifestations.

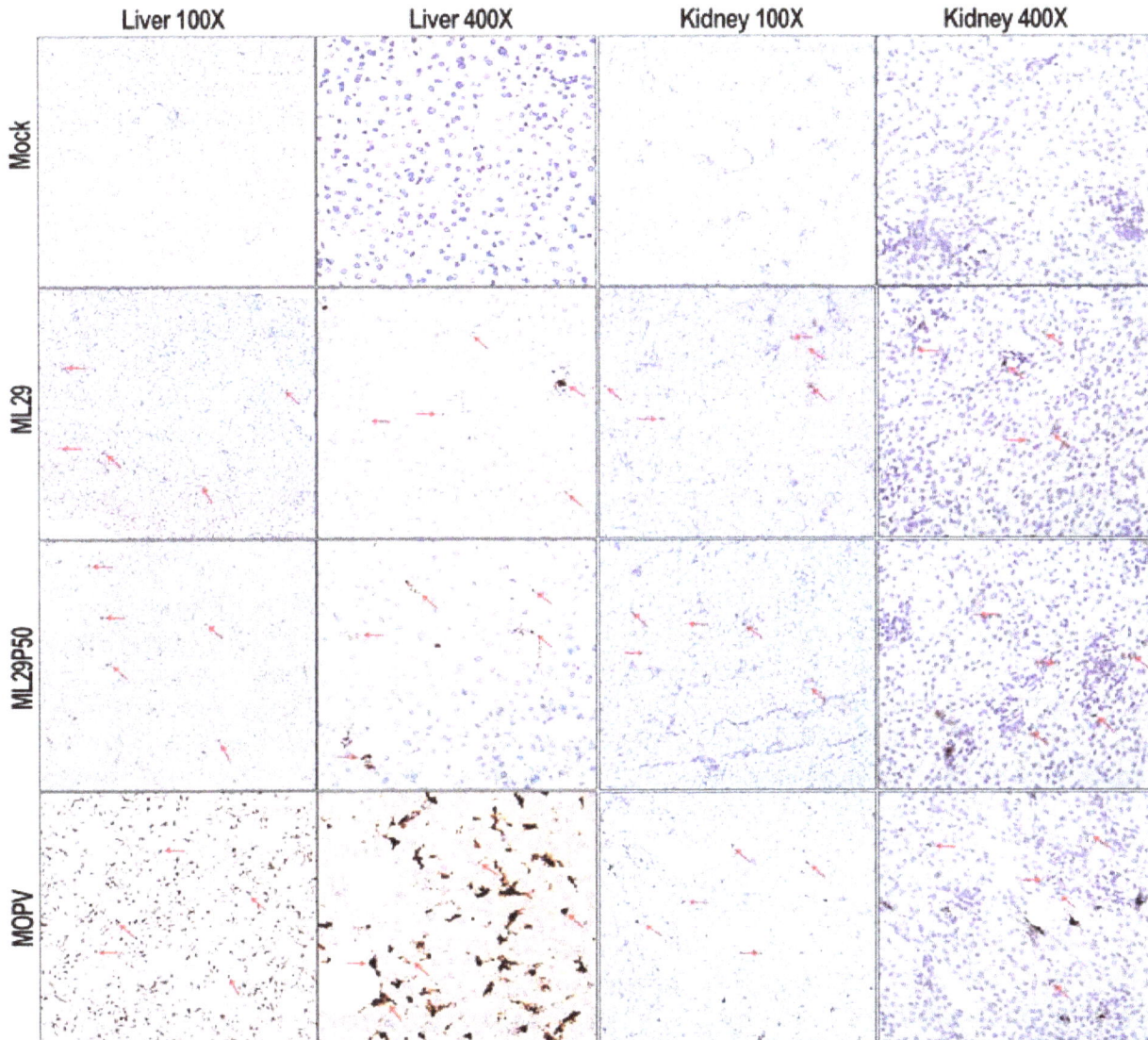

Figure 3. RNAscope in situ hybridization. Representative images at two different magnifications (100× and 400×) of RNAscope in situ hybridization (brown spots, arrowed) targeting the MOPV-L gene in the liver and kidney of STAT1$^{-/-}$ mice.

2.4. Host Responses in Mice Infected with MOPV and ML29

Cell-mediated immune responses in infected mice were assessed by ELISPOT using stimulation of spleen cells isolated on day 3, 7, and 21 after infection with peptide cocktails derived from LASV/JOS GPC and MOPV GPC as previously described [62,63]. At day 3, virus-specific T cells secreting IFN-γ, IL-2 or both were barely detectable in all groups of mice (not shown). By day 7, in STAT-1$^{-/-}$ mice, comparable levels of IFN-γ-secreting cells (~0.4% of total spleen cells) were observed in spleens from ML29- and ML29P50-infected mice (Figure 4a). In wild-type mice, ML29 and ML29P50 infection induced slightly lower T-cell responses Notably, in wild-type and STAT-1$^{-/-}$ mice infected either with ML29 or with ML29P50, similar levels of IFN-γ-secreting cells were induced after stimulation with GPC cocktails derived from LASV or MOPV. Infection with MOPV induced comparatively diminished T cell responses in wild-type and in STAT-1$^{-/-}$ mice, predominantly after stimulation with homologous MOPV GPC-derived peptides. After stimulation with GPC cocktails, spleen cells isolated from mice infected with ML29 and ML29P50, but not with MOPV, also secreted IL-2 cytokine, ~0.1% of total spleen cells. Cells secreting both cytokines were easily detectable at day 7 in ML29 and ML29P50 mice after stimulation with homologous antigens. In MOPV infected STAT-1$^{-/-}$ mice, this cells population was barely detectable.

Survival of ML29P50-infected mice was clearly associated with strong cell-mediated responses. As seen in Figure 4, in spleens isolated from STAT-1$^{-/-}$ mice on day 21, cells secreting IFN-γ, IL2, or both were strongly upregulated after stimulation with GPC cocktails, >0.3–0.6%. In wild-type mice inoculated with ML29P50, these responses had declined by this time point. Interestingly enough, in both groups of mice infected with ML29P50 humoral responses were similar (Figure 4g).

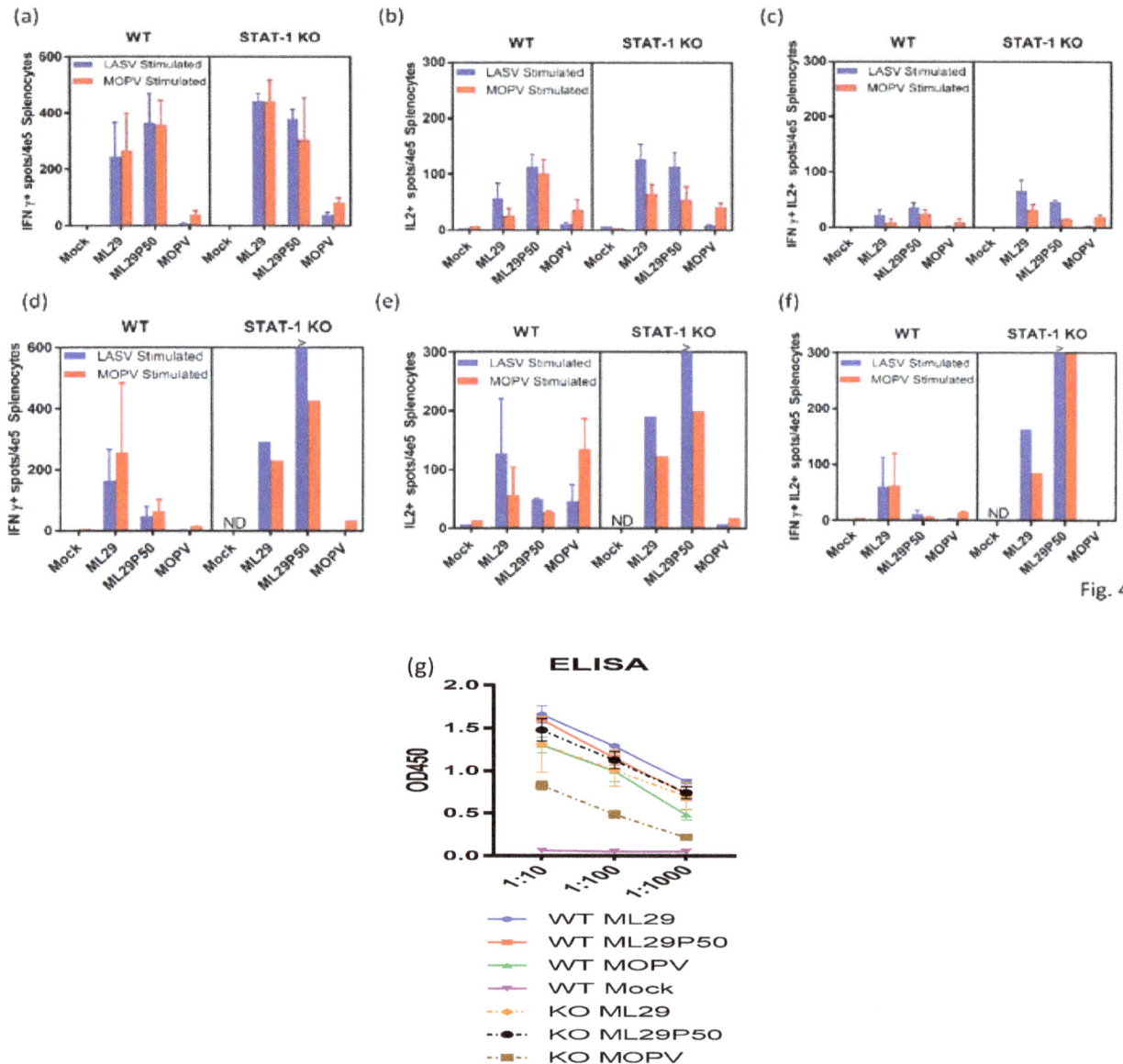

Fig. 4

Figure 4. Adaptive immune responses of STAT-1$^{-/-}$ mice. ELISPOT counts per 4×10^5 splenocytes from STAT-1$^{-/-}$ mice or wild-type (WT) controls collected (**a–c**) 7 days post-infection or (**d–f**) at endpoint criteria or 21 days post-infection. Splenocytes were stimulated with LASV GPC or MOPV GPC-derived peptide cocktails for 24 h. (**a,d**) IFN-γ-secreted cells, (**b,e**) IL-2-secreted cells, or (**c,d**) poly-functional IFN-γ/IL-2-secreting cells. (**g**) Antibody responses measured by IgG ELISA in the serum of STAT-1$^{-/-}$ mice or wild-type controls collected at 21 days post-infection or endpoint criteria. >, Too numerous to count.

Measurement of pro-inflammatory cytokine expression in spleen of STAT-1$^{-/-}$ mice infected with MOPV revealed upregulation of IL-6 and IL-1β at early stages of the infection and rapidly declined at later time points while TNF-α was downregulated for all viruses except the early stages of MOPV and the late stage of ML29P50 (Figure 5, Appendix A, Figure A3). Levels of IL-1β and IL-6 mRNA in spleens of the mice infected with ML29 and ML25P50 were upregulated at day 3 and day 7, respectively. At the later time point, the infection had minimal if any effect on TNF-α and IL-1β expression in STAT-1$^{-/-}$ and control mice. In MOPV-infected wild-type mice, IL-6 mRNA levels had similar kinetics with those in STAT-1$^{-/-}$ mice, with downregulation in the liver and spleen tissues during the infection.

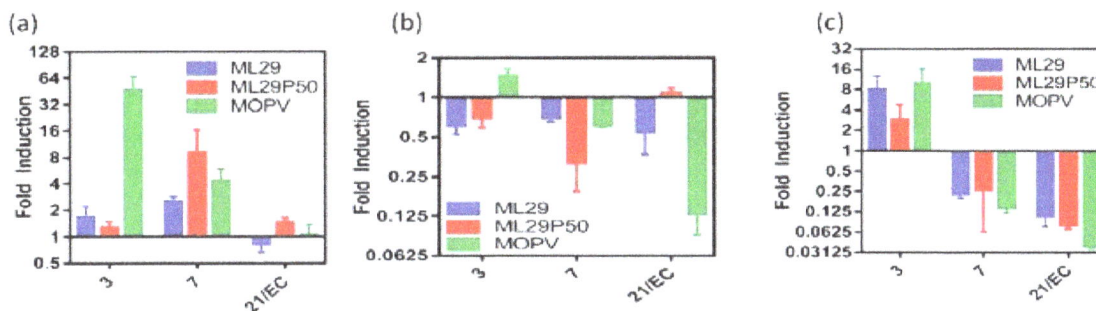

Figure 5. Cytokine responses of STAT-1$^{-/-}$ mice. (**a**) IL-6, (**b**) TNF-α, or (**c**) IL-1β expression in splenocytes of STAT-1$^{-/-}$ mice relative to mock infected by qRT-PCR.

3. Discussion

The first aim of this study was to determine if STAT-1$^{-/-}$ mice provide a reliable small animal model to assess level of attenuation of LASV-related arenaviruses. LASV and MOPV share a common reservoir, *M. natalensis*, found in the western and southeastern regions of Africa [16,17,64]. In Mozambique and Tanzania, areas where MOPV and MORV are prevalent, there is a marked absence of clinical cases of LF. Additionally, MOPV does not cause clinical signs in guinea pigs and NHPs [35]. These observations, combined with ability of MOPV to generate in vitro replication-competent reassortants with LASV [24], and to protect experimentally infected NHPs against fatal LF [65], suggests that MOPV is a "naturally attenuated" genetic relative of LASV.

Studies to assess virulence of human LASV isolates in NHPs are very limited [66]. LASV isolates from LF patients with different clinical outcome showed a weak correlation between severity of human disease and virulence in guinea pigs [35,37]. Meanwhile, in STAT-1$^{-/-}$ mice, outcome of the disease correlated with virulence of human LASV isolates. Four out of 5 mice infected with a lethal isolate met euthanasia criteria between days 7 and 8, while mice infected with nonlethal LASV isolates developed chronic disease [41,42]. In our experiments, MOPV infection of STAT-1$^{-/-}$ mice induced manifested disease that met euthanasia criteria 11–17 days post-infection (Figure 2a). The delayed euthanasia time-point of 11–17 days versus 7–8 days indicates some level of attenuation of MOPV infection in STAT-1$^{-/-}$ mice. However, high levels of viremia and viral load in target tissues, comparable with those in animals infected with virulent LASV isolates [41,42], and poor adaptive immune responses (Figure 4) resulted in aggravated disease. In contrast to MOPV, ML29 infection in STAT-1$^{-/-}$ mice was more attenuated, and 33% of animals survived in this group (Figure 2a). Compared to MOPV-infected mice, ML29 infection notably resulted in more than a thousand-fold reduction in viremia and viral load in tissues by plaque assay (Figure 2d–f). Strong T cell responses contributed to viral control in this experimental group (Figure 4). It is well documented that strong T cell-mediated immunity correlates with protection and positive clinical outcomes in experimentally infected NHPs and LF patients [33,67–69].

The second aim of this study was to assess the contribution of IPs generated by ML29-persistently infected cells to the attenuation and modulation of immune responses. Similar to many other RNA viruses, mammalian arenaviruses can generate IPs during acute infection of cells at high MOI, or during persistent infection. The defective IPs: (i) are antigenically identical to parental viruses and contain the same structural proteins; (ii) preserve 5′ and 3′ terminal sequences of parental genome but have extensive internal deletions; (iii) can only replicate with help of standard virus; and (iv) strongly compete for replication machinery with the parental virus [70–74]. Historically, arenavirus IPs were observed following in vitro infection at high MOI, and masked the cell-killing potential of standard viruses. Earlier studies suggested the contribution of IPs in the establishment and/or maintenance of LCMV persistent infection in vitro, and in inhibition of virus-induced immunopathology in mice [52–58]. Similarly, LASV IPs generated by persistently infected cells strongly interfered with replication of standard LASV in vitro, were attenuated in C3H mice, and partially protected mice against wild-type LASV challenge [59,60,75,76]. In contrast to IPs generated from VSV, Sendai, Sindbis, and other RNA viruses, arenavirus IPs are difficult to separate from standard virions [55]. The unique ability of mammalian arenaviruses to incorporate host ribosomes and RNAs during the late stage of virus maturation [15] seems to be responsible for failure of density-based methods to purify arenavirus IPs. Nevertheless, LCMV defective IPs partially purified from culture medium of persistently infected cells lacked the S-RNA segment [77], compared to LASV defective IPs where the L RNA segment was not detectable [61]. In line with these results, UV inactivation experiments confirmed "smaller" genomes for LCMV [54] and LASV defective IPs [61]. The LCMV L-RNA segment was much less abundant and not detectable during the early stage of persistent infection. However, RNA deletions were not found among virus-specific RNA species in brain tissue of LCMV persistently infected mice. During the progression of persistence, an accumulation of terminally truncated RNA species was documented [78].

In our experiments, we were able to demonstrate the basic features of ML29 IPs generated by persistently infected cells (gradual infectivity loss during passages, antigenic identity and persistence, GP/NP ratio fluctuation, interference with homologous and closely related viruses) (Appendix A, Figure A1). However, we failed to detect genomic deletions among virus-specific RNA species extracted from persistently infected cells or among viral RNA extracted from concentrated supernatants by RT-PCR methods using different sets of primers to amplify the genomic L and S RNA segments. By using qRT-PCR quantification of the LASV(ML29) NP gene, we demonstrated that S-RNA copies rapidly declined during the first five cell culture passages of infected cells and the number of copies persisted at roughly same levels during passages 10–25 (Figure 1b). These levels remain relatively constant for all subsequent passages tested through passage 50 (not shown). In contrast to the permanent level of the S-RNA replication and protein expression detected by IF assay (Figure 1d), the infectivity of particles produced by persistently infected cells dropped dramatically during the first 10 passages, was below the threshold of detection by passage 15 (Figure 1a), and was not detectable at the final passage 50.

The inability of ML29-persistently infected cells to generate infectious plaques after homologous superinfection with ML29, or infection with LASV/JOS or MOPV, can be partially explained by arenavirus Z-mediated "superinfection exclusion" [79]. However, the replication of the NW mammalian arenavirus TCRV was not affected in ML29/Vero cells (Figure 1f). Recent study documented the capability of LCMV, LASV and MACV mammalian arenaviruses to replicate and disseminate without the Z protein providing evidence that NP can play role as potential surrogate of the Z protein [80]. We assume that ML29 IPs-induced interference was unlikely to be related to Z protein. Nevertheless, the contribution of the Z protein to innate immune responses cannot be fully excluded. ML29 has Z protein derived from MOPV. Interestingly enough, Z protein of pathogenic arenaviruses (including LASV,) but not that of nonpathogenic viruses, including the MOPV Z, inhibit RIG-I-like receptor-dependent IFN type I production [81].

In this study, we failed to provide evidence that ML29 IPs produced by ML29/Vero cells are "classical" defective IPs and the nature of ML29 IP-based interference has to be further elucidated. Nevertheless, ML29 IPs seem to be very attractive for vaccine formulation and development. First, as seen in Figure 2a, ML29P50 generated by ML29/Vero cells, passage 50, were completely attenuated in STAT-1$^{-/-}$ mice. These particles were not detectable by plaque assay (test on infectivity) in blood and tissues of mice. However, the level of ML29P50 RNA replication was similar or only slightly reduced in comparison with "wild-type" ML29 RNA replication (Figure 2g–i). Second, while ML29P50 and ML29 induced comparable T cell responses at day 7, at the late stage of the infection ML29P50 generated much stronger T cell immunity as assessed by IFN-ɣ/IL-2 ELISPOT in line with the strong immunomodulation potency of defective IPs [82]. While the mechanism of LASV protection can be dependent on the vaccine platform itself, as well as the animal challenge protocol—in the case of the ML29 vaccine, T cell immunity, but not antibody production—was associated with protection of NHPs [83]. Third, ML29 is the only vaccine with documented evidence of T-cell-mediated cross-protection against Nigerian LASV strains from clade II, among currently available LASV vaccine candidates [84]. This is critical considering the Nigerian LASV strains from clade II are responsible for causing the current unprecedented LF outbreak. LASV genetic diversity is the greatest challenge for vaccine development. The formulation of ML29 with IPs will improve the breadth of the host's immune responses [85] and further contribute to the development of a pan-LASV vaccine with full coverage meeting the WHO requirements [13].

4. Materials and Methods

4.1. Viruses and Cells

Generation of MOPV An20410, LASV/Josiah, and MOP/LAS reassortant (ML29) LCMV (WE and ARM) stocks in Vero cells and plaque titration technique was previously described [25]. Freeze-dried Tacaribe virus (TCRV-11573, ATCC® VR-1272CAF™) was purchased from ATCC and the virus stock was prepared by low MOI passage in Vero cells. Infectious plaques for all viruses, except MOPV, were counted at 5 days after infection by treatment of infected cell monolayers under agarose overlay with 4% paraformaldehyde and staining with 1% crystal violet. For MOPV, neutral red stain staining was used for plaque development. Vero C1008 cells (Vero 76, clone E6, ATCC® CRL1586) were maintained in DMEM/F-12 supplemented with 10% fetal calf serum, 1X antibiotic-antimycotic (ThermoFisher), and 1X Glutamax (ThermoFisher). ML29 persistent infection in Vero cells was established by using a previously described protocol [59,61]. In brief, after the initial infection of Vero cell monolayers with an MOI of 1.0, at weekly intervals, cells were detached from cell tissue flasks by treatment with 0.05% trypsin-EDTA (ThermoFisher) and subcultured at a 1:10 ratio. Culture medium was changed at 3–4-day intervals. Samples of cells and/or culture medium were used for plaque titration, antigen detection assays (IF, Western) and for RNA isolation. To titrate ML29 IPs produced by persistently infected Vero/ML29 cells, monolayers of naïve Vero cells were pretreated with dilutions of Vero/ML29 passage 5, 20 and 30 supernatants for 1 h followed by infection with ML29 and detection of plaques as described above. LASV/JOS or EBOV plaque titrations were performed in BSL-4 facilities using maximum containment practices at the University of Texas Medical Branch with the assistance of Dr. Slobodan Paessler's lab.

4.2. Immunofocus Assay

Vero E6 cells or ML29 persistently infected cells (Vero/ML29) were plated at a density of 2×10^4 cells/well in 96-well tissue culture plates. Twenty-four hours later, cells were overlaid with methylcellulose media. Naïve or Vero/ML29 cells were infected with 0.1 MOI of ML29 for 1 h prior to being overlaid with methylcellulose. After 3 days, the methylcellulose was removed and cells were then fixed with an acetone methanol mixture. Residual endogenous peroxidase was blocked by hydrogen peroxide and cells were incubated overnight in 10% FBS. After washing, cells were treated with either polyclonal monkey-anti-ML29 antibody (1:400), monoclonal mouse-anti-LASV/JOS-NP, 1:100 (GenScript, Piscataway, NJ, USA) or polyclonal rabbit-anti-LASV-GP 1:400 (IBT Bioservices, Rockville, MD, USA) followed by HRP linked appropriate secondary antibody. TrueBlue Peroxidase Substrate (SeraCare, Milford, MA, USA) was used for detection. Quantification of staining from high-quality images of scanned plates was performed using Adobe Photoshop to reduce background and threshold images followed by ImageJ counting of pixels.

4.3. Animal Protocols

Four-to-five week-old female STAT-1$^{-/-}$ mice (129S6/SvEv-Stat1tm1Rds) and wild-type controls (129SVE-F) were purchased from Taconic (Hudson, NY, USA). During a 1-week acclimation, a temperature and identification transponder was implanted subcutaneously and the mice were transferred to ABSL-3 housing at the NIH Regional Biocontainment Laboratory on the University of Louisville campus. For infection, 1×10^3 PFU of MOPV, ML29 or ML29P50 (quantitated as a qRT-PCR equivalent dose) was administered (i.p.) in 100 µL of PBS. Mice were monitored daily during 21 days and any animal with 25% weight loss was determined to have met the humane euthanasia criteria. Plasma samples from infected mice that had been euthanized were collected in EDTA tubes (BD). Tissue sample homogenates (10% w/v) were prepared with an Omni TH Tissue Homogenizer in DMEM/F12 followed with centrifugation at 4500× g for 20 min. Clarified tissue homogenates were tested in the plaque assay described above. All animal protocols were approved by the University of Louisville Institutional Animal Care and Use Committee.

4.4. qRT-PCR and RNAscope In Situ Hybridization

Tissue samples were placed into 2-mL screw-top tubes with 1 mL TRIzol Reagent (ThermoFisher) and glass beads, processed in a bead homogenizer, and tissue homogenates were stored at −80 °C until RNA isolation by phenol-chloroform extraction and ethanol precipitation. The qScript cDNA super mix (Quanta Biosciences) was used to make cDNA with an input of 1000 ng of RNA. qRT-PCR with TaqMan primers targeting the MOPV L gene, the LASV NP gene, IL-6, TNF-α, or IL-1β were used with a 18S housekeeping probe on a StepOnePlus qRT-PCR analyzer (Applied Biosystems). All IL-6, TNF-α, IL-1β and 18S primer/probe sets were commercially purchased through ThermoFisher Scientific through the Applied Biosystems division. Primer/probe set for MOPV amplified a region of the L segment (FWD 5′-TCCTCAATTAGG CGTGTGAA-3′; REV 5′-TACACATCCTTGGGTCCTGA-3′; probe 6FAM-CCCTGTTCCCTCCAACTTGTTCTT TG-TAMRA). Primer/probe set for LASV (ML29) amplified the NP gene segment (FWD 5′-TCC AACATATTGCCACCATC-3′; REV 5′- GCT GAC TCA AAG TCA TCC CA-3′; probe 6FAM TGCCTTCACAGCTGCACCCA-TAMRA). The qRT-PCR reaction contained 5 µM of each primer and 2 µM of probe for each primer/probe set, 5 µL of cDNA and TaqMan Fast Advanced Master Mix (ThermoFisher) in a final reaction volume of 20 µL. The reaction conditions were as follows: 50 °C for 2 min, 95 °C for 20 s then 40 cycles alternating between 95 °C for 3 s and 60 °C for 30 s. For RNAscope hybridization, fixed tissue sections were embedding in paraffin, cut on a Leica RM2125 RTS microtome, and mounted on glass slides. Custom designed target probes, preamplifier, amplifier, and label probe targeting MOPV L RNA were synthesized by Adanced Cell Diagnostics (Hayward, CA, USA) and RNAscope assay was performed according to the manufacturer's manual. Chromogenic detection was performed using DAB followed by counterstaining with hematoxylin.

4.5. EISPOT and IgG ELISA

Assessment of T cell responses in infected mice by the murine IFN-γ/IL-2 Double-Color Enzymatic ELISPOT (Cellular Technology Ltd., Cleveland, OH, USA) has been recently described [63]. In brief, erythrocyte-free splenocytes were added to 96-well filter plates (Millipore, MSIPS4510) pre-coated with anti-mouse cytokine antibody in triplicate at a density of 4×10^5 cells/well. Cells were stimulated overnight at 37 °C with cocktails of 10 µM LASV/JOS or MOPV GPC peptides (Mimotopes Ltd, Melbourne, Australia). Each cocktail contained 69 overlapping 20-mer peptides. As positive and negative controls, Conconavalin A (ThermoFisher) and CLT media alone was added to quality control wells. After stimulation, plates were developed according to the manufacturer's protocol and cells secreting individual cytokines IFN-γ or IL-2 or both were counted using C.T.L. Ltd. Immunospot® S5 Micro-analyzer and Immunospot® V 4.0 software. Quality control analysis was provided by C.T.L. Ltd.

IgG ELISA was performed as previously described [62]. In brief, microtiter plates were coated with 5×10^6 PFU/well of sonicated virus suspension in carbonate buffer (Sigma) overnight. Plates were washed, blocked with 10% milk for 2 h, washed again, and coated with dilutions of mouse serum for 1 h. Plates were washed and secondary HRP linked rabbit-anti-mouse IgG (Sigma) was added at a 1:2500 dilution for 1 h. Plates were washed and SureBlue TMB peroxidase substrate (SeraCare) was added for 15 min before the addition of TMB Stop Solution (SeraCare).

4.6. Statistics Analysis

Results are reported as means ± SEM (n = 4–5). ANOVA with Bonferroni's post-hoc test (for parametric data) or the Mann–Whitney rank-sum test (for nonparametric data) was used for the determination of statistical significance among treatment groups, as appropriate. Statistical analysis (mean, SD, T-test) and graphics were performed using the GraphPad Prism version 7 for Windows package (GraphPad Software, LaJolla, CA, USA).

Author Contributions: Conceptualization, I.S.L.; Methodology, I.S.L., D.M.J., J.D.J.; Animal Studies, D.M.J., J.D.J.; Data Analysis, I.S.L., D.M.J., J.D.J.; Visualization, D.M.J., J.D.J.; Writing, I.S.L., D.M.J.; Funding Acquisition, I.S.L.; Supervision, I.S.L.

Acknowledgments: We thank the University of Louisville Center for Predictive Medicine for Biodefense and Emerging Infectious Diseases for the support of animal studies as well as Dr. Slobodan Paessler (The University of Texas Medical Branch at Galveston) for titration of Lassa and Ebola samples using Vero/ML29 cells.

Appendix A

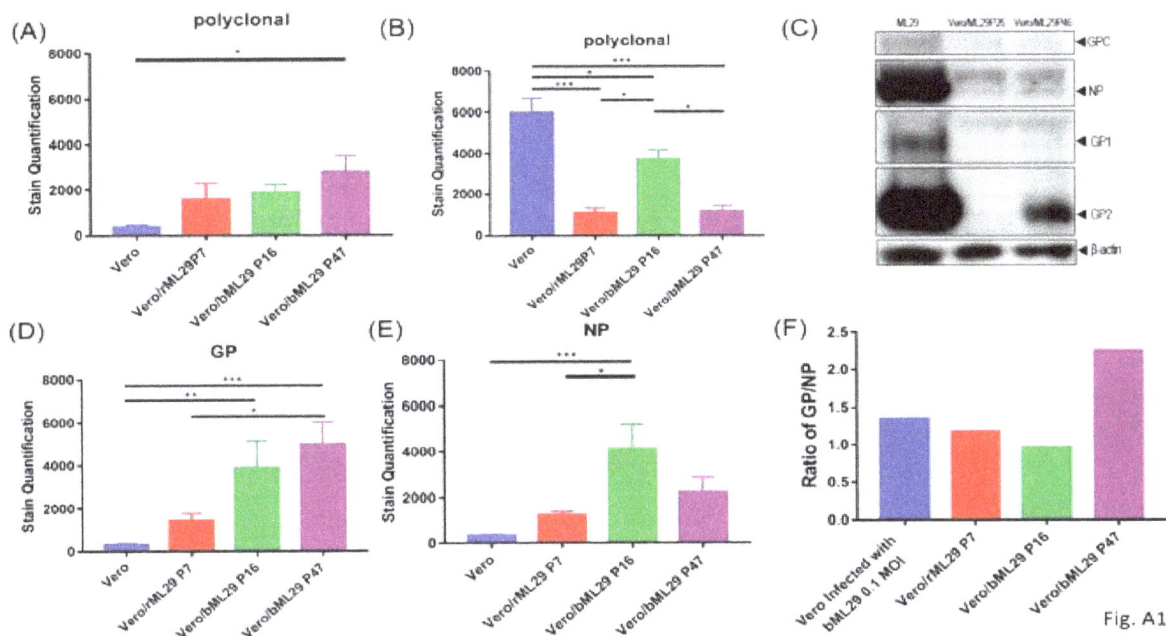

Figure A1. Quantification of immunofocus staining using polyclonal moneky-anti-ML29 on the indicated cell lines (**A**) without additional treatment, or (**B**) 3 days following infection with a 0.1 MOI of ML29. (**C**) Western blot of cell lysates from ML29, Vero/ML29P26, and Vero/ML29P46 detected with polyclonal monkey-anti-ML29 antibody. (**D–E**) Quantification of immunofocus staining using (**D**) polyclonal rabbit-anti-LASV-GP 1:400, or (**E**) mouse-anti-LASV/Jos-NP 1:100 antibodies. (**F**) The calculated ratio between staining quantified in (**D**) and (**E**). * $p < 0.05$, ** $p < 0.01$, *** $p < 0.001$.

Fig. A2

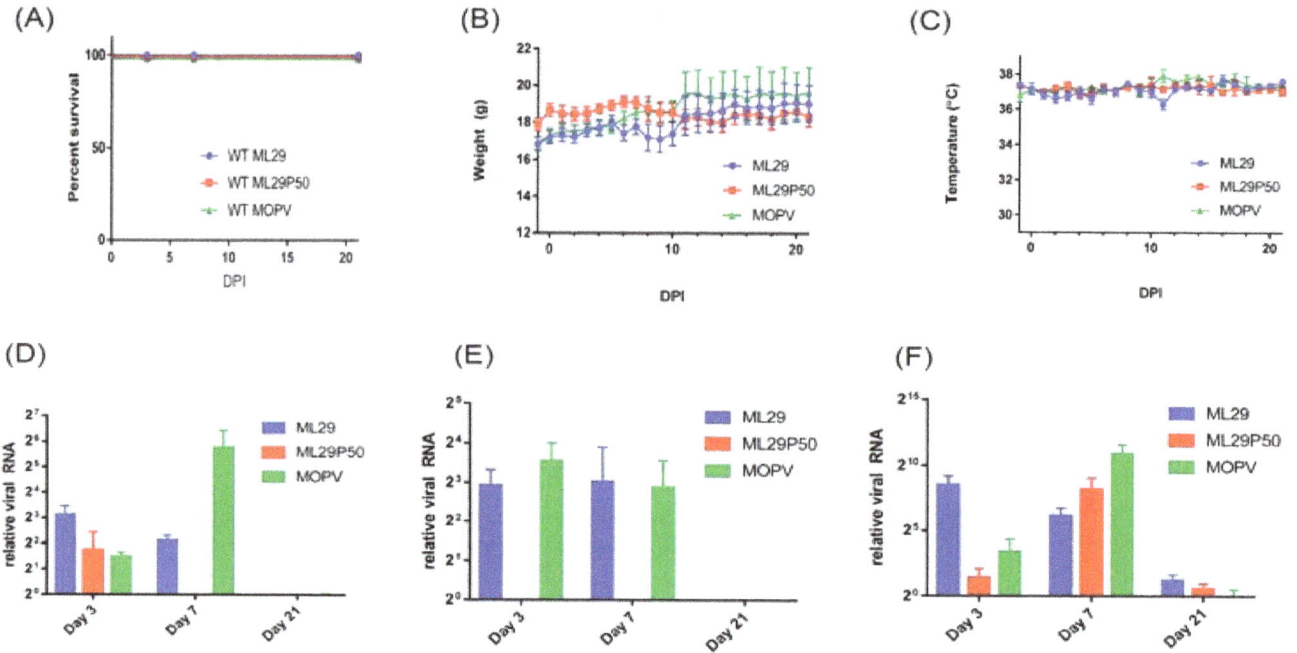

Figure A2. (**A**) Survival of wild-type 129S6 mice infected IP with 1×10^3 PFU of ML29, 1×10^3 PFU of MOPV, or a MOPV L gene qRT-PCR equivalent dose of supernatant from passage 50 Vero/ML29 cells. Daily (**B**) weight and (**C**) temperature of mice from (**A**). (**D–F**) Relative expression of MOPV L gene by qRT-PCR in the (**D**) liver, (**E**) spleen, and (**F**) kidney of wild-type 129S at the time points indicated post-infection.

Fig. A3

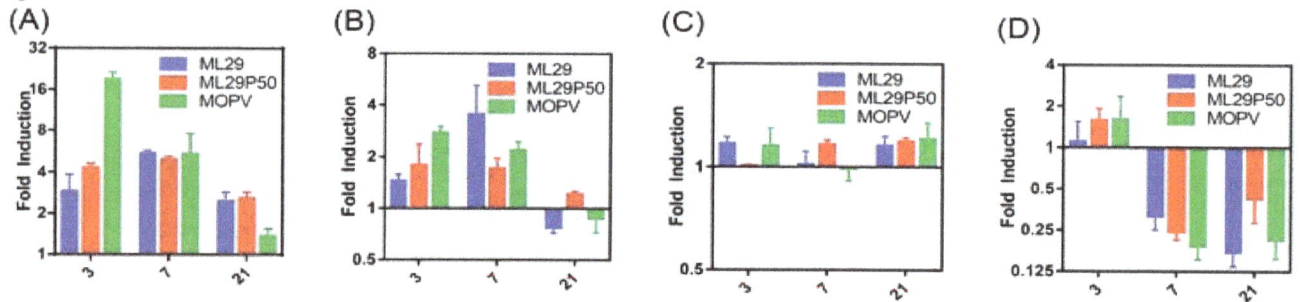

Figure A3. qRT-PCR analysis showing IL-6 expression in the (**A**) liver and (**B**) spleen, (**C**) TNF-α in the spleen, or (**D**) IL-1β expression in the spleen of wild-type 129S6 mice infected with the indicated viruses relative to mock infected at days 3, 7, and 21 post-infection.

Supplemental Materials and Methods

Quantification of immunofocus staining from high-quality images of scanned plates was performed using Adobe Photoshop to reduce background and threshold images followed by ImageJ counting of pixels. Statistical significance was tested with a one-way ANOVA using GraphPad Prism version 7.

For western blotting, a T-75 cell culture flask with a confluent monolayer of either Vero cells was infected with a 1 MOI of ML29 5 days prior, or Vero/ML29, was harvested in Tris-buffer containing 1.0% NP-40, protease inhibitors and 0.1% SDS. Protein content was standardized based on a pierce modified Lowry protein assay (ThermoFisher) denatured by boiling in Laemmli's buffer and run on a 10% acrylamide gel at 120 V for 1 h. The proteins were transferred to a nitrocellulose membrane, blocked with 5% milk, and detected with a 1:1000 dilution of polyclonal monkey-anti-ML29 antibody.

References

1. Frame, J.D.; Baldwin, J.M., Jr.; Gocke, D.J.; Troup, J.M. Lassa fever, a new virus disease of man from West Africa. I. Clinical description and pathological findings. *Am. J. Trop. Med. Hyg.* **1970**, *19*, 670–676. [CrossRef] [PubMed]

2. McCormick, J.B. Epidemiology and control of Lassa fever. *Curr. Top. Microbiol. Immunol.* **1987**, *134*, 69–78.

3. Fichet-Calvet, E.; Rogers, D.J. Risk Maps of Lassa Fever in West Africa. *PLoS Negl. Trop. Dis.* **2009**, *3*, e388. [CrossRef] [PubMed]

4. Richmond, J.K.; Baglole, D.J. Lassa fever: Epidemiology, clinical features, and social consequences. *BMJ* **2003**, *237*, 1271–1275. [CrossRef] [PubMed]

5. Sogoba, N.; Feldmann, H.; Safronetz, D. Lassa Fever in West Africa: Evidence for an Expanded Region of Endemicity. *Zoonoses Public Health* **2012**, *59*, 43–47. [CrossRef] [PubMed]

6. Bowen, M.; Rollin, P.E.; Ksiazek, T.G.; Hustad, H.L.; Buasch, D.G.; Demby, A.H.; Bjani, M.D.; Peters, C.J.; Nichol, S.T. Genetic diversity among Lassa virus strains. *J. Virol.* **2000**, *74*, 6992–7004. [CrossRef] [PubMed]

7. Andersen, K.G.; Shapiro, B.J.; Matranga, C.B.; Sealfon, R.; Lin, A.E.; Moses, L.M.; Floarin, O.A.; Goba, A.; Oida, I.; Ehiane, P.E.; et al. Clinical Sequencing Uncovers Origins and Evolution of Lassa Virus. *Cell* **2015**, *162*, 738–750. [CrossRef] [PubMed]

8. Emmerich, P.; Gunter, S.; Schmitz, H. Strain-specific antibody response to Lassa virus in the local population of West AFrica. *J. Clin. Virol.* **2008**, *42*, 40–44. [CrossRef] [PubMed]

9. Falzarano, D.; Feldmann, H. Vaccines for viral hemorrhagic fevers—Progress and shortcomings. *Curr. Opin. Virol.* **2013**, *3*, 1–9. [CrossRef] [PubMed]

10. Buba, M.I.; Dalhat, M.M.; Nguku, P.M.; Waziri, N.; Mohammad, J.O.; Bomoi, I.M.; Onyiah, A.P.; Balogun, M.S.; Bashorun, A.T.; et al. Mortality Among Confirmed Lassa Fever Cases During the 2015–2016 Outbreak in Nigeria. *Am. J. Public Health* **2017**, *108*, 262–264. [CrossRef] [PubMed]

11. Roberts, L. Nigeria hit by unprecedented Lassa fever outbreak. *Science* **2018**, *359*, 1201–1202. [CrossRef] [PubMed]

12. WHO. *Annual Review of Diseases Prioritized under the Research and Development Blueprint*; WHO: Geneva, Switzerland, 24–25 January 2017. Available online: http://www.who.int/blueprint/what/research-development/2017-Prioritization-Long-Report.pdf?ua=1 (accessed on 14 January 2019).

13. WHO. WHO Target Product Profile for Lassa Virus Vaccine. June 2017. Available online: http://www.who.int/blueprint/priority-diseases/key-action/LassaVirusVaccineTPP.PDF?ua=1 (accessed on 14 January 2019).

14. WHO. Lassa Fever. 2018. Available online: http://www.who.int/csr/don/20-april-2018-lassa-fever-nigeria/en/ (accessed on 14 January 2019).

15. Radoshitzky, S.R.; Bào, Y.; Buchmeier, M.J.; Charrel, R.N.; Clawson, A.N.; Clegg, C.S.; DeRisi, J.L.; Emonet, S.; Gonzalez, J.P.; Kuhn, J.H.; et al. Past, present, and future of arenavirus taxonomy. *Arch. Virol.* **2015**, *160*, 1851–1874. [CrossRef] [PubMed]

16. Wulff, H.; McIntosh, B.M.; Hamner, D.B.; Johnson, K.M. Isolation of an arenavirus closely related to Lassa virus from Mastomys natalensis in South-East Africa. *Bull. World Health Organ.* **1977**, *55*, 441–444. [PubMed]

17. Günther, S.; Hoofd, G.; Charrel, R.; Röser, C.; Becker-Ziaja, B.; Lloyd, G.; Sabuni, C.; Verhagen, R.; van der Groen, G.; Kennis, J.; Katakweba, A.; et al. Mopeia virus-related arenavirus in Natal multimammate mice, Morogoro, Tanzania. *Emerg. Infect. Dis.* **2009**, *15*, 2008–2010. [CrossRef] [PubMed]

18. Ishii, A.; Thomas, Y.; Moonga, L.; Nakamura, I.; Ohnuma, A.; Hang'ombe, B.; Takada, A.; Mweene, A.; Sawa, H. Novel arenavirus, Zambia. *Emerg. Infect. Dis.* **2011**, *17*, 1921–1924. [CrossRef]

19. Gryseels, S.; Rieger, T.; Oestereich, L.; Cuypers, B.; Borremans, B.; Makundi, R.; Leirs, H.; Günther, S.; Goüy de Bellocq, J. Gairo virus, a novel arenavirus of the widespread Mastomys natalensis: Genetically divergent, but ecologically similar to Lassa and Morogoro viruses. *Virology* **2015**, *476*, 249–256. [CrossRef]

20. Radoshitzky, S.R.; Kuhn, J.H.; Jahrling, P.B.; Bavari, S. Hemorrhagic Fever-Causing Mammarenaviruses. In *Medical Aspects of Biological Warfare*; Bozue, J., Cote, C.K., Glass, P.J., Eds.; Office of the Surgeon General: Fort Sam Houston, TX, USA, 2018; Chapter 21; pp. 517–545.

21. Riviere, Y.; Ahmed, R.; Southern, P.J.; Buchmeier, M.J.; Oldstone, M.B. Genetic mapping of lymphocytic choriomeningitis virus pathogenicity: Virulence in guinea pigs is associated with the L RNA segment. *J. Virol.* **1985**, *55*, 704–709.

22. Zhang, L.; Marriott, K.A.; Harnish, D.G.; Aronson, J.F. Reassortant analysis of guinea pig virulence of Pichinde virus variants. *Virology* **2001**, *290*, 30–38. [CrossRef]

23. Lukashevich, I.S.; Vasiuchkov, A.D.; Stel'makh, T.A.; Scheslenok, E.P.; Shabanov, A.G. The isolation and characteristics of reassortants between the Lassa and Mopeia arenaviruses. *Vopr. Virusol.* **1991**, *36*, 146–150.

24. Lukashevich, I.S. Generation of reassortants between African arenaviruses. *Virology* **1992**, *188*, 600–605. [CrossRef]

25. Lukashevich, I.S.; Patterson, J.; Carrion, R.; Moshkoff, D.; Ticer, A.; Zapata, J.; Brasky, K.; Geiger, R.; Hubbard, G.B.; Bryant, J.; et al. A Live Attenuated Vaccine for Lassa Fever Made by Reassortment of Lassa and Mopeia Viruses. *J. Virol.* **2005**, *79*, 13934–13942. [CrossRef]

26. Cohen, J. Unfilled Vials. *Science* **2016**, *351*, 16–19. [CrossRef] [PubMed]

27. Moshkoff, D.A.; Salvato, M.S.; Lukashevich, I.S. Molecular characterization of a reassortant virus derived from Lassa and Mopeia viruses. *Virus Genes* **2007**, *34*, 169–176. [CrossRef]

28. Lukashevich, I.; Carrion, R., Jr.; Salvato, M.S.; Mansfield, K.; Brasky, K.; Zapata, J.; Cairo, C.; Goicochea, M.; Hoosien, GE.; Ticer, A.; Bryant, J.; et al. Safety, immunogenicity, and efficacy of the ML29 reassortant vaccine for Lassa fever in small non-human primates. *Vaccine* **2008**, *26*, 5246–5254. [CrossRef] [PubMed]

29. Zapata, J.C.; Carrion, R., Jr.; Patterson, J.L.; Crasta, O.; Zhang, Y.; Mani, S.; Jett, M.; Poonia, B.; Djavani, M.; White, D.M.; et al. Transcriptome Analysis of Human Peripheral Blood Mononuclear Cells Exposed to Lassa Virus and to the Attenuated Mopeia/Lassa Reassortant 29 (ML29), a Vaccine Candidate. *PLoS Negl. Trop. Dis.* **2013**, *7*, e2406. [CrossRef]

30. Iwasaki, M.; Cubitt, B.; Jokinen, J.; Lukashevich, I.S.; de la Torre, J.C. Use of recombinant ML29 platform to generate polyvalent live-attenuated vaccines against lassa fever and other infectious diseases. In Proceedings of the 66th Annual Meeting of Japanese Society for Virology, Kyoto, Japan, 28–30 October 2018. Available online: http://www.c-linkage.co.jp/jsv66/data/pro_workshop_day1.pdf (accessed on 14 January 2019).

31. Lukashevich, I.S. The search for animal models for Lassa fever vaccine development. *Expert Rev. Vaccines* **2013**, *12*, 71–86. [CrossRef]

32. Fisher-Hoch, S.P.; Hutwagner, L.; Brown, B.; McCormick, J.B. Effective Vaccine for Lassa Fever. *J. Virol.* **2000**, *74*, 6777–6783. [CrossRef] [PubMed]

33. Prescott, J.B.; Marzi, A.; Safronetz, D.; Robertson, S.; Feldmann, H.; Best, S.M. Immunobiology of Ebola and Lassa virus infections. *Nat. Rev. Immunol.* **2017**, *17*, 195–207. [CrossRef] [PubMed]

34. Jahrling, P.B.; Smith, S.; Hesse, R.A.; Rhoderick, J.B. Pathogenesis of Lassa virus infection in guinea pigs. *Infect. Immunity* **1982**, *37*, 771–778.

35. Peters, C.; Jahrling, P.B.; Lui, C.T.; Kenyon, R.H.; McKee, K.T., Jr.; Barrera Oro, J.G. Experimental studies of arenaviral hemorrhagic fevers. *Curr. Top. Microbiol. Immunol.* **1987**, *134*, 5–68.

36. Bell, T.M.; Shaia, C.I.; Bearss, J.J.; Mattix, M.E.; Koistinen, K.A.; Honnold, S.P.; Zeng, X.; Blancett, C.D.; Donnelly, G.C.; Shamblin, J.D.; et al. Temporal Progression of Lesions in Guinea Pigs Infected with Lassa Virus. *Vet. Pathol.* **2017**, *54*, 549–562. [CrossRef] [PubMed]

37. Jahrling, P.B.; Frame, J.D.; Smith, S.B.; Monson, M.H. Endemic Lassa fever in Liberia. III. Characterization of Lassa virus isolates. *Trans. R. Soc. Trop. Med. Hyg.* **1985**, *79*, 374–379. [CrossRef]

38. Morrison, H.; Bauer, S.P.; Lange, J.V.; Esposito, J.J.; McCormick, J.B.; Auperin, D.D. Protection of guinea pigs from Lassa fever by vaccinia virus recombinants expressing the nucleoprotein or the envelope glycoproteins of Lassa virus. *Virology* **1989**, *171*, 179–188. [CrossRef]

39. Pushko, P.; Geisbert, J.; Parker, M.; Jarling, P.; Smith, J. Individual and bivalent vaccines based on alphavirus replicons protect guinea pigs against infection with Lassa and Ebola viruses. *J. Virol.* **2001**, *75*, 11677–11685. [CrossRef] [PubMed]

40. Golden, J.W.; Hammerbeck, C.D.; Mucker, E.M.; Brocato, R.L. Animal Models for the Study of Rodent-Borne Hemorrhagic Fever Viruses: Arenaviruses and Hantaviruses. *BioMed Res. Int.* **2015**, *2015*, 793257. [CrossRef] [PubMed]

41. Yun, N.E.; Seregin, A.V.; Walker, D.H.; Popov, V.L.; Walker, A.G.; Smith, J.N.; Miller, M.; de la Torre, J.C.; Smith, J.K.; Borisevich, V.; et al. Mice lacking functional STAT1 are highly susceptable to lethal infection with Lassa virus. *J. Virol.* **2013**, *87*, 10908–10911. [CrossRef] [PubMed]

42. Yun, N.E.; Ronca, S.; Tamura, A.; Koma, T.; Seregin, A.V.; Dineley, K.T.; Miller, M.; Cook, R.; Shimizu, N.; Walker, A.G.; et al. Animal Model of Sensorineural Hearing Loss Associated with Lassa Virus Infection. *J. Virol.* **2016**, *90*, 2920–2927. [CrossRef]

43. López, C.B. Defective Viral Genomes: Critical Danger Signals of Viral Infections. *J. Virol.* **2014**, *88*, 8720–8723. [CrossRef]

44. Rezelj, V.V.; Levi, L.I.; Vignuzzi, M. The defective component of viral populations. *Curr. Opin. Virol.* **2018**, *33*, 74–80. [CrossRef]

45. Baltes, A.; Akpinar, F.; Inankur, B.; Yin, J. Inhibition of infection spread by co-transmitted defective interfering particles. *PLoS ONE* **2017**, *12*, e0184029. [CrossRef]

46. McLaren, L.; Holland, J. Defective interfering particles from poliovirus vaccine and vaccine reference strains. *Virology* **1974**, *60*, 579–583. [CrossRef]

47. Frensing, T. Defective interfering viruses and their impact on vaccines and viral vectors. *Biotechnol. J.* **2015**, *10*, 681–689. [CrossRef] [PubMed]

48. Gould, P.S.; Easton, A.J.; Dimmock, N.J. Live Attenuated Influenza Vaccine contains Substantial and Unexpected Amounts of Defective Viral Genomic RNA. *Viruses* **2017**, *9*, 269. [CrossRef] [PubMed]

49. Calain, P.; Roux, L. Generation of measles virus defective interfering particles and their presence in a preparation of attenuated live-virus vaccine. *J. Virol.* **1988**, *62*, 2859–2866. [PubMed]

50. Whistler, T.; Bellini, W.J.; Rota, P.A. Generation of Defective Interfering Particles by Two Vaccine Strains of Measles Virus. *Virology* **1996**, *220*, 480–484. [CrossRef] [PubMed]

51. Ho, T.H.; Kew, C.; Lui, P.Y.; Chan, C.P.; Satoh, T.; Akira, S.; Jin, D.Y.; Kok, K.H. PACT- and RIG-I-Dependent Activation of Type I Interferon Production by a Defective Interfering RNA Derived from Measles Virus Vaccine. *J. Virol.* **2016**, *90*, 1557–1568. [CrossRef] [PubMed]

52. Dutko, F.J.; Pfau, C.J. Arenavirus Defective Interfering Particles Mask the Cell-Killing Potential of Standard Virus. *J. Gen. Virol.* **1978**, *38*, 195–208. [CrossRef]

53. Popescu, M.; Schaefer, H.; Lehmann-Grube, F. Homologous interference of lymphocytic choriomeningitis virus: Detection and measurement of interference focus-forming units. *J. Virol.* **1976**, *20*, 1–8.

54. Welsh, R.M.; Connell, C.M.; Pfau, C.J. Properties of Defective Lymphocytic Choriomeningitis Virus. *J. Gen. Virol.* **1972**, *17*, 355–359. [CrossRef]

55. Welsh, R.M.; Burner, P.A.; Holland, J.J.; Oldstone, M.B.; Thompson, H.A.; Villarreal, L.P. A comparison of biochemical and biological properties of standard and defective lymphocytic choriomeningitis virus. *Bull. World Health Organ.* **1975**, *52*, 403–408.

56. Welsh, R.; Lampert, P.W.; Oldstone, M.B. Prevention of virus-induced cerebellar diseases by defective-interfering lymphocytic choriomeningitis virus. *J. Infect. Dis.* **1977**, *136*, 391–399. [CrossRef] [PubMed]

57. Welsh, R.; Oldstone, M.B.A. Inhibition of immunologic injury of cultered cells infected with lymphocytic choriomeningitis virus: Role of defective interfering virus in regulating viral antigen expression. *J. Exp. Med.* **1977**, *145*, 1449–1468. [CrossRef] [PubMed]

58. Popescu, M.; Lehmann-Grube, F. Defective interfering particles in mice infected with lymphocytic choriomeningitis virus. *Virology* **1977**, *77*, 78–83. [CrossRef]

59. Lukashevich, I.S.; Mar'iankova, R.F.; Fidarov, F.M. Acute and chronic Lassa virus infection of Vero cells. *Vopr. Virusol.* **1981**, *4*, 452–456.

60. Lukashevich, I.S.; Mar'iankova, R.F.; Lemeshko, N.N. Autointerfering activity of Lassa virus. *Vopr. Virusol.* **1983**, *1*, 96–101.

61. Lukashevich, I.S.; Trofimov, N.M.; Golibev, V.P.; Maryankova, R.F. Sedimentation analysis of the RNAs isolated from interfering particles of Lassa and Machupo viruses. *Acta Virol.* **1985**, *29*, 455–460. [PubMed]

62. Goicochea, M.A.; Zapata, J.C.; Bryant, J.; Davis, H.; Salvato, M.S.; Lukashevich, I.S. Evaluation of Lassa virus vaccine immunogenicity in a CBA/J-ML29 mouse model. *Vaccine* **2012**, *30*, 1445–1452. [CrossRef]

63. Wang, M.; Jokinen, J.; Tretyakova, I.; Pushko, P.; Lukashevich, I.S. Alphavirus vector-based replicon particles expressing multivalent cross-protective Lassa virus glycoproteins. *Vaccine* **2018**, *36*, 683–690. [CrossRef] [PubMed]

64. Kiley, M.P.; Swanepoel, R.; Mitchell, S.W.; Lange, J.V.; Gonzalez, J.P.; McCormick, J.B. Serological and biological evidence that Lassa-complex arenaviruses are widely distributed in Africa. *Med. Microbiol. Immunol.* **1986**, *175*, 161–163. [CrossRef] [PubMed]

65. Kiley, M.P.; Lange, J.V.; Johnson, K.M. Protection of rhesus monkeys from Lassa virus by immunisation with closely related Arenavirus. *Lancet* **1979**, *2*, 738. [CrossRef]

66. Safronetz, D.; Strong, J.E.; Feldmann, F.; Haddock, E.; Sogoba, N.; Brining, D.; Geisbert, T.W.; Scott, D.P.; Feldmann, H. A Recently Isolated Lassa Virus from Mali Demonstrates Atypical Clinical Disease Manifestations and Decreased Virulence in Cynomolgus Macaques. *J. Infect. Dis.* **2013**, *207*, 1316–1327. [CrossRef] [PubMed]

67. Russier, M.; Pannetier, D.; Baize, S. Immune Responses and Lassa Virus Infection. *Viruses* **2012**, *4*, 2766–2785. [CrossRef] [PubMed]

68. Hallam, H.J.; Hallman, S.; Rodriguez, S.E.; Barrett, A.D.T.; Beasley, D.W.C.; Chau, A.; Ksiazek, T.G.; Milligan, G.N.; Sathiyamoorthy, V.; Reece, L.M. Baseline mapping of Lassa fever virology, epidemiology and vaccine research and development. *NPJ Vaccines* **2018**, *3*, 11. [CrossRef] [PubMed]

69. McElroy, A.K.; Akondy, R.S.; Harmon, J.R.; Ellebedy, A.H.; Cannon, D.; Klena, J.D.; Sidney, J.; Sette, A.; Mehta, A.K.; Kraft, C.S. A Case of Human Lassa Virus Infection with Robust Acute T-Cell Activation and Long-Term Virus-Specific T-Cell Responses. *J. Infect. Dis.* **2017**, *215*, 1862–1872. [CrossRef] [PubMed]

70. Huang, A.S.; Baltimore, D. Defective interfering particles of animal viruses. *Comput. Virol.* **1977**, *10*, 73–116.

71. Huang, A.S. Defective Interfering Viruses. *Annu. Rev. Microbiol.* **1973**, *27*, 101–118. [CrossRef] [PubMed]

72. Barrett, A.D.; Dimmock, N.J. Defective interfering viruses and infections of animals. *Curr. Top. Microbiol. Immunol.* **1986**, *128*, 55–84.

73. Perrault, J. Origin and replication of defective interfering particles. *Curr. Top. Microbiol. Immunol.* **1981**, *93*, 151–207.

74. Roux, L.; Simon, A.E.; Holland, J.J. Effects of defective interfering viruses on virus replication and pathogenesis in vitro and in vivo. *Adv. Virus Res.* **1991**, *40*, 181–211.

75. Lukashevich, I.S.; Salvato, M.S. Lassa Virus Genome. *Curr. Genet.* **2006**, *7*, 351–379. [CrossRef]

76. Lukashevich, I.S.; Vela, E.M. Pathogenesis of Lasa virus infection in experimentl animals. In *Molecular Pathogenesis of Viral Hemorrhagic Fevers*; Vela, E.M., Ed.; Transworld Research Network: Kerala, India, 2010; pp. 101–142.

77. Peralta, L.M.; Bruns, M.; Lehmann-Grube, F. Biochemical composition of lymphocytic choriomeningitis virus interfering particles. *J. Gen. Virol.* **1981**, *55*, 475–479. [CrossRef] [PubMed]

78. Meyer, B.; Southern, P. A novel type of defective viral genome suggests a unique strategy to establish and maintain persistent lymphocytic choriomeningitis virus infections. *J. Virol.* **1997**, *71*, 6757–6764. [PubMed]

79. Cornu, T.I.; Feldmann, H.; de la Torre, J.C. Cells Expressing the RING Finger Z Protein Are Resistant to Arenavirus Infection. *J. Virol.* **2004**, *78*, 2979–2983. [CrossRef] [PubMed]

80. Zaza, A.D.; Herbreteau, C.H.; Peyrefitte, C.N.; Emonet, S.F. Mammarenaviruses deleted from their Z gene are replicative and produce an infectious progeny in BHK-21 cells. *Virology* **2018**, *518*, 34–44. [CrossRef] [PubMed]

81. Xing, J.; Ly, H.; Liang, Y. The Z Proteins of Pathogenic but Not Nonpathogenic Arenaviruses Inhibit RIG-i-Like Receptor-Dependent Interferon Production. *J. Virol.* **2015**, *89*, 944–2955. [CrossRef] [PubMed]

82. Sun, Y.; Jain, D.; Koziol-White, C.J.; Genoyer, E.; Gilbert, M.; Tapia, K.; Panettieri, R.A., Jr.; Hodinka, R.L.; López, C.B. Immunostimulatory Defective Viral Genomes from Respiratory Syncytial Virus Promote a Strong Innate Antiviral Response during Infection in Mice and Humans. *PLoS Pathog.* **2015**, *11*, e1005122. [CrossRef] [PubMed]

83. Lukashevich, I.S.; Pushko, P. Vaccine platforms to control Lassa fever. *Expert Rev. Vaccines* **2016**, *15*, 1135–1150. [CrossRef] [PubMed]

84. Carrion, R., Jr.; Patterson, J.L.; Johnson, C.; Gonzales, M.; Moreira, C.R.; Ticer, A.; Brasky, K.; Hubbard, G.B.; Moshkoff, D.; Zapata, J.; et al. A ML29 reassortant virus protects guinea pigs against a distantly related Nigerian strain of Lassa virus and can provide sterilizing immunity. *Vaccine* **2007**, *25*, 4093–4102. [CrossRef] [PubMed]

85. Zapata, J.; Medina-Moreno, S.; Guzmán-Cardozo, C.; Salvato, M.S. Improving the Breadth of the Host's Immune Response to Lassa Virus. *Pathogens* **2018**, *7*, 84. [CrossRef]

14

Risk Factors for *Brucella* Seroprevalence in Peri-Urban Dairy Farms in Five Indian Cities

Johanna F. Lindahl [1,2,3] 🆔, **Jatinder Paul Singh Gill** [4], **Razibuddin Ahmed Hazarika** [5], **Nadeem Mohamed Fairoze** [6], **Jasbir S. Bedi** [4], **Ian Dohoo** [7], **Abhimanyu Singh Chauhan** [8,9] 🆔, **Delia Grace** [1] **and Manish Kakkar** [8,*]

[1] Department of Biosciences, International Livestock Research Institute, Nairobi 00100, Kenya; J.lindahl@cgiar.org (J.F.L.); D.Randolph@cgiar.org (D.G.)

[2] Department of Clinical Sciences, Swedish University of Agricultural Sciences, PO Box 7054, SE-750 07 Uppsala, Sweden

[3] Zoonosis Science Centre, Department of Medical Biochemistry and Microbiology, Uppsala University, Po Box 582, SE-751 23 Uppsala, Sweden

[4] Guru Angad Dev Veterinary and Animal Sciences University, Ludhiana 141004, Punjab, India; gilljps@gmail.com (J.P.S.G.); bedijasbir78@gmail.com (J.S.B.)

[5] Department of Veterinary Public Health, Assam Agricultural University, Khanapara Campus, Guwahati-781022, India; rah1962@rediffmail.com

[6] Department of LPT, Veterinary College, Karnataka Veterinary Animal & Fisheries Sciences University Bangalore, Bangalore 560024, India; prof.nadeem@gmail.com

[7] Atlantic Veterinary College, University of Prince Edward Island, Charlottetown, C1A 4P3, Canada; dohoo@upei.ca

[8] Public Health Foundation India, Gurgaon 122002, India; abhimanyu.hm@gmail.com

[9] Department of Public Health Sciences, Faculty of Medicine, University of Liège, 4000 Liege, Belgium

* Correspondence: manish.kakkar@phfi.org.

Abstract: Brucellosis is endemic among dairy animals in India, contributing to production losses and posing a health risk to people, especially farmers and others in close contact with dairy animals or their products. Growing urban populations demand increased milk supplies, resulting in intensifying dairy production at the peri-urban fringe. Peri-urban dairying is under-studied but has implications for disease transmission, both positive and negative. In this cross-sectional study, five Indian cities were selected to represent different geographies and urbanization extent. Around each, we randomly selected 34 peri-urban villages, and in each village three smallholder dairy farms (defined as having a maximum of 10 dairy animals) were randomly selected. The farmers were interviewed, and milk samples were taken from up to three animals. These were tested using a commercial ELISA for antibodies against *Brucella abortus*, and factors associated with herd seroprevalence were identified. In all, 164 out of 1163 cows (14.1%, 95% CI 12.2–16.2%) were seropositive for *Brucella*. In total, 91 out of 510 farms (17.8%, 95% CI 14.6–21.4%) had at least one positive animal, and out of these, just seven farmers stated that they had vaccinated against brucellosis. In four cities, the farm-level seroprevalence ranged between 1.4–5.2%, while the fifth city had a seroprevalence of 72.5%. This city had larger, zero-grazing herds, used artificial insemination to a much higher degree, replaced their animals by purchasing from their neighbors, were less likely to contact a veterinarian in case of sick animals, and were also judged to be less clean. Within the high-prevalence city, farms were at higher risk of being infected if they had a young owner and if they were judged less clean. In the low-prevalence cities, no risk factors could be identified. In conclusion, this study has identified that a city can have a high burden of infected animals in the peri-urban areas, but that seroprevalence is strongly influenced by the husbandry system. Increased intensification can be associated with increased risk, and thus the practices associated with this, such as artificial insemination, are also associated with increased risk. These results may be important to identify high-risk areas for prioritizing interventions and for policy decisions influencing the structure and development of the dairy industry.

Keywords: zoonoses; prevalence; *Brucella abortus*; urban livestock keeping; smallholder farming

1. Introduction

Infectious diseases cause a major burden on both human health and society as a whole. Zoonotic diseases inflict a double burden, since they also affect animal health, with associated costs and reduced productivity. Brucellosis is a very common but frequently neglected zoonosis that occurs globally, except for in a few countries that have managed to eradicate it, and the disease is often underreported and uncontrolled in low and middle-income countries, which may have the highest burden of the disease [1–4].

The disease can be caused by different bacteria of the genus *Brucella*, of which most species are pathogenic to multiple mammals, including cattle and humans [5,6]. Cattle are most frequently infected by *Brucella abortus* or *Brucella melitensis* [5,6]. These bacteria cause a chronic infection with preferred localization in the reproductive system, where they can cause abortion in pregnant cows or other reproductive problems, as well as reduced milk production in lactating animals and orchitis in bulls [1,7]. Although most infected animals only abort once, they may remain infected their entire life [8]. After the first abortion, as well as in non-pregnant animals, the disease can be asymptomatic [5]. Infected male cattle can spread the disease sexually, and both sexes may become infertile. Joint hygromas are another common manifestation of brucellosis [3].

Milk consumption has been increasing in low and middle-income countries, a trend likely to continue as the demand for animal-source food trends upwards due to population growth, changing lifestyles, and increasing wealth [9]. In India, the large vegetarian population increases the dependence on dairy products for high quality proteins. India has the world's largest dairy herd at around 300 million and is the world's leading milk producer, contributing around 17% of the world's total milk production, with more than 70 million households engaged in milk production [10,11]. Milk consumption is higher in urban areas and while the majority of the Indian population still live in rural areas, urbanization is increasing. Cities require a constant supply of fresh milk, and peri-urban dairy production plays an important role in meeting this demand.

The health of livestock, humans and livelihoods are closely linked, with zoonotic diseases such as brucellosis causing not only human and animal morbidity, but also reduced animal production and hence reduced incomes [12,13]. In India, awareness of brucellosis is low among livestock-keepers and healthcare staff, and because of the non-specific symptoms and the limited availability of laboratory facilities in many rural hospitals, diagnosis is seldom feasible [14,15]. Multiple studies have found seropositivity in humans in India, indicating the need to have an OneHealth approach for controlling this disease [16].

2. Materials and Methods

2.1. Ethical Approval

The study received ethical approval from the ethics committee of the Public Health Foundation of India [TRC-IEC-219/14, 27 May 2014; amended 12 October 2015]. Ethical approval was also obtained by Institutional Ethics Committees of Guru Angad Dev Veterinary and Animal Sciences University (GADVASU), Assam Agricultural University (AAU), Karnataka Veterinary, Animal and Fisheries Sciences University (KVAFSU), Rajasthan University of Veterinary and Animal Sciences (RAJUVAS) and School of Biotechnology, Kalinga Institute of Industrial Technology (KSBT) at the Ludhiana, Guwahati, Bangalore, Udaipur and Bhubaneswar study sites, respectively. Before a farmer was interviewed, they were informed about the purpose of the study and gave their consent to participate.

2.2. Farm Selection

Five Indian cities were selected purposively to represent different parts of the country (Figure 1). Peri-urban was defined as within 5 km of the official city boundaries, and all villages in that circle were mapped. For the purpose of this study, smallholder farms were defined as a dairy farm with a herd size of less than 10 cattle/buffaloes at the time of the survey and at least one milking animal, with dairy constituting a source of livelihood with or without domestic consumption. A systematic selection of 34 of these villages was done by identifying the proportion that needed to be sampled, and then systematically choosing these in a clockwise fashion around the city. The selected villages were then visited to identify all farms, using local village leaders as guides. The methodology of the creation of this sampling frame has been described elsewhere [17]. Out of this sampling frame, three smallholder farmers per village were randomly selected.

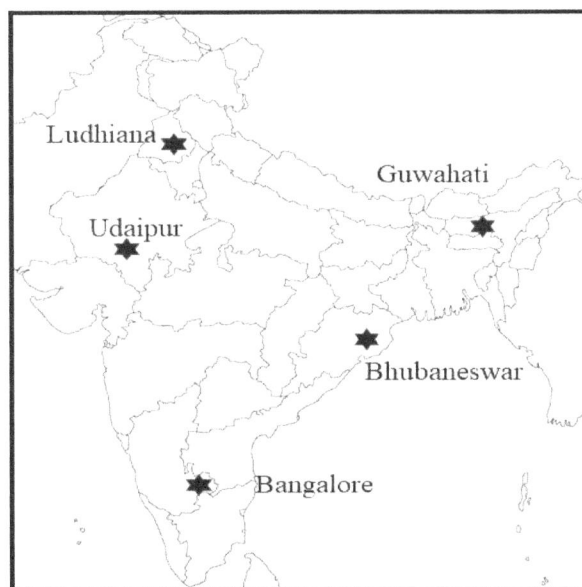

Figure 1. Location of selected cities in India.

2.3. Data Collection

Data collection was done between June 2015 and January 2016. A questionnaire was developed and piloted on farms in each site before starting the sampling. The tool was uploaded into electronic format and data collection was conducted using tablets, from which the data was uploaded into a central server. Data was collected by different data collection teams in each city, but all teams were trained by the same trainers, who joined in the first days of data collection. The data was collected through interviews in the local language, after the participants had been read the information about the project and given their written consent. Observations about cleaning practices and hygienic status were done during milking using an observation checklist. Cleanliness and drainage scores were standardized using pictures to guide the grading, and the scoring was assessed during the training to make sure it was consistent. Knowledge about antibiotics was assessed based on if the farmer reported to know the word (in the local language).

2.4. Sample Collection

In each farm, up to three milking cows or buffaloes were selected for sampling. In the 33% of farms where the number of milking cattle exceeded three, all cows were given a unique number, and then three numbers were selected randomly. The data collection teams were trained on aseptic collection of milk from the selected cows, and 40 mL of milk was collected in sterile vials and immediately kept chilled until they were transported to the laboratory on the same day of collection. The samples were thereafter stored in deep freezer at −80 °C. Samples were kept frozen when transported to the laboratory of microbiology at GADVASU and stored at −80 °C until analysis.

2.5. Serological Analysis

Milk was analyzed for the presence of antibodies using a commercial indirect enzyme-linked immunosorbent assay (iELISA) developed for use with milk samples (IDEXX Brucellosis Milk X2 Ab Test, IDEXX, Westbrook, ME, USA). The protocol of the manufacturer was followed, and all samples were done in duplicates. In brief, 50 µL of milk was diluted into 200 µL of sample diluent on a microplate precoated with *Brucella* lipopolysaccharide (LPS). The plate was incubated for 90 min, before being washed and the subsequent addition of conjugated anti-bovine IgG antibodies. After 30 min of incubation and washing, the tetramethylbenzidine (TMB) substrate was added and incubated for 20 min before the stop solution was added and the plate read at 450 nm.

The ratio of the optical density of the samples (mean) to the mean positive control was calculated after subtracting the mean of the negative controls from both. A ratio of above 55% was considered positive, while between 45 and 55% was considered suspected positive. In the analysis, only one sample was suspected positive, and since all other animals tested at the same farm were also positive, this animal is considered positive in the analyses and results. The specificity for this kit used on milk samples has been found to be very high [18], and a meta-analysis suggest a specificity of 96% for ELISA conducted on milk [19].

2.6. Data Analysis

An initial screening of all information collected was carried out with only the variables listed in Table 1 being retained for analysis, after identifying the variables with potential causal association with brucellosis. Analysis of the retained data proceeded in four steps. First, multiple correspondence analysis (MCA) was used to investigate relationships among all the predictors recorded. All predictors were initially recoded to di- or trichotomous variables. An MCA was carried out using all predictors and those having a contribution to either the first or second dimension that exceeded 0.02 were retained. The process was repeated sequentially with the required contribution being raised by 0.01 at each step (to a maximum of 0.06). At this point, the six variables that best explained the information content of the full set had been identified and these were plotted on a two-dimensional MCA plot (Figure 2).

One site (Guwahati) had a dramatically higher farm prevalence (72%) than the other four sites (4%), so the second step in the analysis was to evaluate the unconditional associations between each of the predictors and a variable representing Guwahati compared to the other sites. Either two-sample *t*-tests or cross-tabulations with chi-square statistics were used to determine if the regions were different. Results are presented in Table 1. Guwahati was also added as a supplemental variable (s51 vs s50 in Figure 2) to the MCA plot in Figure 2 to show which predictors were most associated with Guwahati vs other sites.

The third step was to use logistic regression models to identify factors associated with the risk of a farm being *Brucella* spp. positive within Guwahati, using backward elimination among variables with unconditional associations with $p < 0.15$. A random effect for village was included in all models. The linearity of continuous predictors was evaluated using lowess smoothed curves and a quadratic term was added to the model if there was significant evidence of curvature in the relationship. Initially, unconditional associations were determined with predictors having $p < 0.15$ retained for further consideration. A manual backward elimination was used to remove non-significant (at $p > 0.05$) predictors. Age of farmer and farm size (number of animals) were forced into all models as potential confounders. In addition to age and number of animals, two factors (cleanliness of floor and level of vaccination) were identified as potentially important. An MCA plot was generated (using trichotomous versions of each of the predictors) with *Brucella* spp. added as a supplemental variable to the final plot to see which predictors were generally associated with being *Brucella* spp. positive or negative.

Table 1. Potential risk factors for brucellosis given as either mean (standard deviation), or proportion (95% confidence interval).

	All Sites	Guwahati	Bangalore	Bhubaneswar	Ludhiana	Udaipur	p-Value *
Age of farmer	46.2 (12.3)	43.9 (12.9)	44.8 (13.2)	51.1 (10.8)	46.6 (12.7)	44.6 (10.2)	0.035
Female respondents	21.8% (18.3–25.6)	15.7% (9.2–24.2)	41.2% (31.5–51.4)	11.8% (6.2–19.6)	14.7% (8.5–23.1)	25.5% (17.4–35.1)	0.096
Illiterate respondents	35.4% (31.0–39.9)	51.1% (40.2–61.9)	41.1% (30.8–52.0)	23.5% (15.7–33.0)	15.7% (8.6–25.3)	44.9% (34.8–55.3)	0.001
Number of dairy animals	7.7 (4.0)	10.3 (4.1)	5.4 (2.7)	8.1 (3.6)	7.2 (3.7)	7.5 (4.0)	<0.001
Zero-grazing	53.3% (48.9–57.7)	95.1% (88.9–98.3)	9.8% (4.8–17.2)	4.9% (1.6–11.1)	93.1% (86.4–97.2)	63.7% (53.6–73.0)	<0.001
Using AI	76.0% (72.1–79.7)	92.2% (85.1–96.6)	98.0% (93.1–99.8%)	47.5% (37.5–57.7)	69.6% (59.7–78.3)	72.5% (62.8–80.9)	<0.001
Purchasing cows from neighboring farms	57.6% (52.8–62.3)	98.9% (94.0–100)	71.7% (57.7–83.2)	21.1% (13.4–30.6)	34.4% (24.9–45.0)	69.0% (59.0–77.9)	<0.001
Dirty floors in cow sheds	11.1% (8.5–14.2)	24.8% (16.7–34.3)	11.0% (5.6–18.8)	10.8% (5.5–18.5)	6.1% (2.3–12.7)	3.0% (0.6–8.4)	<0.001
Well-drained floors	19.8% (16.4–23.6)	8.9% (4.2–16.2)	22.8% (15.2–32.5)	23.5% (15.7–33.0)	35.4% (26.0–45.6)	8.9% (4.2–16.2)	0.007
Never vaccinate animals	15.5% (12.4–18.9)	25.5% (17.4–35.1)	0% (0–3.6)	2.0% (0.2–6.9)	7.8% (3.4–14.9)	42.42% (32.4–52.3)	<0.001
Vaccinate young animals routinely	26.7% (22.9–30.7)	61.8% (51.6–71.2)	2.9% (0.6–8.4)	44.1% (34.3–54.3)	0% (0–3.6)	24.5% (16.5–34.0)	<0.001
Records of sick animals	11.6% (8.0–14.7)	0% (0–3.6)	8.8% (4.1–16.1)	24.5% (16.5–34.0)	1.0% (0–5.3)	23.5% (15.7–33.0)	<0.001
Alpha score for cleaning routines	2.19 (0.28)	2.14 (0.23)	2.10 (0.28)	2.16 (0.08)	2.06 (0.13)	2.50 (0.34)	0.034
Alpha score for observed hygiene	0.32 (0.28)	0.10 (0.11)	0.31 (0.21)	0.60 (0.31)	0.25 (0.21)	0.35 (0.23)	<0.001
Regular health checks	23.9% (20.3–27.9)	3.9% (1.1–9.7)	14.7% (8.5–23.1)	33.3% (24.3–43.4)	46.1% (36.2–56.2)	21.6% (14.0–30.8)	<0.001
Let veterinarian check animals before purchase, or test the animal	25.9% (22.1–29.9)	2.9% (0.6–8.4)	35.3% (26.1–45.4)	58.8% (48.6–68.5)	9.8% (4.8–17.3)	22.6% (14.9–31.9)	<0.001
Quarantine new animals	24.6% (20.8–28.4)	17.7% (10.8–26.4)	19.6% (12.4–28.6)	41.4% (31.6–51.8)	19.6% (12.4–28.6)	24.5% (16.5–34.0)	0.074

* Comparing Guwahati with the four other sites.

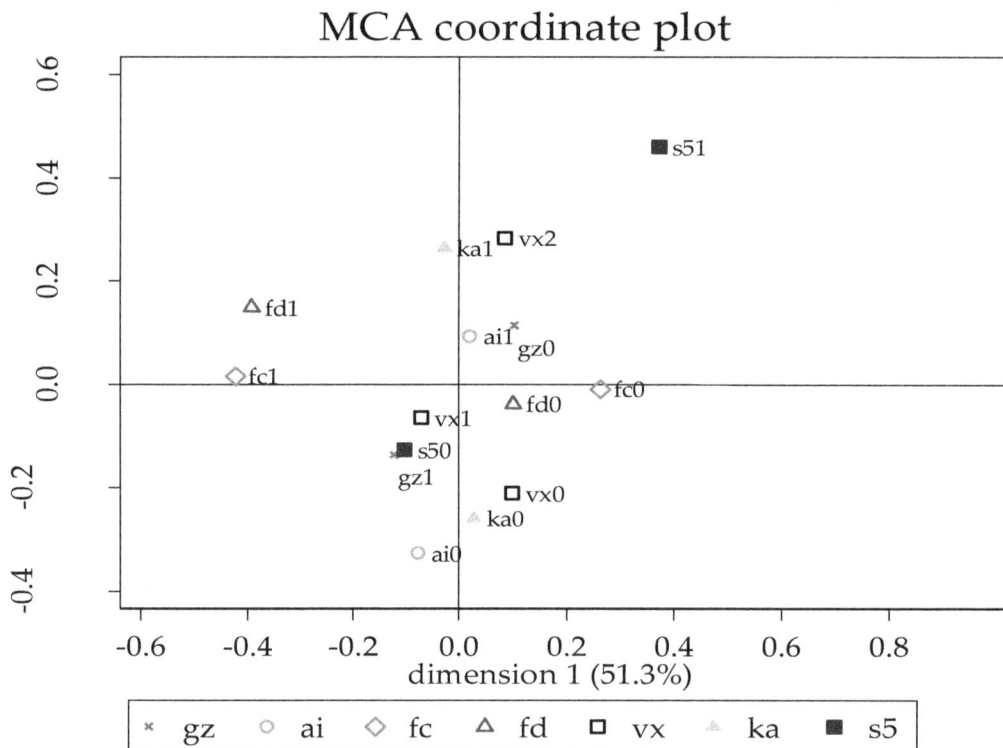

Figure 2. Multiple correspondence analysis (MCA) plot for the factors associated with the high seroprevalence site. Gz = grazing, where gz0 is zero-grazing and gz1 is grazing. Ai = artificial insemination, where ai0 is no artificial insemination and ai1 is use of artificial insemination. Fc = floor cleanliness, where fc0 is clean or moderately clean floor and fc1 is dirty floor. Fd = drainage, where fd0 equals insufficient drainage and fd1 is good drainage. Vx = vaccination, where vx0 means no vaccination done, vx1 means vaccination when there is an outbreak or when given free vaccines, and vx2 means vaccinating animals as young. Ka = knowledge about antibiotics, where ka0 is no knowledge and ka1 is the farmer reporting to know about antibiotics. S5 = site Guwahati, where s50 means any other site and s51 means Guwahati.

Finally, the model building process was repeated to determine which factors most influenced the risk of being *Brucella* spp. positive in sites 1 to 4. Only two predictors (farm size and use of *Haemorrhagic septicemia* vaccine) had unconditional associations with $p < 0.15$, but neither of these was significant in a final model so no results are presented.

3. Results

3.1. Brucella Seroprevalence

In total, 164 out of 1163 cows (14.1%, 95% CI 12.2–16.2%) were seropositive for *Brucella*.

A farm was considered positive for *Brucella* if at least one out of the three tested animals tested positive. In total, 91 farms out of 510 (17.8%, 95% CI 14.6%–21.4%) had at least one positive animal (see Table 2), and out of these, 23 farms had two positive animals and 25 (all in Guwahati) had all three animals positive. There were large differences in farm prevalence between the five different cities (Table 2). Guwahati had significantly higher seroprevalence ($p < 0.001$) than the other sites, and the odds ratio for a farm being positive in Guwahati was 44.4 (95% CI 7.5–113.2) times higher than in Udaipur and 138.9 (95% CI 32.0–602.3) times higher than in Bhubaneswar.

Table 2. Farm level *Brucella* seroprevalence (95% confidence interval) in the five different cities.

	Brucella Farm Positivity	*Brucella* Farm Positivity Excluding Farms with Vaccination
Bangalore	2.9% (0.6–8.4)	3.0% (0.6–8.6)
Bhubaneswar	2.0% (0.2–6.9)	1.4% (0–7.4)
Guwahati	73.5% (63.9–81.8)	72.5% (62.5–81.0)
Ludhiana	4.9% (1.6–11.1)	4.3% (1.2–10.6)
Udaipur	5.9% (2.2–12.4)	5.2% (1.7–11.6)
Overall	17.8% (14.6–21.34)	18.3% (14.8–22.1)

3.2. Risk Factor Analyses for Herds with No Previous Vaccination

The presence of different stipulated risk factors varied across the five cities. After exclusion of farms that reported having vaccinated against *Brucella* earlier, 460 farms from 162 villages in five sites (geographic regions) were included. Missing values were observed in 0 to 15.6% of observations within a variable and 62% of farms had complete data for all variables. *Brucella* prevalence ranged from 1.4 to 5.2% across four sites, while the prevalence in Guwahati was 72.5%.

The MCA analysis for investigating relationships among predictors identified pasture grazing, use of artificial insemination (AI) (vs natural breeding), routine (vs irregular) vaccination, floor cleanliness, adequacy of floor drainage, and owner knowledge of antibiotics as the six variables most useful in discriminating among farms. Floor cleanliness and drainage contributed most to the first dimension (explaining 51.3% of inertia (information) in the data) while level of vaccination, knowledge of antibiotics and AI contributed most to the second dimension (45.0% of inertia). Farmers that had knowledge of antibiotics also used routine vaccination, and they tended to be farms that did not pasture (graze) animals but did use AI. Farms with good floor cleanliness also had good floor drainage.

Evaluation of unconditional associations between the recorded predictors and Guwahati vs the other sites showed many statistically significant differences. With the exception of three of the four demographic variables and the quarantining of new entries into the herd, all predictors showed significant differences at $p < 0.05$. Compared to the other cities, Guwahati had larger non-pastured herds, used AI for breeding, purchased their replacements from neighbors, were less likely to have good stable cleanliness or drainage scores, were more likely to have dirty stable floors, had a lower composite hygiene score, and were less likely to have veterinarians regularly check their animals or check animals before purchase. However, they were more likely to use routine vaccinations of young animals and to know what antibiotics were.

3.3. Risk Factors for Brucella Seropositivity in Guwahati

In addition to age and herd size, which were included as potential confounders, two management factors (floor cleanliness and level of vaccine use) were identified as being associated with *Brucella* spp. A multiple correspondence analysis (MCA) plot was generated (using trichotomous versions of each of the predictors) with *Brucella* spp. added as a supplemental variable to the final plot to see which predictors were generally associated with being *Brucella* spp. positive or negative (Figure 3). Being *Brucella* positive (B1) was most common in farms that had a younger age owner (ag0 or ag1) and had a lower floor cleanliness scores (fc1 or fc2). Being *Brucella* negative (B0) was most strongly associated with the cleanest floors (fc3) and the smallest herds (na0). Table 3 shows the odds ratios associated with seropositivity for risk factors in Guwahati from the multivariable model. The high village level variance indicates a very high intra-cluster correlation.

MCA coordinate plot

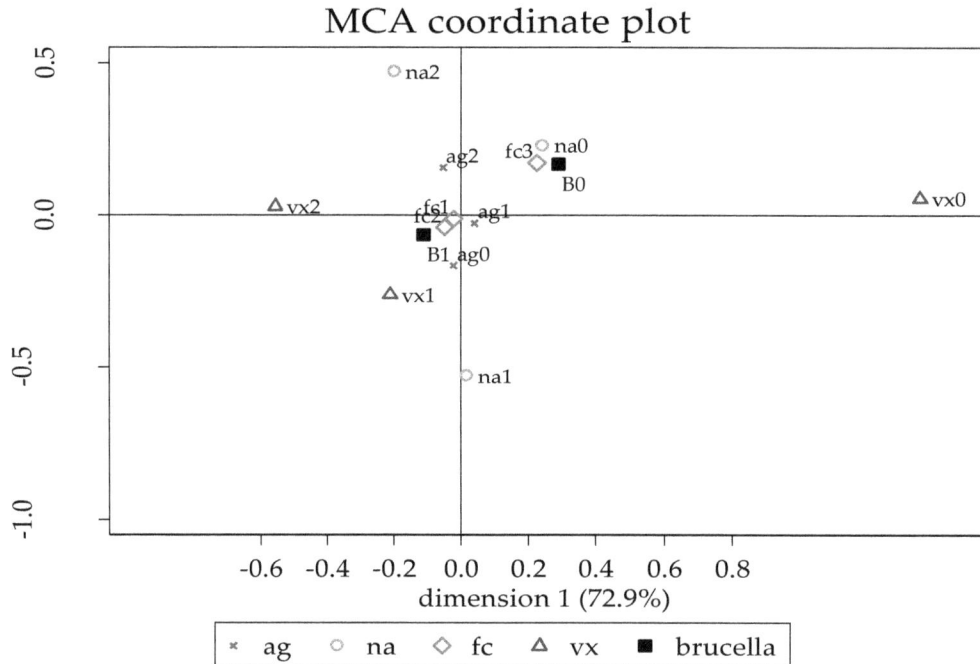

Figure 3. MCA plot of risk factors for *Brucella* seropositivity in Guwahati, India. Ai = Artificial insemination, where ai0 is no artificial insemination and ai1 is use of artificial insemination. Na = number of animals, where na0 is less than 7 animals and na1 is 7–10 animals. Fc = floor cleanliness, where fc0 is clean or moderately clean floor and fc1 is dirty floor. Vx = vaccination, where vx0 means no vaccination done, vx1 means vaccination when there is an outbreak or when given free vaccines, and vx2 means vaccinating animals as young. B = *Brucella*, where B0 = seronegative farm and B1 = seropositive farm.

Table 3. Risk factors for *Brucella* seropositivity within Guwahati, India, using a mixed logistic regression model.

Risk Factor	Odds Ratio	95% Confidence Interval	Standard Error	*p*-Value
Farmer age (year)	0.96	0.90–1.02	0.03	0.20
Floor cleanliness				
Clean	Reference			
Average	11.6	1.29–105.18	13.1	0.03
Dirty	42.8	1.87–978.57	68.3	0.02
Vaccination				
No vaccination	Reference			
Vaccinate irregularly	44.1	0.73–2669.57	92.3	0.07
Vaccinate routinely	12.8	1.40–116.80	14.4	0.02
Number of animals	1.0	0.85–1.30	0.4	0.7
Quadratic term of number of animals	0.95	0.90–0.999	0.02	0.05
Constant	2.2	0.05–91.5	4.1	
Village level variance	4.2	0.65–26.84	4.0	

3.4. Risk Factors for Brucella Seropositivity in Bangalore, Bhubaneswar, Ludhiana, and Udaipur

Logistic models were also used to investigate risk factors for *Brucella* spp. positivity within the low-prevalence sites. However, no risk factors had significant associations, so no results are presented.

4. Discussion

This study found high variation in the seroprevalence between the different peri-urban sites. In general, our findings were comparable with the literature on bovine brucellosis in India. A recent review concluded that most studies using probabilistic sampling and not targeting cows with a clinical history suggesting brucellosis, reported a prevalence of 5–12%, which is above what was detected in the four other cities but considerably less than that we found in Guwahati [20]. While this study could not identify many risk factors in the peri-urban farms, it was found that keeping floors clean was important. Risk of *Brucella* exposure was also associated with herd size, which has been shown previously [21–24]. Vaccinating (for other diseases than brucellosis), either routinely or when there were vaccination campaigns in the face of outbreaks or vaccines provided for free, was associated with a higher risk of exposure, which could potentially be explained as farmers with more experience with disease being more positive to vaccination.

The peri-urban seroprevalence in Ludhiana, Punjab, was lower than previously reported in the state. Here 21% and 18% seroprevalence was found by Aulakh et al. [25] and Ul-Islam et al. [26]. Gill et al. [23] and Dhand et al. [27] also found more than 10% prevalence in cattle. This may indicate that reducing prevalence is associated with better control or changing husbandry, or may reflect a more systematic approach to sampling in our study, which focused only on smallholder peri-urban dairying.

The high seropositivity in Guwahati is in accordance with results from the same area using a milk ring test, where 88% of farms were found positive [28]. Chakraborty et al. [29] found 60% seropositivity among lactating cows in Guwahati, whereas Gogoi et al. [30] found 30% seroprevalence in Kamrup metropolitan district of Guwahati. It is worth noting that Renukaradhya et al. [31] did not find any seropositive animals in Assam, using their own developed ELISA. Given the results of our research and the earlier research from the state, it seems that the peri-urban belt around Guwahati may have a higher than average burden of brucellosis. Brucellosis in humans has not been extensively studied, but in one previous study, three (all with animal husbandry background) out of 52 humans tested positive in Assam [32]. In people with animal contact, more than 24% seropositivity was found in Ludhiana as well [33], indicating the need to include brucellosis as a potential diagnosis in febrile cases with occupational risk factors.

The study shows how MCA can be used when data are collected on quite a large number of predictors and many of these are potentially related (weakly or strongly). In this context, it is useful to visualize these inter-relationships in order to get a better understanding of how farms could be grouped. The MCA identified a set of key variables which could be used to discriminate among farms, and these should be considered as important to collect information on in any future research undertaken in this region of India. Another methodological issue was presented because one site (Guwahati) had an extremely high herd prevalence of *Brucella* spp. compared to the other four sites. The strong collinearity between the outcome of interest (seropositivity against *Brucella*) and the site meant that the risk factor analyses could not utilize the full data set in one analysis. It would have been impossible to tell if any significant predictor was actually associated with *Brucella* spp. positivity or whether it just strongly differed between Guwahati and the other sites (with no effect on *Brucella* spp. risk). Consequently, risk factors were evaluated in Guwahati separately from the other study sites, which reduced the power of the study. For the four low-prevalence sites, there were only 14 positive farms (out of 362) while in Guwahati there were only 27 negative farms (out of 98). This lack of power limited our ability to identify risk factors for *Brucella* spp.

Raising awareness, training farmers, and modern techniques are often recommended for improving livestock disease control. In our study, the evidence for this was ambiguous. Guwahati, which had the highest prevalence in this study, was characterized by greater knowledge and higher use of modern animal health care inputs, such as vaccination and AI. On the other hand, hygiene appeared to be poor. Overall, a picture emerges of larger, less well managed herds with more reliance on vaccines and antibiotics for disease control. Other studies in Guwahati found that while training interventions had some impact on both hygiene and knowledge, there was no impact on the seropositivity for brucellosis [28]. This indicates caution in assuming intensification, even with improving knowledge and training, will lead to better disease control. It should be noted, however, that overall use of vaccination was low, indicating considerable scope for improvement. There seemed to be a high dependency on vaccinations in the face of outbreaks or when they were provided for free, with two of the sites having less than 3% of farms reporting routine vaccinations. Poor vaccination coverage can have different explanations, including poor access to vaccines, limited extension services, or poor understanding of farmers as to the benefits of using vaccines. In other studies in India, low knowledge about the function of vaccines and low willingness to pay has been associated with low uptake of vaccination [34,35], which could possibly also explain the low adoption here. Studying the use of vaccines in chickens, it has been shown that having active support promotes vaccination and also makes people understand the function of vaccines better, which makes for more positive attitudes, and hence better uptake [36]. Even though farms that reported having used *Brucella* vaccines were excluded from analyses, it is possible that there might be farms where the farmer did not know which disease the animals were vaccinated against, which could have affected the results, but considering the low vaccination against *Brucella* overall, this is deemed a low risk. India has a government sponsored control program for brucellosis in cattle, with planned use of the S19 vaccine [31], but still vaccination is seldom performed in the field.

Many sero-surveys have been carried out for brucellosis in India, but these are typically conducted in one area, and differing methods make it hard to compare results from different areas, including the frequent targeting of animals with clinical symptoms [20]. Using the same, probabilistic study approach contemporaneously in five widely dispersed cities allowed us to confidently detect important and likely real differences between cities and to link this with some risk factors. An important finding of the study was that brucellosis can be very prevalent in some peri-urban areas and have very low presence in others. Moreover, disease transmission risk factors are different in scenarios with a high or a low infection pressure, and a habit, such as purchasing cows from neighbors is likely a protective factor when living in a low-risk area, but a high-risk practice in an area with a very high prevalence. Within Guwahati, the mixed effects model suggested a very high village level variance and a high intra-cluster correlation, indicating that future studies need to include as many villages as possible, which could be explained by the habit of purchasing animals from nearby farms, spreading the disease within a village, but less so between villages.

5. Conclusions

This study emphasizes the need to systematically identify disease hotspots for zoonotic diseases; the importance of considering intensifying peri-urban dairy belts in disease surveillance and control; the high degree to which structural factors may influence disease risk in peri-urban dairy, and the need for targeted, effective interventions. In light of the brucellosis control program in India, this study highlights the lack of sufficient vaccination coverage among smallholder dairy farmers in different parts of India, and also the high variability in prevalence. Knowledge about the prevalence in different areas can guide the control efforts, and improved information about local risk factors as well as the extent of farmers' understanding about the disease, can aid in creating better extension campaigns.

Author Contributions: J.F.L., M.K. & D.G. conceptualized and designed the project, J.F.L. & I.D. conducted the data analyses, J.S.B. & J.P.S.G. conducted laboratory analyses, A.S.C., R.A.H., N.M.F. & M.K. coordinated data collection, J.F.L. drafted the manuscript & all authors contributed to critically revise the manuscript.

Acknowledgments: The authors would like to acknowledge all participating farmers, the data collection teams and other collaborators.

References

1.   WHO FAO OIE; Corbel, M.J. *Brucellosis in Humans and Animals*; WHO: Rome, Italy, 2006.

2.   Pappas, G.; Papadimitriou, P.; Akritidis, N.; Christou, L.; Tsianos, E.V. The new global map of human brucellosis. *Lancet. Infect. Dis.* **2006**, *6*, 91–99. [CrossRef]

3.   OIE. *Bovine Brucellosis: OIE Terrestrial Manual 2009*; Office International de Epizootie: Paris, France, 2009.

4. McDermott, J.J.; Grace, D.; Zinsstag, J. Economics of brucellosis impact and control in low-income countries. *Sci. Tech. Rev. Off. Int. Des Epizoot.* **2013**, *32*, 249–261. [CrossRef]

5. Godfroid, J.; Nielsen, K.; Saegerman, C. Diagnosis of brucellosis in livestock and wildlife. *Croat. Med. J.* **2010**, *51*, 296–305. [CrossRef] [PubMed]

6. OIE. Infection with Brucella abortus, Brucella melitensis and Brucella suis. In *OIE Terrestrial Manual 2016*; OIE (World Organisation for Animal Health): Rome, Italy, 2016.

7. Seleem, M.N.; Boyle, S.M.; Sriranganathan, N. Brucellosis: A re-emerging zoonosis. *Vet. Microbiol.* **2010**, *140*, 392–398. [CrossRef] [PubMed]

8. Millar, M.; Stack, J. Brucellosis—What every practitioner should know. *Practice* **2012**, *34*, 532–539. [CrossRef]

9. Delgado, C.L. Rising Consumption of Meat and Milk in Developing Countries Has Created a New Food Revolution. *J. Nutr.* **2003**, *133*, 3907S–3910S. [CrossRef]

10. FAOSTAT. Milk Total Production in India. 2015. Available online: http://faostat3.fao.org/browse/Q/QL/E (accessed on 12 April 2015).

11. Douphrate, D.I.; Hagevoort, G.R.; Nonnenmann, M.W.; Lunner Kolstrup, C.; Reynolds, S.J.; Jakob, M.; Kinsel, M. The dairy industry: A brief description of production practices, trends, and farm characteristics around the world. *J. Agromed.* **2013**, *18*, 187–197. [CrossRef] [PubMed]

12. Thumbi, S.M.; Njenga, M.K.; Marsh, T.L.; Noh, S.; Otiang, E.; Munyua, P.; Ochieng, L.; Ogola, E.; Yoder, J.; Audi, A.; et al. Linking Human Health and Livestock Health: A "One-Health" Platform for Integrated Analysis of Human Health, Livestock Health, and Economic Welfare in Livestock Dependent Communities. *PLoS ONE* **2015**, *10*, e0120761. [CrossRef]

13. Grace, D.; Wanyoike, F.; Lindahl, J.; Bett, B.; Randolph, T.; Rich, K.M. Poor livestock keepers: Ecosystem-poverty-health interactions. *Philos. Trans. R. Soc. B-Econ.* **2017**, *372*, 20160166. [CrossRef]

14. Omemo, P.; Ogola, E.; Omondi, G.; Wasonga, J.; Knobel, D. Knowledge, attitude and practice towards zoonoses among public health workers in Nyanza province, Kenya. *J. Public Health Afr.* **2012**, *3*, 22. [CrossRef]

15. de Glanville, W.A.; Conde-Álvarez, R.; Moriyón, I.; Njeru, J.; Díaz, R.; Cook, E.A.J.; Morin, M.; de, C.; Bronsvoort, B.M.; Thomas, L.F.; Kariuki, S.; et al. Poor performance of the rapid test for human brucellosis in health facilities in Kenya. *PLoS Negl. Trop. Dis.* **2017**, *11*, e0005508. [CrossRef]

16. Lindahl, J.F.; Vrentas, C.E.; Ram, P.; Deka, R.A.; Hazarika, H.; Rahman, R.G.; Bambal, J.S.; Bedi, C.; Pallab Chaduhuri, B.; Fairoze, N.M.; et al. Brucellosis in India: Results of a collaborative workshop to define One Health priorities. *Trop. Anim. Health Prod.* **2019**. (submitted).

17. Lindahl, J.F.; Chauhan, A.; Gill, J.P.S.; Hazarika, R.A.; Fairoze, N.M.; Grace, D.; Kakkar, M. The extent and structure of peri-urban smallholder dairy farming in five cities in India. *Trop. Anim. Health Prod.* **2019**. (submitted).

18. Emmerzaal, A.; de Wit, J.J.; Dijkstra, T.; Bakker, D.; van Zijderveld, F.G. The Dutch *Brucella abortus* monitoring programme for cattle: The impact of false-positive serological reactions and comparison of serological tests. *Vet. Q.* **2002**, *24*, 40–46. [CrossRef] [PubMed]

19. Gall, D.; Nielsen, K. Serological Diagnosis of Bovine Brucellosis: A Review of Test Performance and Cost Comparison. *Rev. sci. tech. Off. int. Epiz.* **2004**, *23*, 3. [CrossRef]

20. Deka, R.P.; Magnusson, U.; Grace, D.; Lindahl, J. Bovine brucellosis: Prevalence, risk factors, economic cost and control options with particular reference to India—A review. *Infect. Ecol. Epidemiol.* **2018**, *8*, 1556548. [CrossRef]

21. Makita, K.; Fèvre, E.M.; Waiswa, C.; Eisler, M.C.; Thrusfield, M.; Welburn, S.C. Herd prevalence of bovine brucellosis and analysis of risk factors in cattle in urban and peri-urban areas of the Kampala economic zone, Uganda. *BMC Vet. Res.* **2011**, *7*, 60. [CrossRef]

22. Mugizi, D.R.; Boqvist, S.; Nasinyama, G.W.; Waiswa, C.; Ikwap, K.; Rock, K.; Lindahl, E.; Magnusson, U.; Erume, J. Prevalence of and factors associated with Brucella sero-positivity in cattle in urban and peri-urban Gulu and Soroti towns of Uganda. *J. Vet. Med. Sci.* **2015**, *77*, 557–564. [CrossRef]

23. Gill, J.; Kaur, S.; Joshi, D.; Sharma, J. Epidemiological studies on brucellosis in farm animals in Punjab state of India and its public health significance. In Proceedings of the 9th International Symposium on Veterinary Epidemiology and Economics, Breckenridge, CO, USA, 6–11 August 2000.

24. Patel, M.; Patel, P.; Prajapati, M.; Kanani, A.N.; Tyagi, K.K.; Fulsoundar, A.B. Prevalence and risk factor's analysis of bovine brucellosis in peri-urban areas under intensive system of production in Gujarat, India. *Vet. World* **2014**, *7*, 509–516. [CrossRef]

25. Aulakh, H.K.; Patil, P.K.; Sharma, S.; Kumar, H.; Mahajan, V.; Sandhu, K.S. A study on the epidemiology of bovine brucellosis in Punjab (India) using milk-ELISA. *Acta Vet. Brno.* **2008**, *77*, 393–399. [CrossRef]
26. Ul-Islam, M.R.; Gupta, M.P.; Filia, G.; Sidhu, P.K.; Shafi, T.A.; Bhat, S.A.; Hussain, S.A.; Mustafa, R.; Verma, A.K.; Sinha, D.K. Sero-epidemiology of brucellosis in organized cattle and buffaloes in Punjab (India). *Adv. Anim. Vet. Sci.* **2013**, *1*, 5–8.
27. Dhand, N.K.; Gumber, S.; Singh, B.B.; Aradhana; Bali, M.S.; Kumar, H.; Sharma, D.R.; Singh, J.; Sandhu, K.S. A study on the epidemiology of brucellosis in Punjab (India) using Survey Toolbox. *Rev. Sci. Tech.* **2005**, *24*, 879–885. [CrossRef]
28. Lindahl, J.F.; Deka, R.P.; Melin, D.; Berg, A.; Lundén, H.; Lapar, M.L.; Asse, R.; Grace, D. An inclusive and participatory approach to changing policies and practices for improved milk safety in Assam, northeast India. *Glob. Food Sec.* **2018**, *17*, 9–13. [CrossRef]
29. Chakraborty, M.; Patgiri, G.P.; Barman, N.N. Application of delayed-type hypersensitivity test (DTH) for the diagnosis of bovine brucellosis. *Indian Vet. J.* **2000**, *77*, 849–851.
30. Gogoi, S.B.; Hussain, P.; Sarma, P.C.; Barua, A.G.; Mahato, G.; Bora, D.P.; Konch, P.; Gogoi, P. Prevalence of bovine brucellosis in Assam, India. *J. Entomol. Zool. Stud.* **2017**, *5*, 179–185.
31. Renukaradhya, G.; Isloor, S.; Rajasekhar, M. Epidemiology, zoonotic aspects, vaccination and control/eradication of brucellosis in India. *Vet. Microbiol.* **2002**, *90*, 183–195. [CrossRef]
32. Hussain, S.A.; Rahman, H.; Pal, D.; Ahmed, K. Sero-prevalence of bovine and human brucellosis in Assam. *Indian J. Comp. Microbiol. Immunol. Infect. Dis.* **2000**, *21*, 165–166.
33. Yohannes Gemechu, M.; Paul Singh Gill, J. Seroepidemiological survey of human brucellosis in and around Ludhiana, India. *Emerg. Health Threat. J.* **2011**, *4*, 1–7. [CrossRef]
34. Heffernan, C.; Thomson, K.; Nielsen, L. Caste, livelihoods and livestock: An exploration of the uptake of livestock vaccination adoption among poor farmers in India. *J. Int. Dev.* **2011**, *23*, 103–118. [CrossRef]
35. Basunathe, V.K.; Sawarkar, S.W.; Sasidhar, P.V.K. Adoption of Dairy Production Technologies and Implications for Dairy Development in India. *Outlook Agric.* **2010**, *39*, 134–140. [CrossRef]
36. Lindahl, J.F.; Young, J.; Wyatt, A.; Young, M.; Alders, R.; Bagnol, B.; Kibaya, A.; Grace, D. Do vaccination interventions have effects? A study on how poultry vaccination interventions change smallholder farmer knowledge, attitudes, and practice in villages in Kenya and Tanzania. *Trop. Anim. Health Prod.* **2018**, *51*, 213–220. [CrossRef] [PubMed]

15

Improving the Breadth of the Host's Immune Response to Lassa Virus

Juan Carlos Zapata *, Sandra Medina-Moreno, Camila Guzmán-Cardozo⬛ and Maria S. Salvato

Institute of Human Virology, School of Medicine, University of Maryland, Baltimore, MD 21201, USA; smmoreno@ihv.umaryland.edu (S.M.-M.); mcguzmanc13@gmail.com (C.G.-C.); MSalvato@ihv.umaryland.edu (M.S.S.)
* Correspondence: jczapata@ihv.umaryland.edu.

Abstract: In 2017, the global Coalition for Epidemic Preparedness (CEPI) declared Lassa virus disease to be one of the world's foremost biothreats. In January 2018, World Health Organization experts met to address the Lassa biothreat. It was commonly recognized that the diversity of Lassa virus (LASV) isolated from West African patient samples was far greater than that of the Ebola isolates from the West African epidemic of 2013–2016. Thus, vaccines produced against Lassa virus disease face the added challenge that they must be broadly-protective against a wide variety of LASV. In this review, we discuss what is known about the immune response to Lassa infection. We also discuss the approaches used to make broadly-protective influenza vaccines and how they could be applied to developing broad vaccine coverage against LASV disease. Recent advances in AIDS research are also potentially applicable to the design of broadly-protective medical countermeasures against LASV disease.

Keywords: Lassa virus disease (LVD); vaccine breadth; mimicry; B cell anergy; conserved antigens; Fc-gamma receptors; conformational antigens; broadly-neutralizing antibodies; focused immunity; dominant and subdominant epitopes; cross-restriction

1. Introduction

Lassa virus (LASV) is a zoonotic pathogen endemic to West Africa. Annual outbreaks occur primarily during the dry season amongst the rural population [1]. In December 2013, West Africa experienced an outbreak of Ebola virus that quickly grew into an epidemic, revealing that much of this part of the world was unprepared to handle such a disaster. The Ebola epidemic was a more terrifying version of the annual Lassa disease outbreaks, and was characterized by high person-to-person transmission, the deaths of medical personnel, popular hysteria and occasional transmission outside West Africa [2]. It became clear that the unchecked spread of such infections could endanger the rest of the world.

In 2017, the global Coalition for Epidemic Preparedness (CEPI) declared Lassa virus disease to be one of the world's foremost biothreats [3]. In January 2018, the World Health Organization (WHO) convened a "Lassa Roadmap" panel lead by Mike Osterholm, an epidemiologist and expert in biosecurity [4]. As the panel considered the technical obstacles to Lassa vaccine production, one of the more important obstacles was "breadth of vaccine protection". Breadth refers to the variety of infections suppressed by one vaccine. If the vaccine is broadly protective, it might shield vaccinees from all of the genetically diverse Lassa lineages identified in patient samples [5]. Sequencing studies of blood from infected West African patients showed an almost 50-fold greater variation of LASV isolates than of Ebola virus isolates [6,7]. This means that a Lassa vaccine needs to be more broadly protective than an Ebola vaccine because it needs to cover a greater genetic variation. This variation is presumably due to the fact that most of the Lassa patients are infected directly through the rodent reservoir, whereas most Ebola patients are infected by contact with other human patients. Hence, the high variation of Lassa outbreaks is due to multiple introductions from the rodents and not to any changes in viral mutation rate. Another contributing factor may be that LASV replication in culture generates 10–1000-fold fewer virus particles per infectious particle than Ebola virus Zaire or Sudan isolates [8]. This means Ebola virus produces an excess of viral products and only a few of them assemble to become infectious particles.

Vaccine cross-protection reflects the genetic diversity covered by a vaccine. If a Lassa vaccine is "narrowly protective", it will only protect against one or two Lassa lineages: two closely-related lineages differ in 5–7% of their nucleotide sequence. If the vaccine is more broadly protective, it could protect against all Lassa lineages (the most divergent LASV lineages differ by as much as 27% of their nucleotides) [9]. If the vaccine is even broader, it should protect against other arenavirus species. The genetic diversity between LASV species and a closely related Old World arenavirus species such as LCMV ranges 30–50% difference between their nucleotide sequences [9].

The last 50 years of LASV research shed some light on its pathogenesis and effects on the host immune response. During the early innate response, LASV infection seems to affect dendritic cell function, resulting in poor antigen-presentation, partial immunosuppression and unchecked virus replication [10–12]. In monkeys and in Lassa-infected people, neutralizing antibodies are slow to develop, partially due to glycans on the viral envelope (GP) that mimic self-glycans and anergize the B cell response [13].

Several LASV vaccine candidates have demonstrated efficacy in animal models. A live attenuated MOP/LAS reassortant vaccine (clone ML29), designed by Lukashevich and further developed to pre-clinical studies in our laboratory, has shown sterilizing protection against Lassa disease in mice, guinea pigs, and non-human primates [14–18]. Additionally, this vaccine elicits immune responses to LASV glycoprotein (GP) and nucleoprotein (NP), even in primates chronically-infected with SIV [19]. In this review, we discuss the Lassa vaccine candidates that have demonstrated broad cross-protection and the key properties contributing to their breadth.

The goal of this review is to discuss possible ways to improve the immune response to LASV. In the first part, we discuss what is known about the development of immune responses to Lassa virus and the current vaccine candidates used to confer antiviral immunity, then we describe the approaches used to obtain "universal flu vaccines" and broadly protective AIDS vaccines, and how these approaches could possibly be applied to medical countermeasures against Lassa fever.

2. Clinical Manifestations and Pathogenesis of Lassa Virus Disease

LASV pathogenesis and its failure to develop strong immune responses remain a mystery. Although there is a strong correlation between the level of viremia and the disease outcome (Figure 1), the damage is not caused directly by viral-cell lysis and seems to depend on the initial host immune response [20–22]. The first symptoms are poorly differentiated from other diseases. In addition, the incubation period can be as long as two weeks. Those two situations make the initial diagnosis difficult and cause a delay in the initiation of the treatment. Twenty percent of the infected patients develop symptoms of muscle fatigue, facial edema, and sore throat, and a few of these progress to systemic disease with mucosal, conjunctival, gastrointestinal or genital bleeding. Platelet dysfunction and endothelial damage seem to play a role in the characteristic vascular leakage.

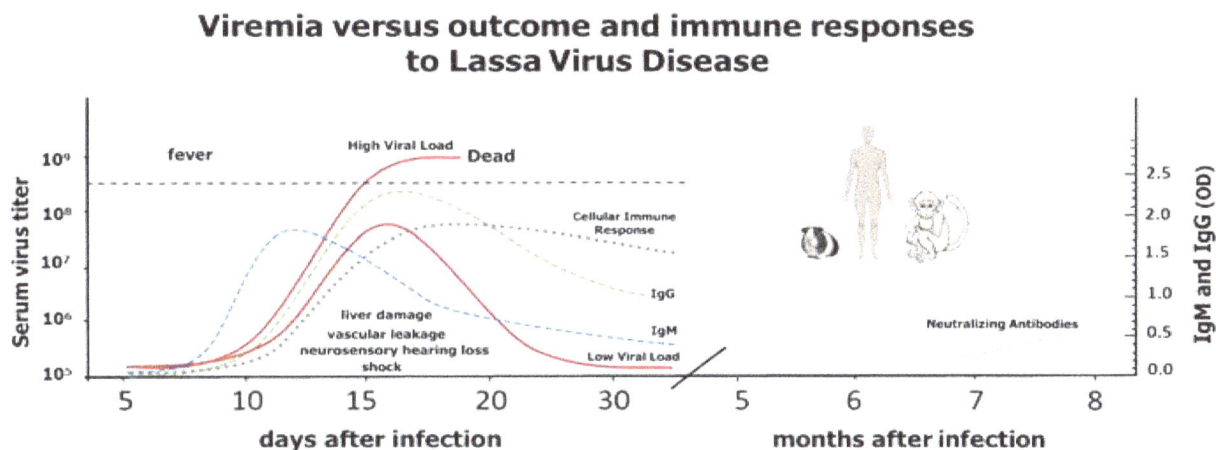

Figure 1. This is a representation of LASV viremia in relation to Lassa virus disease outcomes and immune responses to Lassa virus based on published data about rodent, non-human primate and human infections. When the immune system fails to control the virus, disease is more acute and leads to death. Those individuals with moderate viral replication (~80%) are either asymptomatic or, if they develop symptoms, they have higher possibilities to survive (low solid red line), while those patients with high viral loads suffer severe disease that can lead to death (high solid red line) [21,23]. Dotted lines represent cellular and humoral immune responses. Solid blue line represents the rise of neutralizing antibodies.

Fatal cases are associated with myocarditis, pulmonary edema, acute respiratory distress, and a hypovolemic shock; in addition, elevated plasma aminotransferases (AST and ALT), uncontrolled viremia, and high levels of IL-6 are pathognomonic for LF [22]. Massive viral replication in the liver and spleen leads to progressive hemorrhagic manifestations and increased mortality. It is common to find hepatocellular necrosis and foci of hepatocyte proliferation [24–26]. A recent description of arenavirus-induced liver pathology was characterized by hepatocytes with increased cell death, upregulated cell cycling factor p21, IFN-γ, and LASV receptor Axl-1, but aborted cell cycling. Whereas mature hepatocytes had low alpha-dystroglycan (α-DG; a LSV receptor) expression, oval cells had high expression of α-DG [27]. Coagulation disorders are not common in LF; however, when they happen, platelet counts could be normal with little disseminated intravascular coagulation, while platelet aggregation is impaired and loss of liquids [28–32]. Neuropathological manifestations include disorientation, motor and sensory abnormalities, convulsions, hiccups, and in advanced stages coma. Brain dysfunctions are associated with poor prognosis and it is not clear if they are the result of the direct effect of LASV, nonspecific metabolites, or immune-mediated effects. LASV infection is responsible for the high prevalence of hearing loss in West Africa: around 30% of LF patients develop hearing problems and 17% of LF survivors suffer permanent hearing loss [33–37].

3. Early Immune Response to Lassa Virus Infection

LF survivors are able to control viral loads early during the infection. In contrast, fatal cases show poor inflammatory responses characterized by lymphopenia, that affects all lymphocyte subpopulations, including CD4+ and CD8+ T cells, B cells, and NK cells, along with necrosis of lymphoid organs [29,38–41]. This immuno-suppressive state appears to be induced early during the infection. In vitro LASV infection of macrophages, dendritic cells (DC), and endothelial cells down-regulated the production of inflammatory mediators [10,11,42]. In vivo, antigen presenting cells (APC; macrophages (MP) and dendritic cells (DC)) are the primary targets of LASV. In monkeys, by seven days after infection, infected DC were found in a variety of tissues. MP were also infected to a lesser extent. Kupffer cells, hepatocytes, adreno-cortical cells and endothelial cells were more frequently infected in the tissues of terminal animals. In lymph nodes, LASV antigen was detected in

DC located in the marginal zone and to a lesser extent in monocytes and MP in the marginal zone and red pulp [40].

Most RNA viruses activate DC and MP while replicating due to the production of dsRNA genomic intermediates and other viral sub-products presenting pathogen molecular patterns (PAMPs), which are recognized by specialized pattern recognition receptors (PRR). LASV PAMPs activate several signaling cascades that lead to the secretion of chemokines and cytokines, including interferon (IFN) responses that inhibit virus replication and induce cellular genes involved in innate and adaptive immunity [43,44]. Although sensitive to the antiviral effects of IFN-α and IFN-γ, LASV has been shown to regulate IFN production in vitro and in vivo [10,11,42,45]. In lethally-infected animals, IFN-γ levels were moderately elevated [46] and, in human fatal cases, IFN-γ levels were increased in some individuals [47]. In macaques, IFN type I was detected very early in survivors but only in the late stages of fatal cases [38]. The inhibition of IFN by LASV affects plasmacytoid DC maturation and reduces production of cytokines and chemokines by these cells [43,48]. Another function inhibited by the block to DC maturation is their capacity to migrate to the secondary lymphoid organs, to express CCR7, and thus to activate T cells [11].

A common feature of the viral nucleoprotein (NP) of mammalian arenaviruses is its ability to prevent nuclear translocation of interferon regulatory factor 3 (IRF-3), IFN type I activation, and the downstream induction of the interferon stimulated genes (ISG) [48–51]. The anti-IFN activity of NP is located in its C-terminus that is structurally homologous to the DEDDH family of 3′-5′ exoribonucleases [52]. The NP crystal structure and its interaction with RIG-I and MDA-5 suggest that NP ribonuclease activity is able to remove viral PAMP RNA, thereby avoiding recognition by PRRs and inhibiting IFN production [52,53]. The LASV Z matrix protein also binds RIG-I and MDA-5 to inhibit type I IFN induction [54]. In contrast to NP, Z proteins of some arenaviruses do not bind RIG-I/MDA-5 and fail to inhibit IFN production [54]. The authors suggest that Z-mediated anti-IFN activity is more frequently associated with pathogenic arenaviruses. Another group, showing that the L polymerase is subject to more positive selection events (>dN/dS) during evolution than any other arenaviral gene, argues that the polymerase might be central to viral pathogenesis [55].

LASV infection of monocyte and endothelial cell cultures suppressed TNF-α and IL-8, an effect that in vivo would be predicted to inhibit inflammation and neutrophil migration [10]. In contrast, infected monocyte-derived DC showed an increase in IL-8 secretion with a reduction in the expression of co-stimulatory molecules such as CD86, CD80, and CD40. Additionally, LASV-infected DC failed to produce pro-inflammatory cytokines and to stimulate T cells [42]. Although both MP and DC are susceptible to LASV infection, immature DC supported virus replication without being destroyed or activated. Neither the infection of human DC and MP nor their stimulation with inactivated virus induced the production of TNF-α, IL-1β, IL-2, IL-6, IL-8, IL-10, IL-12p35, TGF-β, IFN-γ, or CD25 [11,42].

In line with the cell culture results, LF fatal cases see a reduction in IL-8 and IP-10 in comparison to survivors [11,42]. Similar results were seen in vivo in cynomolgus macaques [40]. IL-8 was the only cytokine that peaked in infected people who did not develop LASV disease [56]. In addition, primates and human PBMC exposed to LCMV-WE (a virus causing hemorrhagic fever) showed that virulent infection was associated with undetectable levels of TNF-α, low levels of IL-8 in plasma and inhibition of IL-8 mRNA expression [46,57].

In vitro, LASV and LCMV-WE down-regulated IL-6 and other pro-inflammatory cyto/chemokines in human MP and epithelial cells. In contrast, MOPV and LCMV-ARM strongly up-regulated pro-inflammatory responses in a TLR-2/Mal-dependent manner [58]. Meanwhile, a high level of IL-6 in plasma is a biomarker of progressing LF in humans and in primates experimentally infected with LASV or LCMV-WE. This high level of IL-6 during the last stages of severe LF could result from hepatic regeneration and may be associated with neutrophilia [22,24,38,46,59]. We speculate that the in vitro studies model the earliest events in LASV infection, whereas the IL-6 in infected macaque plasma is a late event of LASV infection; hence, severe pathology would be marked by early suppression of IL-6 and late abundance of IL-6.

Taken together, the above evidence suggests that LASV targets monocytes and DC, inhibits the initial immune response and suppresses the migration of activated cells to the primary infection site resulting in higher viral replication, greater virulence, and a delay in the induction of the acquired immune response.

4. Acquired Immunity to Lassa Virus Infection

LASV-specific IgM and IgG are detected during peak viremia, and appear unrelated to recovery from disease [20]. Primate immunization with gamma-irradiated LASV, an inactivation procedure that preserves the natural structure of antigens, induced strong antibody responses to NP and GP antigens, but failed to protect immunized animals from fatal LF [60]. Notably, NP is the earliest antigen detected by antigen-capture assays in infected individuals, most likely because it is the most abundant structural component of each virion [61]. In addition, ELISA to detect NP antibody was used in early seroprevalence studies [62]. Due to the structural importance of NP, it is likely to contribute to the breadth of the acquired immune response to LASV (see arguments in Section 6).

In cynomolgus macaques experimentally infected with LASV, the antibody titers against GP1, GP2, and NP increased more rapidly in survivors than in fatal cases [38]. Neutralizing antibodies (nAbs) in convalescing people can be detected only in low titers, several months after the initial infection and have been LASV strain-specific [23,63]. These findings suggest that the antibody response may not be responsible for the patient's recovery. However, antibodies could be playing an important role in attenuating acute infection, as suggested by its early appearance in surviving monkeys, the high seroprevalence in endemic areas without clinically overt disease, the lack of disease in infected contacts or the high mortality rate in individuals from LASV-free regions [38,56,64].

Treatment of human beings and animals with immune-antiserum showed a range of results [23,65–67]. A study testing a cocktail of human nAbs, generated in vitro from $LASV_{Josiah}$-infected individuals, was able to rescue late-stage infected macaques from death. In those experiments, viremic macaques were treated with a single dose of the cocktail at Days 6 and 8 after LASV infection leading to virus clearance and survival [68]. Although antibody cocktails of 15 mg nAb /kg macaque constitute an expensive treatment, their success is an important proof-of-concept. Recent structural studies revealed that artificially-generated nAbs recognized a metastable pre-fusion GP complex and blocked changes required for engagement with the intracellular receptor LAMP-1 and fusion with host membrane in late endosomes [69]. However, LASV infection induces predominantly non-nAbs against conserved NP and GP2 antigens and with a few exceptions these antibodies become undetectable after several months [62,70]. Seronegative survivors (approximately 18% of total within the LASV endemic areas) were not resistant to LASV re-infection but were protected from clinical LF [71].

After acute LF recovery, patients overcome the initial lymphopenia and develop a strong CD4+ immune response against NP and GP2. The NP-CD4+ response is only partially strain-specific since it cross-reacts with other LASV strains [72]. The LASV-GP2-CD4+-specific response recognizes a conserved epitope that is common in the Old World (100% similarity with LCMV) and New World arenaviruses (>90% similarity) [73]. In animal models, T cell responses are more important than B cells responses, and the CTL-mediated protection seems to rely more on CD8+ cells than on CD4+ cells [19]. In LASV-infected monkeys T-cell activation was delayed in fatal cases and in vitro stimulation of lymphocytes from those animals did not result in proliferation [38]. There were also decreases in CD20+ cells, and down-regulation of class II MHC antigens [25]. In contrast to fatal cases, survivors showed activation and proliferation after exposure to inactivated LASV, as well as an increase in circulating monocytes [38]. Similarly, ML29 immunization of marmosets increased the number of CD3+ and CD14+ cells [25].

The LASV-infection of one health care worker gave the USA Centers for Disease Control the rare opportunity to monitor blood cells during disease progression in a human patient [74]. During the acute phase, CD4 and CD8 T cells peaked in conjunction with virus clearance. During convalescence, the CD4 T cells waned while CD8 T cell activation and degranulation peaked for a second time. The patient was ultimately able to generate long-term, polyfunctional, Lassa virus-specific T cells, with approximately 66% of the CD4 T cells and 75% of the CD8 T cells expressing more than one cytokine. Taken together, these results suggest strong participation of T cell responses in protection and recovery during natural LASV infection. However, despite recent successful recoveries, the mechanism of protection remains unknown and more studies of human cases are needed to characterize the role of T cells in LF protection [15,41,70,75–77]. The evidence suggests that the inhibition of pattern recognition receptors (PRR) by LASV at the beginning of the infection, and the failure to induce early pro-inflammatory cytokines results in a temporary immunosuppression and uncontrolled virus replication. An early and strong immune response that controls virus replication is more likely to promote recovery from LASV disease.

5. A comparison of Promising Lassa Vaccine Candidates

Immunization of monkeys and guinea pigs with LCMV, MOBV, MOPV, and other non-pathogenic Old-World viruses can all confer some protection against LF disease [15,19,41,70,75,76,78] (Figure 2). Mopeia virus (MOPV), an arenavirus species found in rodents of eastern and southern Africa, serves as a naturally attenuated vaccine, protecting non-human primates from a lethal challenge with LASV [78,79]. The fact that MOPV and LASV can cross-protect, even though they belong to different species shows that broadly-protective vaccines are feasible. Knowledge that MOPV is a widespread, cross-protecting and non-pathogenic virus led to the production of at least two vaccines based on the MOPV platform (ML29 and MOP-VAC).

Phylogenetic relationships of arenaviruses

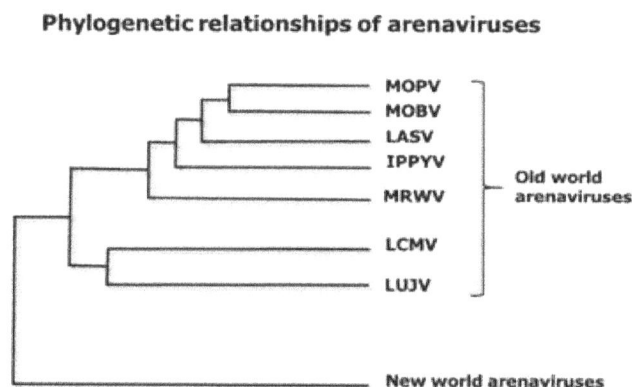

Figure 2. Phylogenetic relationships of some Old-World arenavirus species. LASV is related to several "Old World" arenaviruses. Mopeia virus AN20410 (NC_006574.1) is designated MOPV. Mobala virus (NC_007904.1) is MOBV. Lassa virus (NC_004297.1) is LASV. Ippy virus (NC_007906 is IPPYV. Merino Walk Virus (NC_023763.1) is MRWV. Lymphocytic choriomeningitis virus (NC_004291.1 is LCMV. Lujo virus (NC_012777.1) is LUJV. The family *Arenaviridae* has three genera: *Mammarenaviruses*, *Reptarenaviruses* and *Hartmaniviruses* [80]. Here, we only depict seven species of the Old-World group of the *Mammarenavirus* genus, omitting the New World *Mammarenaviruses* and the other two genera. This is a maximum clade credibility tree of the polymerase region. The tree was constructed from amino acid alignment using Bayesian MCMC method with LG model of substitution.

In this section, we compare five Lassa vaccine candidates with respect to their estimated economy of production, safety for pregnant women, breadth of protection, and capacity to confer sterilizing immunity after a lethal challenge (Table 1). Published claims and extrapolated guesses have been used for these estimates, since no pair of these vaccines has yet been put to a rigorous head-to-head comparison. Such a comparison should eventually be done for the benefit of all stakeholders.

ML29, derived from lineage IV Lassa$_{Josiah}$, is considered a broadly cross-protective Lassa vaccine because it showed sterilizing immunity in guinea pigs challenged with a distantly-related lineage

II strain of Lassa virus [5,16]. Broad cross-protection by ML29 was also observed in SIV-infected rhesus macaques given a lethal challenge with LCMV-WE. Whereas naive macaques given LCMV-WE succumbed to a LF-like febrile illness, four macaques immunized with ML29 survived for a month without increases in plasma AST or ALT (MSS unpublished, with remaining animals from [19]). This finding was consistent with the previous observation that ML29-inoculated rhesus macaques induced strong cross-reactive cell-mediated immunity to LCMV-WE [15].

The VSV-Las vaccine is a rhabdovirus vector expressing a single Lassa gene, the GPC. Guinea pigs vaccinated with VSV-Las$_{Josiah}$ were challenged with two closely-related strains, Liberian Lassa$_{Z-132}$, and a Malian Lassa$_{SorombaR}$. Currently, there is no challenge model for LASV from lineage I LASV$_{Pinneo}$, so in these experiments all animals survived including the challenge controls, making it impossible to justify claims about cross-protection from LASV$_{Pinneo}$. Three cynomolgus macaques vaccinated with VSV-Las$_{GP}$ and challenged with the related lineage IV strain, Lassa$_{Z-132}$, also survived. Monkey challenges with distantly-related strains such as LASV$_{Pinneo}$ were not reported. Thus, in contrast to ML29, the VSV-Las$_{GP}$ has demonstrated only narrow protection against LASV lineages closely-related to the vaccine and has failed to demonstrate sterilizing immunity [81].

Lassa vaccine testing in guinea pigs has given misleading positive results in the past, for example a LasNP vaccine was able to protect guinea pigs but not primates [82]. Cross-protection between LCMV and LASV in guinea pigs was less effective in primates [83]. Vaccines constructed on the yellow fever vaccine platform, YF17D, were found to work well in guinea pigs but were relatively disappointing in primates. It was discovered that the YF-Las$_{GP1}$ and YF-LAS$_{GP2}$ vaccines were more stable than the YF-Las$_{GPC}$ vaccine and protected 80% of guinea pigs [84,85] but failed to protect marmosets (I. Lukashevich, unpublished). We would speculate that the best cross-protection can be achieved only with the most stable and conserved particle structures. Additional Lassa antigens, such as NP or Z, which provide conserved epitopes as well as increase the formation of stable ribonucleoprotein particles, are predicted to increase vaccine breadth. A rigorous test of vaccine cross-protection or breadth must ultimately occur in primates.

Table 1. Comparison of select Lassa vaccine candidates.

Vaccine	Breadth of Cross-Protection [a]	Safety for Pregnant Women and Fetus [b]	Sterilizing Immunity [c]	Production Costs [d]	References
ML29 [e]	High	Low	Yes	Low	[16]
MOPVAC$_{LasGP}$ [f]	ND [g]	Low	Yes	Med	[86]
VSV-LAS$_{GP}$ [h]	Med	Low	No	Med	[81]
MVA-LAS$_{GP+Z}$ [i]	ND	High	ND	Med	[87]
LASV$_{GPC}$ DNA [j]	ND	High	Yes	High	[88]

[a] Refers to protection from distantly-related virus isolates. [b] This is a guess based on the propensity of similar viruses to cause fetal malformations or miscarriage. [c] Sterilizing immunity means that, after immunizing with an effective dose, there is no trace of the vaccine a week after immunization, neither in tissue nor in excreta. [d] Production costs are extrapolated from reported doses and levels of virus (or RNA) production in cell culture. [e] Mopeia/Lassa reassortant 29 (ML29) has the L RNA of Mopeia and the S RNA of Lassa$_{Josiah}$. It was selected from a library of MOPV/LASV reassortants for small-plaque phenotype, attenuation in mice, genotype from MOPV L RNA and LASV S RNA, genetic stability, and efficient replication in Vero cell cultures (~10^8 plaque forming units (pfu)/mL) [14]. The Russian laboratories of Fort, LLC have produced a variety of Mopeia/Lassa reassortants to improve upon the vaccine efficacy and patent protections of the initial isolates (Moshkoff D. and Nasidi A. in preparation). [f] MOPVAC or Mopeia-ExoNb6 (MOPV-ExoNb6) is a recombinant virus expressing the Mopeia genome, six mutations in the MOPV-NP exonuclease, and the LASV GP in place of the MOPV GP [86]. [g] ND means not determined. [h] VSV-LAS$_{GP}$ refers to vaccines using the vesicular stomatitis virus (VSV) platform and expressing the Lassa GP. Both current versions have reduced neurovirulence: the Feldmann/Merck version has been attenuated by replacing the VSV G with the Lassa GP [89], and the Rose/Profectus version has been attenuated by altering the natural VSV gene order [90]. Both have reduced growth capacity compared to VSV, and, from our experience with other VSV pseudotypes, it is likely that they fail to reach titers above 10^7 plaque-forming units (pfu)/mL. [i] The GeoVax-made vaccine replicates well in avian cells but does not replicate in mammals. In mammals, it expresses LASV GP and Z genes, forming virus-like-particles (VLP) in vivo. The Modified Vaccinia Ankara (MVA) vector was developed by B. Moss at NIH and has been used in thousands of human beings in the form of an AIDS vaccine [91]. VLP can be powerful and broadly-protective immunogens. [j] LASV$_{GPC}$ DNA vaccine.

The laboratory of Silvain Baize has recently described a new vaccine (MOPVAC$_{LasGP}$) that is a Mopeia recombinant bearing a Lassa$_{Josiah}$ glycoprotein (GP). It has been genetically engineered to have six missense mutations in the exonuclease portion of its nucleocapsid protein (NP), a portion that is known to suppress the antiviral IFN response by cleavage of PRR-detecting RNA. This MOPVAC has not been tested for cross-protection, but it is seen as a platform for insertion of sequences for each of the Lassa lineages. Whereas the wild-type virus can reach high titers in culture, this attenuated version (MOPV-ExoN6b) reaches titers that are two logs lower [86], so it may not be vigorous enough for scaled production. In addition, it is possible that the altered exonuclease would allow vaccine persistence in vivo.

No live-attenuated RNA virus vaccines are recommended for administration to pregnant women because all replicating RNA viruses tested have been teratogenic for live births from an infected pregnant host. This is likely because viral replication requires host molecules that are also needed for fetal development [92]. Amongst the Lassa vaccines listed above, the first three are live-attenuated RNA viruses, whereas the last two, MVA and DNA vaccines, are not able to replicate in mammals, so are likely to be safe for pregnant human subjects.

All five listed vaccines can be altered by reverse genetics. A recombinant ML29 (rML29) has recently been rescued from cDNA clones. Using rML29 and tri-segmented technology, additional genes of interest (eGFP, Ebola GP, and *Plasmodium berghei* antigens) have been expressed in rML29 [93]. Thus, rML29 can be used as a potent vaccine platform for expressing arenaviral genes (e.g., LASV GP$_{Pinneo}$ from distantly-related lineage I) and non-related antigens and immunomodulators.

At this time, only two Lassa vaccine candidates (ML29 and VSV-Las$_{GP}$) have demonstrated breadth of protection in guinea pigs; and only one, ML29, has shown the ability to protect against challenges from virus outside the lineage IV of Lassa$_{Josiah}$. After a head-to-head comparison, the ML29 and VSV-Las$_{GP}$ candidates should move forward in clinical trials targeting health care workers and other people on the front lines of an outbreak. The two vaccine candidates that do not replicate in mammals, MVA-LAS and LASV-DNA, and would consequently be more expensive to produce, should be reserved for clinical trials with children and pregnant women.

6. Improving the Humoral Immune Response to Lassa Vaccines

The humoral immune response appears late after infection and after experimental vaccination. HIV, LCMV, and Lassa viruses evade antibodies by mimicking self-glycoproteins and cloaking their foreign envelope glycoproteins with self-glycans [94–97]. The development of B cell responses to glycan-cloaked epitopes is a slow process that ultimately depends upon antigen density and the avidity of the antigens for the B cell receptors (BCR). Self-reactivity can be removed from antibodies by V(D)J recombination or hypermutation. For example, binding studies showed that only three mutations in a BCR could confer 50-fold lower binding to self-versus foreign antigens [98]. Helper T cells cooperate with anergic B cells only when BCR cross-linking by foreign antigen is greater than that induced by self-antigen [99]. The higher threshold to activate anergic B cells and recruit them to germinal centers can only be overcome by high antigen density or high affinity for the BCR. This means that low density GP on virions will fail to activate anergic B cells, especially if they have only moderate affinity for self-glycans. Consequently, the B cell arm of the antiviral immune response will only develop after exposure to high-density, high-affinity antigen.

Despite an initial cloaking of B cell antigens during viral infection, survivors acquire memory responses that increase over time. A study of 45 people who survived avian influenza showed that the sickest individuals, presumably those with highest viral titers, were the slowest to develop cell-mediated and humoral responses, but then they also developed the most long-term protective antibody responses [100].

The effort to make "universal flu vaccines" illustrates some approaches that could be used in making broadly-protective antibodies for Lassa virus disease. Initially, influenza researchers tried to increase the vaccine breadth by choosing immunogens such as the influenza hemagglutinin

(HA) stem that are most evolutionarily conserved. By choosing conserved antigens, one could vaccinate against the most stable portions of a pathogen and also achieve the greatest cross-protective immune responses. In one particular effort, a broadly-reactive vaccine was created by engineering a consensus of 2656 HA_{H1N1} protein sequences into one protein, CH1, that bore conserved B and T cell epitopes. A PR8-CH1 influenza virus elicited broadly-protective immunity against heterologous H1N1 viruses [101]. Researchers also considered using the neuraminidase (NA) since it is a less rapidly-evolving protein and thus a good contributor for vaccine antigens. Similarly, for arenaviruses such as LASV, the GP1 is highly variable, but a segment of GP2 and the NP are not very variable and therefore good antigens to include as immunogens.

It was recognized in the 1990s that the three-dimensional structure of an antigen contributed to the B cell response [102]. The contribution of large repetitive structures and conformational antigens to broadening the antigen response is an important approach that has been pursued in the search for universal influenza vaccines. Particulation of an antigen (e.g., putting it on a nanoparticle) leads to significant enhancement of BCR cross-linking and B cell activation [103]. B cell activation also leads to more activated CD4+ T cell responses, and promotion of antigen cross-presentation for CD8+ T cell activation [104]. Particulate antigens tend to cause auto-immunity, they are more frequently taken up by phagocytosis, they are DC-tropic, they are more immunogenic than soluble antigens, and they activate the inflammasome [105]. In agreement with these observations about particulation, vaccines comprised of virus particles or virus-like particles would be predicted to be more immunogenic than DNA vaccines or unstructured assemblages of viral antigens.

The production of VLP also exploits the particulation approach. The MVA-VLP vaccine results in highly structured antigens, in this case the Lassa Z (or matrix protein) in combination with the Lassa GP form VLP in vivo [87]. Stable particle formation for retroviruses also depends on two types of proteins: the envelope (Env) is thought to bear the most variable "type-specific antigens" while the abundant capsid protein "Gag" bears the more evolutionarily-stable "group-specific antigens" [106]. By adding Gag to a vaccine some investigators have been able to introduce evolutionarily-conserved regions that also contribute to a more stable ribonucleoprotein (RNP) structure [107].

The most conserved antigenic regions tend to include many non-linear (conformational) antigens that remain functionally stable during virus evolution. This finding is strengthened by the observation that roughly 60% of the neutralizing antibodies derived from convalescent Lassa patients relied on conformational epitopes [108]. A remarkable effort to characterize nAbs from convalescent human blood revealed that as antibodies matured over time, some antibodies were capable of neutralizing Lassa isolates from all four lineages, and some could neutralize LCMV as well as Lassa [108]. Unfortunately, it is well known that pseudotypes are more sensitive to nAbs than wild-type viruses [109,110], so this conclusion needs corroboration with LASV isolates. In these cases of broadly-neutralizing antibodies, breadth of neutralizing activity was dependent on conformational epitopes. It is a common theme that broadly-neutralizing anti-microbial antibodies bind to conformational epitopes, for example one of the broadest and most potent HIV neutralizing antibodies binds to the gp41–gp120 interface [111].

Leon et al., [112] showed that binding of large structured antigen-antibody complexes to Fc gamma receptor (FcγR) leads to stronger and more broadly cross-reactive B cell responses than antigens that elicit FcγR-independent antibodies. Antibodies that were hemaglutination (HA)-inhibiting tended to be FcγR-independent and antibodies that bound the conserved HA stalk structure tended to be FcγR-dependent. There was a large discrepancy between in vitro and in vivo assays for nAb efficacy: in vitro, HA stalk antibodies were 100–1000 fold weaker than HA-inhibiting antibodies, but in vivo passive transfer studies showed only a five-fold discrepancy between antibody efficacies. By testing a number of HA variants, this group found that the optimal nAb response requires, not only an interaction with FcγR, but also a second molecular bridge between pathogen and innate effector cells, serving perhaps to activate those cells. Antibodies against the influenza HA are more broadly reactive if they simultaneously engage both the FcγR and other pathogen-specific receptors on innate immune cells [112]. To translate this finding to enhancing the breadth of Lassa vaccines, those vaccines that engage both viral entry receptors and FcγR on innate immune cells should be the most broadly cross-protective immunogens. For example, a recent publication illustrates how a beta-propriolactone-inactivated Lassa-Rabies vector elicits lasting humoral responses against LASV and Rabies in mice and guinea pigs [113].

7. Improving the Cell-Mediated Immune Response to Lassa Infection

Memory T cells play a critical role in long-term protection against Lassa fever [74]. Nevertheless, the CD8+ T cell receptor (TCR) interaction with MHC-presented peptides is very constrained. 9mer epitopes in the context of MHC-class I must have a very tight and specific fit to the TCR to activate cytokine secretion or CTL activity. One strategy known as the "string of beads" approach was meant to increase vaccine breadth by including many of the primary epitopes in one expression vector. This was tried for AIDS and for arenavirus vaccines, but it resulted in a competition between similar epitopes so that the immune response became quickly focused but not broader [114]. A slightly different approach, stringing the non-dominant epitopes, succeeded in avoiding focus and developed a broader protective vaccine response [115]. Using adenoviral vectors expressing invariant chain-linked non-dominant LCMV GP antigen, the AR Thomsen and JP Christensen laboratories were able to show that efficient virus control may be obtained by targeting the intrinsically non-dominant GP antigen, and that this allows for a potent CD8 T cell response to be elicited by virus-encoded dominant NP antigen during the chronic phase of a high-dose infection. In contrast, when mice were initially vaccinated using the dominant NP antigen, the subsequent virus-elicited response remained focused on the major NP epitope. During the early period after virus challenge, it was possible to confirm that T cells primed by the Adeno-GP vaccine and boosted by the virus infection were able to protect against a broad array of challenge viruses [115].

Whereas class I peptides present to CD8 T cells and are constrained in size to anchor within the peptide groove of MHC class I molecules, class II peptides present to CD4 T cells and are much less constrained, varying from 11 to 30 amino acids in length [116]. An approach suggested by Dr. M. Patarroyo for synthetic-vaccine development is to determine immune protection-inducing protein structures (IMPIPS) by stringing together class II peptides. This involves defining the three-dimensional interactions which are essential in MHC$_{ClassII}$–peptide–Tcell receptor (TCR) complex formation, a much more promiscuous coupling activity than the interactions of class I peptides and CD8 TCR. After finding an orientation for perfectly fitting into the TCR that induces an appropriate immune response, non-interfering, long-lasting, protective, multi-epitope peptides can be synthesized against many infections [117,118]. Even non-immunogenic epitopes can be converted into immunogens using the Patarroyo TCR-binding selections, thereby avoiding the over-reaction problems caused by pre-existing immunity against microorganisms.

In AIDS vaccine research, there has also been an approach favoring class II epitopes. This is promising because it is well known that CD4+ TCR can be more frequently cross-restrictive than the CD8 TCR [116]. The ability to cross-restrict allowed AIDS Elite Controllers to have both avid TCR interactions with Gag293 epitope in the context of HLA-DR (class II) and to have broad cross-restriction between Gag and Env V2 epitopes. Thus, a broad cross-reactivity of CD4+ T cell responses, similar to that commonly seen in Elite Controllers, could be established by vaccination in ordinary individuals [119]. With respect to Lassa vaccines, it is likely that Lassa disease survivors bear some similarities to AIDS Elite Controllers in their acquired immunity, showing broadly cross-restricted CD4 responses. An understanding of the CD4 TCR alleles determining this response should make it possible to engineer autologous T cells that confer protection.

With high HLA heterogeneity among the West African population, the feasibility of epitope-based vaccines is limited. A safety issue was raised in murine experiments where epitope-based vaccines given to individuals who had previously been exposed to the pathogen can strongly re-activate the pre-existing CD8+ T clones and induce TNF-dependent immunopathology [120], but then this may be a murine problem and not a serious problem for human subjects.

8. Future Directions Combining Immunological and Drug-Therapy Approaches

When health care professionals are getting ready to risk their lives during an epidemic, a strong, fast-acting and broadly-protective vaccine should be available. The poor conditions and shear volume of needy patients makes a dangerous situation for first-responders and they deserve to be armed with protection. In addition to vaccines, broadly-protective antiviral therapies should be available. Both the ML29 and VSV-LAS vaccines have shown antiviral efficacy when used within two days of Lassa infection [16,81], however their action within this brief window of time is lineage-specific rather than broadly protective. It is telling that a repatriated health care worker who ultimately survived was given intravenous fluids and two broadly acting antivirals (ribavirin pn days 6–15 of illness and favipiravir days 8–12 of illness) [74]. Nevertheless, it is still unclear whether the optimum care requires anything more than intravenous fluids and good hospital practices.

Several studies have yielded broadly cross-protective antivirals that could be used against Lassa infection. High-throughput screens for small molecule inhibitors of LASV revealed an inhibitor of arenavirus polymerases (favipiravir) that was recently used on a LASV-infected health care worker along with intravenous fluids and ribavirin [74]. This treatment is so broadly cross-protective it has even been used on Ebola cases [121]. Ribavirin also has broad reactivity against many RNA viruses and at its lowest concentration works by blocking the capped-mRNA-promoting function of eIF4E [122]. Unfortunately, ribavirin resistance is problematic; thus, it is best used in combination with other antivirals [123]. A recent study of the interactome of LCMV gene products with host cell molecules revealed several host-cell molecules essential to the life cycle of viruses including Junin, LASV and Ebola [124,125]. Mining such data will yield a steady pipeline of antiviral approaches that could protect simultaneously against several viruses. The standard of care for patients may eventually include both rapid-acting vaccines and broadly-acting antiviral drugs.

In summary, there is an urgent need for head-to-head comparisons of the current popular vaccine candidates because their relative stabilities, production capacities, and protective breadth in primates remain unknown. Having established such a comparison, two types of vaccines should be developed: a cheaply-produced vaccine (e.g., ML29 or VSV-LAS) for emergency use in endemic areas, and a more expensive vaccine (e.g. the MVA or DNA vaccines) for vulnerable populations such as pregnant women. These two types of vaccines can be further improved by increasing immunity to conformational antigens or by favoring epitopes known to bind tightly to HLA and cross-restrict with conformational antigens. After following this path to improving the current popular Lassa vaccine candidates, treatments combining vaccines and therapeutic drugs should be optimized as well.

Author Contributions: J.C.Z., S.M.-M., C.G.-C. and M.S.S. reviewed the literature and wrote the manuscript.

Acknowledgments: We like to thank I.S. Lukashevich for providing critical remarks and comments.

References

1. Fichet-Calvet, E.; Rogers, D.J. Risk maps of lassa fever in west africa. *PLoS Negl Trop Dis* **2009**, 3, e388. [CrossRef] [PubMed]
2. WHO. Ebola Situation Report-17. 2016. Available online: http://apps.who.int/ebola/ebola-situation-reports (accessed on 20 October 2018).

3.   CEPI. Coalition for Epidemic Preparedness Innovations (Cepi) Inception and Top Bio-Threats. 2017. Available online: http://www.who.int/medicines/ebola-treatment/TheCoalitionEpidemicPreparednessInnovations-an-overview.pdf (accessed on 20 October 2018).

4.   WHO. Lassa Roadmap Meeting. 2018. Available online: http://www.who.int/blueprint/priority-diseases/key-action/lassa-fever/en/ (accessed on 20 October 2018).

5.   Bowen, M.D.; Rollin, P.E.; Ksiazek, T.G.; Hustad, H.L.; Bausch, D.G.; Demby, A.H.; Bajani, M.D.; Peters, C.J.; Nichol, S.T. Genetic diversity among lassa virus strains. *J. Virol.* **2000**, *74*, 6992–7004. [CrossRef] [PubMed]

6.   Andersen, K.G.; Shapiro, B.J.; Matranga, C.B.; Sealfon, R.; Lin, A.E.; Moses, L.M.; Folarin, O.A.; Goba, A.; Odia, I.; Ehiane, P.E.; et al. Clinical sequencing uncovers origins and evolution of lassa virus. *Cell* **2015**, *162*, 738–750. [CrossRef] [PubMed]

7.   Siddle, K.J.; Eromon, P.; Barnes, K.G.; Mehta, S.; Oguzie, J.U.; Odia, I.; Schaffner, S.F.; Winnicki, S.M.; Shah, R.R.; Qu, J.; et al. Genomic analysis of lassa virus during an increase in cases in nigeria in 2018. *N. Engl. J. Med.* **2018**. [CrossRef] [PubMed]

8.   Weidmann, M.; Sall, A.A.; Manuguerra, J.C.; Koivogui, L.; Adjami, A.; Traore, F.F.; Hedlund, K.O.; Lindegren, G.; Mirazimi, A. Quantitative analysis of particles, genomes and infectious particles in supernatants of haemorrhagic fever virus cell cultures. *Virol. J.* **2011**, *8*, 81. [CrossRef] [PubMed]

9.   Emonet, S.; Lemasson, J.J.; Gonzalez, J.P.; de Lamballerie, X.; Charrel, R.N. Phylogeny and evolution of old world arenaviruses. *Virology* **2006**, *350*, 251–257. [CrossRef] [PubMed]

10. Lukashevich, I.S.; Maryankova, R.; Vladyko, A.S.; Nashkevich, N.; Koleda, S.; Djavani, M.; Horejsh, D.; Voitenok, N.N.; Salvato, M.S. Lassa and mopeia virus replication in human monocytes/macrophages and in endothelial cells: Different effects on il-8 and tnf-alpha gene expression. *J. Med. Virol.* **1999**, *59*, 552–560. [CrossRef]

11. Baize, S.; Kaplon, J.; Faure, C.; Pannetier, D.; Georges-Courbot, M.C.; Deubel, V. Lassa virus infection of human dendritic cells and macrophages is productive but fails to activate cells. *J. Immunol.* **2004**, *172*, 2861–2869. [CrossRef] [PubMed]

12. Pannetier, D.; Reynard, S.; Russier, M.; Journeaux, A.; Tordo, N.; Deubel, V.; Baize, S. Human dendritic cells infected with the nonpathogenic mopeia virus induce stronger t-cell responses than those infected with lassa virus. *J. Virol.* **2011**, *85*, 8293–8306. [CrossRef] [PubMed]

13. Sommerstein, R.; Flatz, L.; Remy, M.M.; Malinge, P.; Magistrelli, G.; Fischer, N.; Sahin, M.; Bergthaler, A.; Igonet, S.; Ter Meulen, J.; et al. Arenavirus glycan shield promotes neutralizing antibody evasion and protracted infection. *PLoS Pathog.* **2015**, *11*, e1005276. [CrossRef] [PubMed]

14. Lukashevich, I.S. Generation of reassortants between african arenaviruses. *Virology* **1992**, *188*, 600–605. [CrossRef]

15. Lukashevich, I.S.; Patterson, J.; Carrion, R.; Moshkoff, D.; Ticer, A.; Zapata, J.; Brasky, K.; Geiger, R.; Hubbard, G.B.; Bryant, J.; et al. A live attenuated vaccine for lassa fever made by reassortment of lassa and mopeia viruses. *J. Virol.* **2005**, *79*, 13934–13942. [CrossRef] [PubMed]

16. Carrion, R., Jr.; Patterson, J.L.; Johnson, C.; Gonzales, M.; Moreira, C.R.; Ticer, A.; Brasky, K.; Hubbard, G.B.; Moshkoff, D.; Zapata, J.; et al. A ml29 reassortant virus protects guinea pigs against a distantly related nigerian strain of lassa virus and can provide sterilizing immunity. *Vaccine* **2007**, *25*, 4093–4102. [CrossRef] [PubMed]

17. Moshkoff, D.A.; Salvato, M.S.; Lukashevich, I.S. Molecular characterization of a reassortant virus derived from lassa and mopeia viruses. *Virus Genes* **2007**, *34*, 169–176. [CrossRef] [PubMed]

18. Lukashevich, I.S.; Carrion, R., Jr.; Salvato, M.S.; Mansfield, K.; Brasky, K.; Zapata, J.; Cairo, C.; Goicochea, M.; Hoosien, G.E.; Ticer, A.; et al. Safety, immunogenicity, and efficacy of the ml29 reassortant vaccine for lassa fever in small non-human primates. *Vaccine* **2008**, *26*, 5246–5254. [CrossRef] [PubMed]

19. Zapata, J.C.; Poonia, B.; Bryant, J.; Davis, H.; Ateh, E.; George, L.; Crasta, O.; Zhang, Y.; Slezak, T.; Jaing, C.; et al. An attenuated lassa vaccine in siv-infected rhesus macaques does not persist or cause arenavirus disease but does elicit lassa virus-specific immunity. *Virol. J.* **2013**, *10*, 52. [CrossRef] [PubMed]

20. Johnson, K.M.; McCormick, J.B.; Webb, P.A.; Smith, E.S.; Elliott, L.H.; King, I.J. Clinical virology of lassa fever in hospitalized patients. *J. Infect. Dis.* **1987**, *155*, 456–464. [CrossRef] [PubMed]

21. Oldstone, M.B.; Campbell, K.P. Decoding arenavirus pathogenesis: Essential roles for alpha-dystroglycan-virus interactions and the immune response. *Virology* **2011**, *411*, 170–179. [CrossRef] [PubMed]

22. Schmitz, H.; Kohler, B.; Laue, T.; Drosten, C.; Veldkamp, P.J.; Gunther, S.; Emmerich, P.; Geisen, H.P.; Fleischer, K.; Beersma, M.F.; et al. Monitoring of clinical and laboratory data in two cases of imported lassa fever. *Microbes Infect.* **2002**, *4*, 43–50. [CrossRef]

23. Jahrling, P.B.; Frame, J.D.; Rhoderick, J.B.; Monson, M.H. Endemic lassa fever in liberia. Iv. Selection of optimally effective plasma for treatment by passive immunization. *Trans. R. Soc. Trop. Med. Hyg.* **1985**, *79*, 380–384. [CrossRef]

24. McCormick, J.B.; Walker, D.H.; King, I.J.; Webb, P.A.; Elliott, L.H.; Whitfield, S.G.; Johnson, K.M. Lassa virus hepatitis: A study of fatal lassa fever in humans. *Am. J. Trop. Med. Hyg.* **1986**, *35*, 401–407. [CrossRef] [PubMed]

25. Carrion, R., Jr.; Brasky, K.; Mansfield, K.; Johnson, C.; Gonzales, M.; Ticer, A.; Lukashevich, I.; Tardif, S.; Patterson, J. Lassa virus infection in experimentally infected marmosets: Liver pathology and immunophenotypic alterations in target tissues. *J. Virol.* **2007**, *81*, 6482–6490. [CrossRef] [PubMed]

26. Fedeli, C.; Torriani, G.; Galan-Navarro, C.; Moraz, M.L.; Moreno, H.; Gerold, G.; Kunz, S. Axl can serve as entry factor for lassa virus depending on the functional glycosylation of dystroglycan. *J. Virol.* **2018**, *92*, e01613-17. [CrossRef] [PubMed]

27. Beier, J.I.; Jokinen, J.D.; Holz, G.E.; Whang, P.S.; Martin, A.M.; Warner, N.L.; Arteel, G.E.; Lukashevich, I.S. Novel mechanism of arenavirus-induced liver pathology. *PLoS ONE* **2015**, *10*, e0122839. [CrossRef] [PubMed]

28. Cummins, D.; Fisher-Hoch, S.P.; Walshe, K.J.; Mackie, I.J.; McCormick, J.B.; Bennett, D.; Perez, G.; Farrar, B.; Machin, S.J. A plasma inhibitor of platelet aggregation in patients with lassa fever. *Br. J. Haematol.* **1989**, *72*, 543–548. [CrossRef] [PubMed]

29. Fisher-Hoch, S.; McCormick, J.B.; Sasso, D.; Craven, R.B. Hematologic dysfunction in lassa fever. *J. Med. Virol.* **1988**, *26*, 127–135. [CrossRef] [PubMed]

30. Fisher-Hoch, S.P.; McCormick, J.B. Pathophysiology and treatment of lassa fever. *Curr. Top. Microbiol. Immunol.* **1987**, *134*, 231–239. [PubMed]

31. Knobloch, J.; McCormick, J.B.; Webb, P.A.; Dietrich, M.; Schumacher, H.H.; Dennis, E. Clinical observations in 42 patients with lassa fever. *Tropenmed. Parasitol.* **1980**, *31*, 389–398. [PubMed]

32. Lange, J.V.; Mitchell, S.W.; McCormick, J.B.; Walker, D.H.; Evatt, B.L.; Ramsey, R.R. Kinetic study of platelets and fibrinogen in lassa virus-infected monkeys and early pathologic events in mopeia virus-infected monkeys. *Am. J. Trop. Med. Hyg.* **1985**, *34*, 999–1007. [CrossRef] [PubMed]

33. Cummins, D.; McCormick, J.B.; Bennett, D.; Samba, J.A.; Farrar, B.; Machin, S.J.; Fisher-Hoch, S.P. Acute sensorineural deafness in lassa fever. *JAMA* **1990**, *264*, 2093–2096. [CrossRef] [PubMed]

34. Fisher-Hoch, S.P.; Mitchell, S.W.; Sasso, D.R.; Lange, J.V.; Ramsey, R.; McCormick, J.B. Physiological and immunologic disturbances associated with shock in a primate model of lassa fever. *J. Infect. Dis.* **1987**, *155*, 465–474. [CrossRef] [PubMed]

35. Khan, S.H.; Goba, A.; Chu, M.; Roth, C.; Healing, T.; Marx, A.; Fair, J.; Guttieri, M.C.; Ferro, P.; Imes, T.; et al. New opportunities for field research on the pathogenesis and treatment of lassa fever. *Antivir. Res.* **2008**, *78*, 103–115. [CrossRef] [PubMed]

36. Peters, C.J.; Liu, C.T.; Anderson, G.W., Jr.; Morrill, J.C.; Jahrling, P.B. Pathogenesis of viral hemorrhagic fevers: Rift valley fever and lassa fever contrasted. *Rev. Infect. Dis.* **1989**, *11* (Suppl. 4), S743–S749. [CrossRef]

37. Solbrig, M.V. Headache syndromes in sierra leone, west africa. *Headache* **1991**, *31*, 419. [PubMed]

38. Baize, S.; Marianneau, P.; Loth, P.; Reynard, S.; Journeaux, A.; Chevallier, M.; Tordo, N.; Deubel, V.; Contamin, H. Early and strong immune responses are associated with control of viral replication and recovery in lassa virus-infected cynomolgus monkeys. *J. Virol.* **2009**, *83*, 5890–5903. [CrossRef] [PubMed]

39. Edington, G.M.; White, H.A. The pathology of lassa fever. *Trans. R. Soc. Trop. Med. Hyg.* **1972**, *66*, 381–389. [CrossRef]

40. Hensley, L.E.; Smith, M.A.; Geisbert, J.B.; Fritz, E.A.; Daddario-DiCaprio, K.M.; Larsen, T.; Geisbert, T.W. Pathogenesis of lassa fever in cynomolgus macaques. *Virol. J.* **2011**, *8*, 205. [CrossRef] [PubMed]

41. McCormick, J.B.; Fisher-Hoch, S.P. Lassa fever. *Curr. Top. Microbiol. Immunol.* **2002**, *262*, 75–109. [PubMed]

42. Mahanty, S.; Hutchinson, K.; Agarwal, S.; McRae, M.; Rollin, P.E.; Pulendran, B. Cutting edge: Impairment of dendritic cells and adaptive immunity by ebola and lassa viruses. *J. Immunol.* **2003**, *170*, 2797–2801. [CrossRef] [PubMed]

43. Jacobs, B.L.; Langland, J.O. When two strands are better than one: The mediators and modulators of the cellular responses to double-stranded rna. *Virology* **1996**, *219*, 339–349. [CrossRef] [PubMed]

44. Kell, A.M.; Gale, M., Jr. Rig-i in rna virus recognition. *Virology* **2015**, *479–480*, 110–121. [CrossRef] [PubMed]

45. Asper, M.; Sternsdorf, T.; Hass, M.; Drosten, C.; Rhode, A.; Schmitz, H.; Gunther, S. Inhibition of different lassa virus strains by alpha and gamma interferons and comparison with a less pathogenic arenavirus. *J. Virol.* **2004**, *78*, 3162–3169. [CrossRef] [PubMed]

46. Lukashevich, I.S.; Tikhonov, I.; Rodas, J.D.; Zapata, J.C.; Yang, Y.; Djavani, M.; Salvato, M.S. Arenavirus-mediated liver pathology: Acute lymphocytic choriomeningitis virus infection of rhesus macaques is characterized by high-level interleukin-6 expression and hepatocyte proliferation. *J. Virol.* **2003**, *77*, 1727–1737. [CrossRef] [PubMed]

47. Branco, L.M.; Grove, J.N.; Boisen, M.L.; Shaffer, J.G.; Goba, A.; Fullah, M.; Momoh, M.; Grant, D.S.; Garry, R.F. Emerging trends in lassa fever: Redefining the role of immunoglobulin m and inflammation in diagnosing acute infection. *Virol. J.* **2011**, *8*, 478. [CrossRef] [PubMed]

48. Martinez-Sobrido, L.; Emonet, S.; Giannakas, P.; Cubitt, B.; Garcia-Sastre, A.; de la Torre, J.C. Identification of amino acid residues critical for the anti-interferon activity of the nucleoprotein of the prototypic arenavirus lymphocytic choriomeningitis virus. *J. Virol.* **2009**, *83*, 11330–11340. [CrossRef] [PubMed]

49. Hastie, K.M.; Kimberlin, C.R.; Zandonatti, M.A.; MacRae, I.J.; Saphire, E.O. Structure of the lassa virus nucleoprotein reveals a dsrna-specific 3′ to 5′ exonuclease activity essential for immune suppression. *Proc. Natl. Acad. Sci. USA* **2011**, *108*, 2396–2401. [CrossRef] [PubMed]

50. Martinez-Sobrido, L.; Giannakas, P.; Cubitt, B.; Garcia-Sastre, A.; de la Torre, J.C. Differential inhibition of type i interferon induction by arenavirus nucleoproteins. *J. Virol.* **2007**, *81*, 12696–12703. [CrossRef] [PubMed]

51. Martinez-Sobrido, L.; Zuniga, E.I.; Rosario, D.; Garcia-Sastre, A.; de la Torre, J.C. Inhibition of the type i interferon response by the nucleoprotein of the prototypic arenavirus lymphocytic choriomeningitis virus. *J. Virol.* **2006**, *80*, 9192–9199. [CrossRef] [PubMed]

52. Qi, X.; Lan, S.; Wang, W.; Schelde, L.M.; Dong, H.; Wallat, G.D.; Ly, H.; Liang, Y.; Dong, C. Cap binding and immune evasion revealed by lassa nucleoprotein structure. *Nature* **2010**, *468*, 779–783. [CrossRef] [PubMed]

53. Zhou, S.; Cerny, A.M.; Zacharia, A.; Fitzgerald, K.A.; Kurt-Jones, E.A.; Finberg, R.W. Induction and inhibition of type i interferon responses by distinct components of lymphocytic choriomeningitis virus. *J. Virol.* **2010**, *84*, 9452–9462. [CrossRef] [PubMed]

54. Xing, J.; Ly, H.; Liang, Y. The z proteins of pathogenic but not nonpathogenic arenaviruses inhibit rig-i-like receptor-dependent interferon production. *J. Virol.* **2015**, *89*, 2944–2955. [CrossRef] [PubMed]

55. Forni, D.; Pontremoli, C.; Pozzoli, U.; Clerici, M.; Cagliani, R.; Sironi, M. Ancient evolution of mammarenaviruses: Adaptation via changes in the l protein and no evidence for host-virus codivergence. *Genome Biol. Evol.* **2018**, *10*, 863–874. [CrossRef] [PubMed]

56. Grove, J.N.; Branco, L.M.; Boisen, M.L.; Muncy, I.J.; Henderson, L.A.; Schieffellin, J.S.; Robinson, J.E.; Bangura, J.J.; Fonnie, M.; Schoepp, R.J.; et al. Capacity building permitting comprehensive monitoring of a severe case of lassa hemorrhagic fever in sierra leone with a positive outcome: Case report. *Virol. J.* **2011**, *8*, 314. [CrossRef] [PubMed]

57. Djavani, M.M.; Crasta, O.R.; Zapata, J.C.; Fei, Z.; Folkerts, O.; Sobral, B.; Swindells, M.; Bryant, J.; Davis, H.; Pauza, C.D.; et al. Early blood profiles of virus infection in a monkey model for lassa fever. *J. Virol.* **2007**, *81*, 7960–7973. [CrossRef] [PubMed]

58. Hayes, M.W.; Carrion, R., Jr.; Nunneley, J.; Medvedev, A.E.; Salvato, M.S.; Lukashevich, I.S. Pathogenic old world arenaviruses inhibit tlr2/mal-dependent proinflammatory cytokines in vitro. *J. Virol.* **2012**, *86*, 7216–7226. [CrossRef] [PubMed]

59. Lukashevich, I.S.; Rodas, J.D.; Tikhonov, I.I.; Zapata, J.C.; Yang, Y.; Djavani, M.; Salvato, M.S. Lcmv-mediated hepatitis in rhesus macaques: We but not arm strain activates hepatocytes and induces liver regeneration. *Arch. Virol.* **2004**, *149*, 2319–2336. [CrossRef] [PubMed]

60. McCormick, J.B.; Mitchell, S.W.; Kiley, M.P.; Ruo, S.; Fisher-Hoch, S.P. Inactivated lassa virus elicits a non protective immune response in rhesus monkeys. *J. Med. Virol.* **1992**, *37*, 1–7. [CrossRef] [PubMed]

61. Arnold, R.B.; Gary, G.W. A neutralization test survey for lassa fever activity in lassa, nigeria. *Trans. R. Soc. Trop. Med. Hyg.* **1977**, *71*, 152–154. [CrossRef]

62. Lukashevich, I.S.; Clegg, J.C.; Sidibe, K. Lassa virus activity in guinea: Distribution of human antiviral antibody defined using enzyme-linked immunosorbent assay with recombinant antigen. *J. Med. Virol.* **1993**, *40*, 210–217. [CrossRef] [PubMed]

63. Tomori, O.; Fabiyi, A.; Sorungbe, A.; Smith, A.; McCormick, J.B. Viral hemorrhagic fever antibodies in nigerian populations. *Am. J. Trop. Med. Hyg.* **1988**, *38*, 407–410. [CrossRef] [PubMed]

64. McCormick, J.B.; Webb, P.A.; Krebs, J.W.; Johnson, K.M.; Smith, E.S. A prospective study of the epidemiology and ecology of lassa fever. *J. Infect. Dis.* **1987**, *155*, 437–444. [CrossRef] [PubMed]

65. Fisher-Hoch, S.P.; McCormick, J.B. Towards a human lassa fever vaccine. *Rev. Med. Virol.* **2001**, *11*, 331–341. [CrossRef] [PubMed]

66. Leifer, E.; Gocke, D.J.; Bourne, H. Lassa fever, a new virus disease of man from west africa. Ii. Report of a laboratory-acquired infection treated with plasma from a person recently recovered from the disease. *Am. J. Trop. Med. Hyg.* **1970**, *19*, 677–679. [CrossRef] [PubMed]

67. McCormick, J.B.; King, I.J.; Webb, P.A.; Scribner, C.L.; Craven, R.B.; Johnson, K.M.; Elliott, L.H.; Belmont-Williams, R. Lassa fever. Effective therapy with ribavirin. *N. Engl. J. Med.* **1986**, *314*, 20–26. [CrossRef] [PubMed]

68. Mire, C.E.; Cross, R.W.; Geisbert, J.B.; Borisevich, V.; Agans, K.N.; Deer, D.J.; Heinrich, M.L.; Rowland, M.M.; Goba, A.; Momoh, M.; et al. Human-monoclonal-antibody therapy protects nonhuman primates against advanced lassa fever. *Nat. Med.* **2017**, *23*, 1146–1149. [CrossRef] [PubMed]

69. Hastie, K.M.; Saphire, E.O. Lassa virus glycoprotein: Stopping a moving target. *Curr. Opin. Virol.* **2018**, *31*, 52–58. [CrossRef] [PubMed]

70. Fisher-Hoch, S.P.; McCormick, J.B. Lassa fever vaccine. *Expert Rev. Vaccines* **2004**, *3*, 189–197. [CrossRef] [PubMed]

71. Richmond, J.K.; Baglole, D.J. Lassa fever: Epidemiology, clinical features, and social consequences. *Br. Med. J.* **2003**, *327*, 1271–1275. [CrossRef] [PubMed]

72. ter Meulen, J.; Badusche, M.; Kuhnt, K.; Doetze, A.; Satoguina, J.; Marti, T.; Loeliger, C.; Koulemou, K.; Koivogui, L.; Schmitz, H.; et al. Characterization of human CD4(+) t-cell clones recognizing conserved and variable epitopes of the lassa virus nucleoprotein. *J. Virol.* **2000**, *74*, 2186–2192. [CrossRef] [PubMed]

73. Meulen, J.; Badusche, M.; Satoguina, J.; Strecker, T.; Lenz, O.; Loeliger, C.; Sakho, M.; Koulemou, K.; Koivogui, L.; Hoerauf, A. Old and new world arenaviruses share a highly conserved epitope in the fusion domain of the glycoprotein 2, which is recognized by lassa virus-specific human cd4+ t-cell clones. *Virology* **2004**, *321*, 134–143. [CrossRef] [PubMed]

74. McElroy, A.K.; Akondy, R.S.; Harmon, J.R.; Ellebedy, A.H.; Cannon, D.; Klena, J.D.; Sidney, J.; Sette, A.; Mehta, A.K.; Kraft, C.S.; et al. A case of human lassa virus infection with robust acute t-cell activation and long-term virus-specific t-cell responses. *J. Infect. Dis.* **2017**, *215*, 1862–1872. [CrossRef] [PubMed]

75. Goicochea, M.A.; Zapata, J.C.; Bryant, J.; Davis, H.; Salvato, M.S.; Lukashevich, I.S. Evaluation of lassa virus vaccine immunogenicity in a cba/j-ml29 mouse model. *Vaccine* **2012**, *30*, 1445–1452. [CrossRef] [PubMed]

76. Jahrling, P.B.; Peters, C.J. Serology and virulence diversity among old-world arenaviruses, and the relevance to vaccine development. *Med. Microbiol. Immunol.* **1986**, *175*, 165–167. [CrossRef] [PubMed]

77. Pushko, P.; Geisbert, J.; Parker, M.; Jahrling, P.; Smith, J. Individual and bivalent vaccines based on alphavirus replicons protect guinea pigs against infection with lassa and ebola viruses. *J. Virol.* **2001**, *75*, 11677–11685. [CrossRef] [PubMed]

78. Kiley, M.P.; Lange, J.V.; Johnson, K.M. Protection of rhesus monkeys from lassa virus by immunisation with closely related arenavirus. *Lancet* **1979**, *2*, 738. [CrossRef]

79. Walker, D.H.; Johnson, K.M.; Lange, J.V.; Gardner, J.J.; Kiley, M.P.; McCormick, J.B. Experimental infection of rhesus monkeys with lassa virus and a closely related arenavirus, mozambique virus. *J. Infect. Dis.* **1982**, *146*, 360–368. [CrossRef] [PubMed]

80. Maes, P.; Alkhovsky, S.V.; Bao, Y.; Beer, M.; Birkhead, M.; Briese, T.; Buchmeier, M.J.; Calisher, C.H.; Charrel, R.N.; Choi, I.R.; et al. Taxonomy of the family arenaviridae and the order bunyavirales: Update 2018. *Arch. Virol.* **2018**, *163*, 2295–2310. [CrossRef] [PubMed]

81. Safronetz, D.; Mire, C.; Rosenke, K.; Feldmann, F.; Haddock, E.; Geisbert, T.; Feldmann, H. A recombinant vesicular stomatitis virus-based lassa fever vaccine protects guinea pigs and macaques against challenge with geographically and genetically distinct lassa viruses. *PLoS Negl. Trop. Dis.* **2015**, *9*, e0003736. [CrossRef] [PubMed]

82. Clegg, J.C.; Lloyd, G. Vaccinia recombinant expressing lassa-virus internal nucleocapsid protein protects guineapigs against lassa fever. *Lancet* **1987**, *2*, 186–188. [CrossRef]

83. Peters, C.J.; Jahrling, P.B.; Liu, C.T.; Kenyon, R.H.; McKee, K.T., Jr.; Barrera Oro, J.G. Experimental studies of arenaviral hemorrhagic fevers. *Curr. Top. Microbiol. Immunol.* **1987**, *134*, 5–68. [PubMed]

84. Bredenbeek, P.J.; Molenkamp, R.; Spaan, W.J.; Deubel, V.; Marianneau, P.; Salvato, M.S.; Moshkoff, D.; Zapata, J.; Tikhonov, I.; Patterson, J.; et al. A recombinant yellow fever 17d vaccine expressing lassa virus glycoproteins. *Virology* **2006**, *345*, 299–304. [CrossRef] [PubMed]

85. Jiang, X.; Dalebout, T.J.; Bredenbeek, P.J.; Carrion, R., Jr.; Brasky, K.; Patterson, J.; Goicochea, M.; Bryant, J.; Salvato, M.S.; Lukashevich, I.S. Yellow fever 17d-vectored vaccines expressing lassa virus gp1 and gp2 glycoproteins provide protection against fatal disease in guinea pigs. *Vaccine* **2011**, *29*, 1248–1257. [CrossRef] [PubMed]

86. Carnec, X.; Mateo, M.; Page, A.; Reynard, S.; Hortion, J.; Picard, C.; Yekwa, E.; Barrot, L.; Barron, S.; Vallve, A.; et al. A vaccine platform against arenaviruses based on a recombinant hyperattenuated mopeia virus expressing heterologous glycoproteins. *J. Virol.* **2018**, *92*, e02230-17. [CrossRef] [PubMed]

87. Salvato, M.S.; Domi, A.; Guzmán-Cardozo, C.; Zapata, J.C.; Medina-Moreno, S.; Hsu, H.; McCurley, N.P.; Basu, R.; Hauser, M.; Hellerstein, M.S.; et al. A single dose of modified vaccinia ankara expressing lassa virus like particles protects mice from lethal intracerebral virus challenge. *Sci. Rep.* **2018**, in preparation.

88. Cashman, K.A.; Wilkinson, E.R.; Shaia, C.I.; Facemire, P.R.; Bell, T.M.; Bearss, J.J.; Shamblin, J.D.; Wollen, S.E.; Broderick, K.E.; Sardesai, N.Y.; et al. A DNA vaccine delivered by dermal electroporation fully protects cynomolgus macaques against lassa fever. *Hum. Vaccin. Immunother.* **2017**, *13*, 2902–2911. [CrossRef] [PubMed]

89. Geisbert, T.W.; Jones, S.; Fritz, E.A.; Shurtleff, A.C.; Geisbert, J.B.; Liebscher, R.; Grolla, A.; Stroher, U.; Fernando, L.; Daddario, K.M.; et al. Development of a new vaccine for the prevention of lassa fever. *PLoS Med.* **2005**, *2*, e183. [CrossRef] [PubMed]

90. Clarke, D.K.; Hendry, R.M.; Singh, V.; Rose, J.K.; Seligman, S.J.; Klug, B.; Kochhar, S.; Mac, L.M.; Carbery, B.; Chen, R.T.; et al. Live virus vaccines based on a vesicular stomatitis virus (vsv) backbone: Standardized template with key considerations for a risk/benefit assessment. *Vaccine* **2016**, *34*, 6597–6609. [CrossRef] [PubMed]

91. Kim, J.H.; Excler, J.L.; Michael, N.L. Lessons from the rv144 thai phase iii hiv-1 vaccine trial and the search for correlates of protection. *Annu. Rev. Med.* **2015**, *66*, 423–437. [CrossRef] [PubMed]

92. Djavani, M.; Topisirovic, I.; Zapata, J.C.; Sadowska, M.; Yang, Y.; Rodas, J.; Lukashevich, I.S.; Bogue, C.W.; Pauza, C.D.; Borden, K.L.; et al. The proline-rich homeodomain (prh/hex) protein is down-regulated in liver during infection with lymphocytic choriomeningitis virus. *J. Virol.* **2005**, *79*, 2461–2473. [CrossRef] [PubMed]

93. Iwasaki, M.; Cubitt, B.; Jokinen, J.; Lukashevich, I.S.; de la Torre, J.C. Use of recombinant ml29 platform to generate polyvalent live-attenuated vaccines against lassa fever and other infectious diseases. In Proceedings of the 66th Annual Meeting of Japanese Society for Virology, Kyoto, Japan, 28–30 October 2018.

94. Haynes, B.F.; Verkoczy, L. Aids/hiv. Host controls of hiv neutralizing antibodies. *Science* **2014**, *344*, 588–589. [CrossRef] [PubMed]

95. Pinschewer, D.D.; Perez, M.; Jeetendra, E.; Bachi, T.; Horvath, E.; Hengartner, H.; Whitt, M.A.; de la Torre, J.C.; Zinkernagel, R.M. Kinetics of protective antibodies are determined by the viral surface antigen. *J. Clin. Investig.* **2004**, *114*, 988–993. [CrossRef] [PubMed]

96. Wyatt, R.; Kwong, P.D.; Desjardins, E.; Sweet, R.W.; Robinson, J.; Hendrickson, W.A.; Sodroski, J.G. The antigenic structure of the hiv gp120 envelope glycoprotein. *Nature* **1998**, *393*, 705–711. [CrossRef] [PubMed]

97. Gristick, H.B.; von Boehmer, L.; West, A.P., Jr.; Schamber, M.; Gazumyan, A.; Golijanin, J.; Seaman, M.S.; Fatkenheuer, G.; Klein, F.; Nussenzweig, M.C.; et al. Natively glycosylated hiv-1 env structure reveals new mode for antibody recognition of the cd4-binding site. *Nat. Struct. Mol. Biol.* **2016**, *23*, 906–915. [CrossRef] [PubMed]

98. Burnett, D.L.; Langley, D.B.; Schofield, P.; Hermes, J.R.; Chan, T.D.; Jackson, J.; Bourne, K.; Reed, J.H.; Patterson, K.; Porebski, B.T.; et al. Germinal center antibody mutation trajectories are determined by rapid self/foreign discrimination. *Science* **2018**, *360*, 223–226. [CrossRef] [PubMed]

99. Cooke, M.P.; Heath, A.W.; Shokat, K.M.; Zeng, Y.; Finkelman, F.D.; Linsley, P.S.; Howard, M.; Goodnow, C.C. Immunoglobulin signal transduction guides the specificity of b cell-t cell interactions and is blocked in tolerant self-reactive b cells. *J. Exp. Med.* **1994**, *179*, 425–438. [CrossRef] [PubMed]

100. Zhao, M.; Chen, J.; Tan, S.; Dong, T.; Jiang, H.; Zheng, J.; Quan, C.; Liao, Q.; Zhang, H.; Wang, X.; et al. Prolonged evolution of virus-specific memory t cell immunity post severe avian influenza a (h7n9) virus infection. *J. Virol.* **2018**. [CrossRef] [PubMed]

101. Ping, X.; Hu, W.; Xiong, R.; Zhang, X.; Teng, Z.; Ding, M.; Li, L.; Chang, C.; Xu, K. Generation of a broadly reactive influenza h1 antigen using a consensus ha sequence. *Vaccine* **2018**, *36*, 4837–4845. [CrossRef] [PubMed]

102. Bachmann, M.F.; Rohrer, U.H.; Kundig, T.M.; Burki, K.; Hengartner, H.; Zinkernagel, R.M. The influence of antigen organization on b cell responsiveness. *Science* **1993**, *262*, 1448–1451. [CrossRef] [PubMed]

103. Ilyinskii, P.O.; Thoidis, G.; Sherman, M.Y.; Shneider, A. Adjuvant potential of aggregate-forming polyglutamine domains. *Vaccine* **2008**, *26*, 3223–3226. [CrossRef] [PubMed]

104. Van Braeckel-Budimir, N.; Haijema, B.J.; Leenhouts, K. Bacterium-like particles for efficient immune stimulation of existing vaccines and new subunit vaccines in mucosal applications. *Front. Immunol.* **2013**, *4*, 282. [CrossRef] [PubMed]

105. Snapper, C.M. Distinct immunologic properties of soluble versus particulate antigens. *Front. Immunol.* **2018**, *9*, 598. [CrossRef] [PubMed]

106. Strand, M.; August, J.T. Structural proteins of mammalian oncogenic rna viruses: Multiple antigenic determinants of the major internal protein and envelope glycoprotein. *J. Virol.* **1974**, *13*, 171–180. [PubMed]

107. Shubin, Z.; Li, W.; Poonia, B.; Ferrari, G.; LaBranche, C.; Montefiori, D.; Zhu, X.; Pauza, C.D. An hiv envelope gp120-fc fusion protein elicits effector antibody responses in rhesus macaques. *Clin. Vaccine Immunol.* **2017**, *24*, 00028-17. [CrossRef] [PubMed]

108. Robinson, J.E.; Hastie, K.M.; Cross, R.W.; Yenni, R.E.; Elliott, D.H.; Rouelle, J.A.; Kannadka, C.B.; Smira, A.A.; Garry, C.E.; Bradley, B.T.; et al. Most neutralizing human monoclonal antibodies target novel epitopes requiring both lassa virus glycoprotein subunits. *Nat. Commun.* **2016**, *7*, 11544. [CrossRef] [PubMed]

109. Provine, N.M.; Cortez, V.; Chohan, V.; Overbaugh, J. The neutralization sensitivity of viruses representing human immunodeficiency virus type 1 variants of diverse subtypes from early in infection is dependent on producer cell, as well as characteristics of the specific antibody and envelope variant. *Virology* **2012**, *427*, 25–33. [CrossRef] [PubMed]

110. Cohen, Y.Z.; Lorenzi, J.C.C.; Seaman, M.S.; Nogueira, L.; Schoofs, T.; Krassnig, L.; Butler, A.; Millard, K.; Fitzsimons, T.; Daniell, X.; et al. Neutralizing activity of broadly neutralizing anti-hiv-1 antibodies against clade b clinical isolates produced in peripheral blood mononuclear cells. *J. Virol.* **2018**, *92*, e01883-17. [PubMed]

111. Huang, J.; Kang, B.H.; Pancera, M.; Lee, J.H.; Tong, T.; Feng, Y.; Imamichi, H.; Georgiev, I.S.; Chuang, G.Y.; Druz, A.; et al. Broad and potent hiv-1 neutralization by a human antibody that binds the gp41-gp120 interface. *Nature* **2014**, *515*, 138–142. [CrossRef] [PubMed]

112. Leon, P.E.; He, W.; Mullarkey, C.E.; Bailey, M.J.; Miller, M.S.; Krammer, F.; Palese, P.; Tan, G.S. Optimal activation of fc-mediated effector functions by influenza virus hemagglutinin antibodies requires two points of contact. *Proc. Natl. Acad. Sci. USA* **2016**, *113*, E5944–E5951. [CrossRef] [PubMed]

113. Abreu-Mota, T.; Hagen, K.R.; Cooper, K.; Jahrling, P.B.; Tan, G.; Wirblich, C.; Johnson, R.F.; Schnell, M.J. Non-neutralizing antibodies elicited by recombinant lassa-rabies vaccine are critical for protection against lassa fever. *Nat. Commun.* **2018**, *9*, 4223. [CrossRef] [PubMed]

114. An, L.L.; Whitton, J.L. A multivalent minigene vaccine, containing b-cell, cytotoxic t-lymphocyte, and th epitopes from several microbes, induces appropriate responses in vivo and confers protection against more than one pathogen. *J. Virol.* **1997**, *71*, 2292–2302. [PubMed]

115. Holst, P.J.; Jensen, B.A.; Ragonnaud, E.; Thomsen, A.R.; Christensen, J.P. Targeting of non-dominant antigens as a vaccine strategy to broaden t-cell responses during chronic viral infection. *PLoS ONE* **2015**, *10*, e0117242. [CrossRef] [PubMed]

116. Rammensee, H.G.; Friede, T.; Stevanoviic, S. Mhc ligands and peptide motifs: First listing. *Immunogenetics* **1995**, *41*, 178–228. [CrossRef] [PubMed]

117. Patarroyo, M.E.; Bermudez, A.; Alba, M.P.; Vanegas, M.; Moreno-Vranich, A.; Poloche, L.A.; Patarroyo, M.A. Impips: The immune protection-inducing protein structure concept in the search for steric-electron and topochemical principles for complete fully-protective chemically synthesised vaccine development. *PLoS ONE* **2015**, *10*, e0123249. [CrossRef] [PubMed]

118. Lozano, J.M.; Varela, Y.; Silva, Y.; Ardila, K.; Forero, M.; Guasca, L.; Guerrero, Y.; Bermudez, A.; Alba, P.; Vanegas, M.; et al. A large size chimeric highly immunogenic peptide presents multistage plasmodium antigens as a vaccine candidate system against malaria. *Molecules* **2017**, *22*, 1837. [CrossRef] [PubMed]

119. Mukhopadhyay, M.; Galperin, M.; Patgaonkar, M.; Vasan, S.; Ho, D.D.; Nouel, A.; Claireaux, M.; Benati, D.; Lambotte, O.; Huang, Y.; et al. DNA vaccination by electroporation amplifies broadly cross-restricted public tcr clonotypes shared with hiv controllers. *J. Immunol.* **2017**, *199*, 3437–3452. [CrossRef] [PubMed]

120. Liu, F.; Feuer, R.; Hassett, D.E.; Whitton, J.L. Peptide vaccination of mice immune to lcmv or vaccinia virus causes serious cd8 t cell-mediated, tnf-dependent immunopathology. *J. C. Investig.* **2006**, *116*, 465–475. [CrossRef] [PubMed]

121. Sissoko, D.; Laouenan, C.; Folkesson, E.; M'Lebing, A.B.; Beavogui, A.H.; Baize, S.; Camara, A.M.; Maes, P.; Shepherd, S.; Danel, C.; et al. Experimental treatment with favipiravir for ebola virus disease (the jiki trial): A historically controlled, single-arm proof-of-concept trial in guinea. *PLoS Med.* **2016**, *13*, e1001967.

122. Kentsis, A.; Volpon, L.; Topisirovic, I.; Soll, C.E.; Culjkovic, B.; Shao, L.; Borden, K.L. Further evidence that ribavirin interacts with eif4e. *RNA* **2005**, *11*, 1762–1766. [CrossRef] [PubMed]

123. Volpon, L.; Culjkovic-Kraljacic, B.; Sohn, H.S.; Blanchet-Cohen, A.; Osborne, M.J.; Borden, K.L.B. A biochemical framework for eif4e-dependent mrna export and nuclear recycling of the export machinery. *RNA* **2017**, *23*, 927–937. [CrossRef] [PubMed]

124. Iwasaki, M.; de la Torre, J.C. A highly conserved leucine in mammarenavirus matrix z protein is required for z interaction with the virus l polymerase and z stability in cells harboring an active viral ribonucleoprotein. *J. Virol.* **2018**, *92*, 02256-17. [CrossRef] [PubMed]

125. Hickerson, B.T.; Westover, J.B.; Jung, K.H.; Komeno, T.; Furuta, Y.; Gowen, B.B. Effective treatment of experimental lymphocytic choriomeningitis virus infection: Consideration of favipiravir for use with infected organ transplant recipients. *J. Infect. Dis.* **2018**, *218*, 522–527. [CrossRef] [PubMed]

16

Respiratory Illness in a Piggery Associated with the First Identified Outbreak of Swine Influenza in Australia: Assessing the Risk to Human Health and Zoonotic Potential

David W. Smith [1,2,*][iD], Ian G. Barr [3,4], Richmond Loh [5], Avram Levy [1], Simone Tempone [6], Mark O'Dea [7][iD], James Watson [8], Frank Y. K. Wong [8] and Paul V. Effler [2,6]

[1]   Department of Microbiology, PathWest Laboratory Medicine WA, Nedlands, WA 6009, Australia;
      avram.levy@health.wa.gov.au
[2]   Faculty of Health and Medical Sciences, University of Western Australia, Nedlands, WA 6009, Australia;
      paul.effler@health.wa.gov.au
[3]   World Health Organization (WHO) Collaborating Centre for Reference and Research on Influenza, at The
      Peter Doherty Institute for Infection and Immunity, Melbourne, VIC 3000, Australia;
      Ian.Barr@influenzacentre.org.au
[4]   Department of Microbiology and Immunology, University of Melbourne, at the Peter Doherty Institute for
      Infection and Immunity, Melbourne, VIC 3000, Australia
[5]   Sustainability and Biosecurity, Department of Primary Industries and Regional Development, Perth,
      WA 6151, Australia; richmond.loh@dpird.wa.gov.au
[6]   Communicable Disease Control Directorate, Department of Health Western Australia, Perth,
      WA 6004, Australia; simone.tempone@health.wa.gov.au
[7]   School of Veterinary Medicine, Murdoch University, Perth, WA 6150, Australia; M.ODea@murdoch.edu.au
[8]   CSIRO Australian Animal Health Laboratory, Geelong, VIC 3219, Australia; James.Watson@csiro.au (J.W.);
      Frank.Wong@csiro.au (F.Y.K.W.)
*   Correspondence: david.smith@health.wa.gov.au.

Abstract: Australia was previously believed to be free of enzootic swine influenza viruses due strict quarantine practices and use of biosecure breeding facilities. The first proven Australian outbreak of swine influenza occurred in Western Australian in 2012, revealing an unrecognized zoonotic risk, and a potential future pandemic threat. A public health investigation was undertaken to determine whether zoonotic infections had occurred and to reduce the risk of further transmission between humans and swine. A program of monitoring, testing, treatment, and vaccination was commenced, and a serosurvey of workers was also undertaken. No acute infections with the swine influenza viruses were detected. Serosurvey results were difficult to interpret due to previous influenza infections and past and current vaccinations. However, several workers had elevated haemagglutination inhibition (HI) antibody levels to the swine influenza viruses that could not be attributed to vaccination or infection with contemporaneous seasonal influenza A viruses. However, we lacked a suitable control population, so this was inconclusive. The experience was valuable in developing better protocols for managing outbreaks at the human–animal interface. Strict adherence to biosecurity practices, and ongoing monitoring of swine and their human contacts is important to mitigate pandemic risk. Strain specific serological assays would greatly assist in identifying zoonotic transmission.

Keywords: influenza; swine; Australia; human; pandemic

1. Introduction

Influenza A viruses (IAV) circulate and evolve continually within bird and swine populations of the world, and are known to be a source of sporadic zoonotic influenza infections, thus presenting a reservoir of potential human pandemic influenza strains. They are known to be present in domestic swine populations internationally, largely as a result of the virus being introduced from humans infected with seasonal influenza viruses [1–3]. Some of these human origin viruses persisted and evolved into stable swine lineages through genetic and antigenic drift and virus gene reassortment. They pose an ongoing potential threat to both animal and human health, as demonstrated by the 2009 pandemic, which arose from swine influenza viruses derived from both human and avian IAV that had undergone long term ongoing reassortment [4].

Human infections with swine IAV have been detected since the 1970s and have caused both sporadic cases and outbreaks, such as those reported in the USA [3,5,6]. These zoonotic viruses are mainly of the A(H3N2) subtype with some A(H1N1) and A(H1N2) viruses, which are referred to as variant viruses with a lower-case "v" placed after the subtype, e.g., A(H3N2)v to denote their swine origin.

Prior to 2012 it was believed that Australian domestic swine populations were free of swine lineages of IAV. This was ascribed to negative results from a few limited serosurveys, and the strict quarantine practices preventing importation of pigs and the use of biosecure breeding facilities for domestic swine within Australia. In 2009, a number of outbreaks due to A(H1N1)pdm09 occurred in domestic Australian swine populations through transmission from infected humans, and these have continued to occur sporadically ever since [7]. The virus had little or no apparent ill effect on the health of infected swine and there was no evidence that this resulted from, or led to, enzootic IAV in Australian swine, and so was not seen to be a threat to human or animal health nor a potential source of pandemic viruses.

However, in 2012 an outbreak of respiratory illness and death occurred amongst pigs in a biosecure piggery near Perth, the capital of Western Australia [8], shown to be due to several previously unidentified swine IAV containing genes of human origin [9]. A mild respiratory illness was also reported by several of the workers. A combined investigation of this outbreak by the Department of Agriculture and Food, Western Australia (DAFWA) and the Communicable Disease Control Directorate (CDCD) of the Department of Health Western Australia led to the detection of a number of genetically distinct divergent IAV in the swine.

An extensive phylogenetic analysis indicated that the IAV in the Western Australian swine contain human origin genes not found in human populations for several decades, and that they are distinct from those identified in swine in the rest of the world, including those subsequently identified in swine in a piggery in Queensland [9], approximately 4000 km distant. This ongoing circulation and evolution of IAV in the Western Australian swine population for up to several decades revealed an unrecognized potential zoonotic threat [9].

In view of the known risk of transmission of IAV from pigs to humans in other countries [2,6], interventions were undertaken to investigate and mitigate the risk of human infection. This paper describes the investigations undertaken into this outbreak to assess the potential risk to human contacts and to determine whether zoonotic transmission had occurred. The importance of these investigations has been further emphasized by the recent description of the first human infection with a variant swine H3N2, acquired within Australia [10]. This occurred outside Western Australia following exposure to exhibition swine at an agricultural fair, and was confirmed to be due to a virus similar to, but distinct from, the swine viruses found in Western Australian and Queensland swine.

2. Materials and Methods

Active surveillance for respiratory illness among the workers at the affected piggery was commenced when the outbreak was notified to the CDCD. Those who developed any respiratory illness were assessed by a medical practitioner, and mid-turbinate nasal and throat swabs were collected using flocked swabs (FLOQSwabs, Copan Diagnostic Inc, Murietta, CA, USA). Swab samples were placed in virus transport medium and transported to PathWest Laboratory Medicine WA (PathWest, Perth, Australia) at 4 °C. Serum samples from symptomatic individuals were collected by standard venipuncture, then stored and transported at 4 °C, with a convalescent sample collected 10–14 days later. Blood samples for the serosurvey were collected in the same manner.

PCR tests at PathWest used an in-house duplex assay which included specific real-time RT-PCRs, respectively, directed at the influenza A matrix gene, the seasonal A(H3N2) HA gene, the seasonal A(H1N1)pdm09 HA gene and the influenza B matrix gene [11]. PCR testing for other respiratory viruses in the human contacts was carried as previously described [12] and swabs were also inoculated onto an MDCK cell monolayer for virus isolation. Rhinovirus speciation was based on 5'NTR sequence [12] and the characterization of matrix, HA and NA genes of influenza A viruses was carried out by conventional Sanger sequencing.

Testing for antibodies to influenza A and B was performed by complement fixation titer (CFT) at PathWest, while haemagglutination inhibition (HI) antibody test for the human sera and the antigenic characterization of the swine IAV isolates was carried out at the World Health Organization Collaborating Centre for Reference and Research on Influenza (WHOCC), Melbourne, Victoria. Comparison of titers used a Kruskal–Wallis test performed on the $\log_2$ converted values.

3. Results

The outbreak of serious illness among swine began in mid-July 2012, and then gradually subsided over the course of a few weeks (Figure 1) [8].

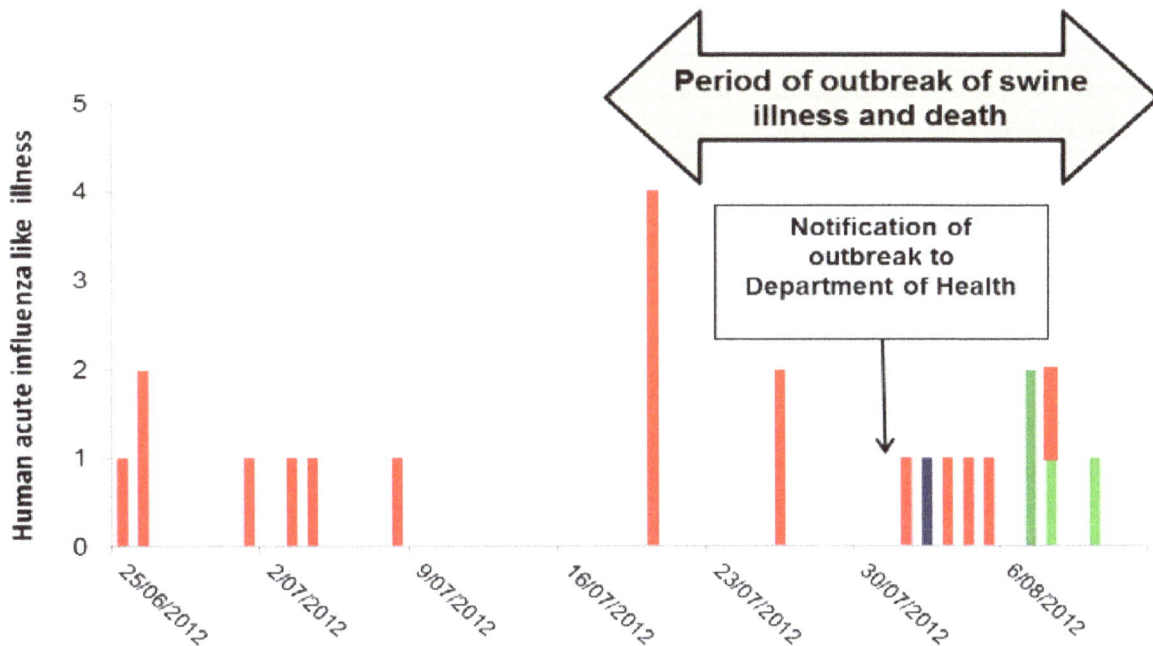

Figure 1. Date of onset of influenza-like illness and respiratory virus detections in 23 workers at a piggery in WA preceding and during an outbreak of respiratory tract illness and deaths in swine. The red columns are those with respiratory illness without laboratory confirmation either because they were not tested (17 workers) or because the results were negative or inconclusive. The blue column is confirmed seasonal A(H3N2) and the green are confirmed RV infections. Initial serologic testing at the DAFWA had suggested influenza infection and on 4 August 2012, a site visit was made by officers from the CDCD and the DAFWA.

No symptomatic humans were present during the initial site visit. However, 20 upper respiratory tract swabs were collected from symptomatic swine for testing by PCR and culture.

Initial PCR testing of the swine samples at PathWest were positive for influenza A matrix gene, but negative for the HA genes of the contemporaneously circulating A(H1N1)pdm09 and A(H3N2) viruses, indicating a possible novel HA type. This was later confirmed by the WHOCC in Melbourne and the Australian Animal Health Laboratories in Geelong, Victoria [9].

Following the initial testing, which indicated that these were likely to be nonseasonal IAV, suggesting a possible swine virus or an exotic human virus, the piggery was placed in quarantine [8] and surveillance for respiratory illness in staff at the piggery was commenced. A protocol was put in place to ensure that staff developing a respiratory illness were assessed and tested urgently by PCR, treatment with oral oseltamivir at 75mg twice daily was immediately provided, and the person was isolated at home until cleared of infection. Acute and convalescent serum samples were collected from these symptomatic workers and arrangements were made for collection of convalescent samples 10–14 days later. The use of personal protective equipment (PPE) by the staff in contact with swine was also emphasized, to reduce respiratory virus transmission.

Phylogenetic analysis of the swine IAVs characterized them as novel reassortant viruses containing only gene segments of human origin: two H1N2 reassortant viruses (H1N2/A/sw/WA/2577899R/2012 and H1N2/A/sw/WA/2577896X/2012) and one H3N2 reassortant virus (H3N2/A/Swine/WA/2577766G/2012) [9]. One of the A(H1N2) viruses (2577899R) and the A(H3N2) virus contained only segments that had not been detected in human populations for up to decades. These were chosen for the comparative serology. The other A(H1N2) virus (2577896X) had the same HA and NA genes as H1N2/2577899R, but the internal genes of the recent A(H1N1)pdm09 virus. The absence of any known matching viruses recently circulating in human populations internationally, and the ongoing circulation and evolution of these viruses within swine populations confirmed them as enzootic swine influenza viruses.

On 10 August, a week after the notification of the outbreak and following confirmation of the virus identification, seasonal influenza vaccination was carried out for the piggery workers, using the 2012 southern hemisphere trivalent influenza vaccine, and prophylaxis with oral oseltamivir 75 mg bd was provided for two weeks while vaccine responses were developing. This was done to reduce the risk of workers being infected with the variant virus, to reduce possible confounding seasonal influenza infections in the workers, to reduce the risk of further introduction of circulating human influenza viruses into the swine population, and to minimize the risk of mixed infections and reassortment between human and pig viruses [13].

Further testing of samples from 131 swine of various ages was carried out at PathWest in order to define the extent of the risk to human contacts. Of these, 43 (32.8%) had IAV detected based on a positive PCR for the matrix gene. Sanger sequencing of the products of the HA and NA genes indicated that six swine had a novel H1N2 virus, three (6.9%) had a novel H3N2 virus, one (2.3%) had A(H1N1)pdm09 infection, and two (4.6%) had likely seasonal A(H3N2) virus. The remainder could not be characterized by this sequencing. These results were consistent with whole genome sequencing result of the reassortant A(H1N2) and A(H3N2) swine viruses [9]. Sanger sequencing of the matrix gene of the six novel H1N2 viruses all matched with seasonal A(H1N1)pdm09 virus sequences, indicating that they were highly likely to be the H1N2/A/sw/WA/2577896X/2012 reassortant.

On 24 August 2012, three weeks after the notification of the outbreak to CDCD and two weeks after the vaccination program, 69 of 70 workers at the piggery completed a survey enquiring about symptoms of influenza-like illness during the period beginning one month prior to the outbreak in swine. Overall 27/69 (39%) of workers reported a mild respiratory illness in the month before or during the swine outbreak, and 23 of these 27 ill workers could recall their onset date. Seven had onset prior to the outbreak, seven during the swine outbreak but prior to notification, and nine after notification of the outbreak (Figure 1). Of those nine cases, eight were swabbed. One yielded a seasonal A(H3N2) virus, and three had a rhinovirus (RV), comprising two RV-C and one RV-A. The remaining four were negative for respiratory viruses.

Paired acute and convalescent serum samples were available for five cases (Table 1), including the individual with PCR-confirmed H3N2 infection who demonstrated an increase in HI antibodies to seasonal A(H3N2) from <1:10 to 1:320 between acute and convalescent sera, compared with an increase from 1:20 to 1:80 to the swine A(H3N2). Two others showed ≥ 4-fold rises in HI titers to A(H1N1)pdm09, one of whom also had a 4-fold rise in antibody titer to seasonal A(H3N2). However, both had been vaccinated between the acute and convalescent sample and this may have accounted for these results. The remaining workers did not show any significant HI changes.

Table 1. Acute and convalescent serum HI titers to swine and vaccine influenza A viruses for five workers with respiratory illness who provided acute and convalescent samples. Significant titer changes are in bolded text.

	Vaccine Given	Respiratory Illness between Samples	Sample	Swine Viruses		Vaccine Viruses	
				H1N2 A/WA/896X/2012	H3N2 A/WA/766G/2012	H1N1pdm09 A/California/7/2009	H3N2 A/Perth/16/2009
1	Yes	No	Acute	<10	10	**<10**	**<10**
			Convalescent	<10	<10	**320**	**40**
2	Yes	Yes [1]	Acute	<10	**20**	10	**<10**
			Convalescent	10	**80**	40	**320**
3	No	No	Acute	40	<10	20	20
			Convalescent	40	<10	40	10
4	Yes	No	Acute	20	20	40	80
			Convalescent	20	20	40	160
5	Yes	No	Acute	**10**	80	**40**	80
			Convalescent	**40**	160	**320**	160

[1] PCR-proven seasonal A(H3N2) infection.

Serum samples were requested at the time of the survey and 57/69 workers, 48 of whom had received the seasonal influenza vaccine two weeks earlier, agreed to provide serum samples. HI titers to swine A(H1N2) and A(H3N2) and to the vaccine A(H1N1) and A(H3N2) were determined (Table S1).

All of the nine unvaccinated workers had HI titers ≤1:80 to the swine A(H1N2) and all of these were lower than or equivalent to the titers to the vaccine A(H1N1). Seven had HI titers <40 to the swine A(H3N2), one had an HI titer of 40 to the swine A(H3N2) but this was lower than the titer to the vaccine A(H3N2). However, the remaining worker had a significantly higher HI titer to the swine A(H3N2) virus (1:320) than to the seasonal A(H3N2) virus (1:80). In summary, we found one unvaccinated worker who had serological evidence of a possible infection with the swine A(H3N2) virus. For the others, we either found no significant titers to the swine viruses or we could not exclude cross-reacting antibody due to infection with seasonal viruses, as represented by the vaccine strains.

The other 48 workers who underwent testing had received the seasonal influenza vaccine as part of the outbreak response. Therefore, we anticipated that we would detect vaccine-induced antibodies that might mask responses to infection with the swine viruses. Therefore we examined the likely effect of vaccination on antibody levels to the swine viruses by comparing HI titers in 48 vaccinated workers with those in the nine unvaccinated workers. Forty-six of the samples from vaccinated workers had sufficient volume to complete the testing for all viruses, while two further workers had sufficient sample to test for antibodies to the swine A(H1N2) and the vaccine A(H1N1) viruses, but not for antibodies to the A(H3N2) viruses (Table 2).

Vaccination had no effect on the HI titers to the swine A(H1N2) virus or the vaccine A(H1N1) strain, so that the antibody titers (Table S1) can be interpreted independent of vaccination. For the combined vaccinated and unvaccinated workers, there were a total of 24 workers who had HI titers ≥40 to the swine A(H1N2) virus, but 23 of these workers had equivalent or higher titers to the vaccine A(H1N1) virus, so that cross-reacting antibody from seasonal influenza A infection or vaccination could not be excluded. However, the remaining worker had a 16-fold higher titer to the swine A(H1N2) virus, suggesting possible infection with that virus.

In contrast, vaccination resulted in significant and similar increases in antibody titers to both the swine and seasonal A(H3N2) viruses. The results for the unvaccinated workers (see above) identified one worker with a possible swine A(H3N2) infection. Among the vaccinated workers, 35/46 had HI titers ≥40 to the swine A(H3N2) virus, of which 17 had higher titers to the swine virus than to the vaccine virus. Eight of these were only two-fold higher and were discounted as this difference was not significant. However, there were nine samples where the HI titer was between four-fold and 32-fold higher to the swine virus, which cannot be attributed to vaccination or seasonal virus infection.

Table 2. A comparison of the mean HI values in vaccinated and unvaccinated workers using a Kruskal–Wallis test on the $\log_2$-transformed HI titer, where HI titers <10 were assigned a notional value of 1. The one worker with a confirmed acute seasonal A(H3N2) infection was excluded.

Virus	Median of the $\log_2$-Converted HI Titers		*p*-Value
	Unvaccinated	Vaccinated [a]	
WA Swine H1N2 [1]	0.00	3.32	0.76
Human vaccine A/H1N1 09pdm [2]	6.32	6.32	0.87
WA Swine H3N2 [3]	3.32	6.32	0.0004
Human vaccine A/H3N2 [4]	5.32	6.32	0.025

[1] A/Swine/WA/2577896X/2012 H1N2, [2] A/California/7/2009 H1N1pdm09, [3] A/Swine/WA/2577766G/2012 H3N2, [4] A/Perth/16/2009 H3N2. [a] Only 46 workers were able to be tested for antibodies to the A(H3N2) viruses due to insufficient sample volume remaining for the final two workers.

These data suggest that, at least in some of the workers, there is evidence that they may have had an infection with one of the swine influenza viruses as their antibody titers could not be explained by cross-reacting antibody from their recent vaccination or seasonal influenza virus infection. However, we cannot exclude higher antibody titers due to past infection with human origin viruses that were serologically closely-related to the swine viruses, as we do not have a demographically matched control group that were not exposed to the swine influenza viruses.

4. Discussion

Influenza A viruses circulate and evolve continually within swine populations and represent a reservoir of potential human pandemic influenza strains. These viruses occasionally cross into human populations following contact with swine, including exhibition swine at agricultural events [6,14,15]. Until 2012 it was thought that Australia was free of this risk, as enzootic influenza had not been detected in local swine populations previously. Characterization of the outbreak described here clearly demonstrated that human influenza viruses have been regularly entering Australian swine populations from humans, probably for decades, and that circulation and reassortment has persisted within swine [9]. Infection of humans with variant influenza viruses arising from piggeries has not yet been documented, but there is a continuing possibility that swine viruses with pandemic potential may spread to humans in contact with swine within Australia. That appears to have happened with the recent first variant influenza virus infection of a human in Australia, associated with exposure to exhibition swine [10].

The Western Australian piggery outbreak was the first to identify enzootic influenza virus infection in swine in Australia [9], and we have described the approach taken to determine whether swine-to-human transmission had occurred and to mitigate the risk of further transmission between swine and humans. That included reinforcing personal hygiene measures and providing seasonal influenza vaccination for previously unvaccinated workers [16]. Active surveillance for respiratory illness in the workers was instituted as soon as the outbreak was notified, but none of the subsequent respiratory illnesses occurring could be attributed to the swine influenza viruses by PCR testing or by serology.

The limitations of using virus detection for assessing infection of human contacts are known, especially where long term exposure is likely and the illness is mild, so that the likelihood of identifying and sampling acute infections is low [17]. Serosurveys have the advantage of detecting past as well as current infections, but are problematic for influenza diagnosis due to the multiple exposures and vaccinations that occur during life and the cross-reactivity of influenza antibodies across different strains of the virus. Adults have diverse immune backgrounds to influenza and therefore have complex serological responses to infections with new influenza viruses. In our study, the interpretation of the results was further complicated by the vaccination program that had been undertaken two weeks prior to the serosurvey. This may have masked antibody responses to the swine viruses, which are difficult to separate from possible cross-reactions from the vaccine response and/or past natural exposure to human viruses.

However, we did not find any evidence that vaccination with the seasonal influenza vaccine influenced the antibody titer to the swine A(H1N2) virus. So the high titer HI antibody to this virus with a low titer to the seasonal A(H1N1)pdm09 virus that we found in one worker could not be explained by vaccination, and indicated possible infection with the swine virus. With the swine A(H3N2) viruses, we did find that vaccination increased titers to both the swine A(H3N2) and the vaccine A(H3N2) viruses, but several workers had HI titers to the swine A(H3N2) virus that were at least fourfold higher than the responses to the vaccine A(H3N2) virus. That result is not consistent with a vaccine response, and again suggests possible infection with a swine A(H3N2) virus. However, the HI titers to the swine A(H1N2) and A(H3N2) viruses could possibly have been due to past natural infection with antigenically similar viruses that circulated within human populations.

The challenges associated with using serosurveys to assess zoonotic influenza infections have been recently reviewed [17]. The authors recommended that, in order to identify antibodies specific to the animal viruses, the protocol should include testing for antibodies to both human and variant viruses for cross-reactivity; the use of two different serological assays, one of which should be a neutralization assay, to improve specificity; and having matched control samples from persons not in contact with the animals. Many of the piggery workers were from overseas, which meant that they had potentially been exposed to a different spectrum of influenza A viruses that may have resulted in antibodies that cross-reacted with the swine influenza viruses. Unfortunately, we could not access satisfactory control sera to exclude that possibility. In view of that limitation, we elected not to proceed with neutralization assays as it was unlikely to provide definitive results.

The ongoing circulation of influenza viruses within swine populations in Australia, with evidence of transmission between humans and swine overseas, and the likely recent human infection acquired within Australia has made us aware of potential for the generation of zoonotic infections. This also raises the possibility, albeit low, of human pandemic strains arising within Australia following zoonotic infection with a swine IAV. While commercial piggeries have not yet been shown to be a source of zoonotic infection with swine IAV, precautions are recommended to mitigate this risk [16]. Further studies are needed to identify the extent and diversity of influenza viruses in swine and other animals in regular contact with humans, and to conduct studies to determine the frequency of transmission to those human contacts.

The animal health sector has recently provided updated recommendations for maintaining biosecurity at piggeries, and for the management of outbreaks [18,19]. In addition it is important to restrict casual contact with swine at agricultural events, to carry out seasonal vaccination programs for piggery workers and others with regular swine contact, to maintain surveillance of people working at the human–animal interface and to have early structured investigation of outbreaks of respiratory illness in the animals or their human contacts [13,16].

Author Contributions: Conceptualization, D.W.S., P.V.E., and R.L.; Methodology, P.V.E., D.W.S., R.L., A.L., and M.O.; Formal Analysis, D.W.S., P.V.E., S.T., and I.J.B.; Investigation, P.V.E., R.L., S.T., and M.O.; Writing—Original Draft Preparation, D.W.S., P.V.E., and I.G.B.; Writing—Review & Editing, D.W.S., P.V.E., I.G.B., A.L., S.T., M.O., J.W. and F.Y.K.W.

Acknowledgments: The authors would like to acknowledge the assistance and cooperation of staff at the Communicable Disease Control Directorate of the Health Department Western Australia, the Surveillance Unit at the Department of Microbiology, PathWest Laboratory Medicine WA at the QEII Medical Centre, the Department of Agriculture and Food Western Australia, and the World Health Organization Collaborating Centre for Reference and Research on Influenza, Melbourne.

References

1.   Myers, K.P.; Olsen, C.W.; Gray, G. Cases of swine influenza in humans: A review of the literature. *Clin. Infect. Dis.* **2007**, *44*, 1084–1088. [CrossRef] [PubMed]

2.   Kitikoon, P.; Vincent, A.L.; Gauger, P.C.; Schlink, S.N.; Bayles, D.O.; Gramer, M.R.; Darnell, D.; Webby, R.; Lager, K.M.; Swenson, S.L.; et al. Pathogenicity and transmission in pigs of the novel A(H3N2)v influenza virus isolated from humans and characterization of swine H3N2 viruses isolated in 2010–2011. *J. Virol.* **2012**, *86*, 6804–6814. [CrossRef] [PubMed]

3.   Baudon, E.; Peyre, M.; Peiris, M.; Cowling, B.J. Epidemiological features of influenza circulation in swine populations: A systematic review and meta-analysis. *PLoS ONE* **2017**, *12*, e0179044. [CrossRef] [PubMed]

4.   Smith, G.J.; Vijaykrishna, D.; Bahl, J.; Lycett, S.J.; Worobey, M.; Pybus, O.G.; Ma, S.K.; Cheung, C.L.; Raghwani, J.; Bhatt, S.; et al. Origins and evolutionary genomics of the 2009 swine-origin H1N1 influenza A epidemic. *Nature* **2009**, *459*, 1122–1125. [CrossRef] [PubMed]

5.   Vijaykrishna, D.; Smith, G.J.; Pybus, O.G.; Zhu, H.; Bhatt, S.; Poon, L.L.; Riley, S.; Bahl, J.; Ma, S.K.; Cheung, C.L.; et al. Long term evolution and transmission dynamics of swine influenza A virus. *Nature* **2011**, *473*, 519–522. [CrossRef] [PubMed]

6.   Biggerstaff, M.; Reed, C.; Epperson, S.; Jhung, M.A.; Gambhir, M.; Bresee, J.S.; Jernigan, D.B.; Swerdlow, D.L.; Finelli, L. Estimates of the number of human infections with influenza A(H3N2) variant virus, United States, August 2011–April 2012. *Clin. Infect. Dis.* **2013**, *57* (Suppl. 1), S12–S15. [CrossRef] [PubMed]

7.   Deng, Y.M.; Iannello, P.; Smith, I.; Watson, J.; Barr, I.G.; Daniels, P.; Komadina, N.; Harrower, B.; Wong, F.Y. Transmission of influenza A(H1N1) 2009 pandemic viruses in Australian swine. *Influenza Respir. Viruses* **2012**, *6*, e42-7. [CrossRef] [PubMed]

8.   Webb, K. State and Territory Reports: Western Australia. *Anim. Health Surveill. Q. Rep.* **2012**, *17*, 19–20.

9.   Wong, F.Y.K.; Donato, C.; Deng, Y.M.; Teng, D.; Komadina, N.; Baas, C.; Modak, J.; O'Dea, M.; Smith, D.W.; Effler, P.V.; et al. Divergent human-origin influenza viruses detected in Australian swine populations. *J. Virol.* **2018**, *92*, e00316-18. [CrossRef] [PubMed]

10. World Health Organization. Influenza at the human-animal interface: Summary and assessment, 22 January to 12 February 2019. 2019. Available online: www.who.int/influenza/human_animal_interface/Influenza_Summary_IRA_HA_interface_12_02_2019.pdf (accessed on 2 April 2019).

11. Chidlow, G.; Harnett, G.; Williams, S.; Levy, A.; Speers, D.; Smith, D.W. Duplex real-time RT-PCR assays for the rapid detection and identification of pandemic (H1N1) 2009 and seasonal influenza viruses A/H1, A/H3 and B. *J. Clin. Microbiol.* **2010**, *48*, 862–866. [CrossRef] [PubMed]

12. Chidlow, G.R.; Laing, I.A.; Harnett, G.B.; Greenhill, A.; Phuanukoonnon, S.; Siba, P.M.; Pomat, W.S.; Shellam, G.R.; Smith, D.W.; Lehmann, D. Respiratory viral pathogens associated with lower respiratory tract disease among young children in the highlands of Papua New Guinea. *J. Clin. Virol.* **2012**, *54*, 235–239. [CrossRef] [PubMed]

13. Centers for Disease Control. Interim Guidance for Workers Who Are Employed at Commercial Swine Farms: Preventing the Spread of Influenza a Viruses. Available online: https://www.cdc.gov/flu/swineflu/guidance-commercial-pigs.htm (accessed on 23 April 2019).

14. Baranovich, T.; Bahl, J. Influenza A virus diversity and transmission in exhibition swine. *J. Infect. Dis.* **2016**, *213*, 169–170. [CrossRef] [PubMed]

15. Wu, J.; Yi, L.; Ni, H.; Zou, L.; Zhang, H.; Zeng, X.; Liang, L.; Li, L.; Zhong, H.; Zhang, X.; et al. Anti-human H1N1pdm09 and swine H1N1 virus antibodies among swine workers in Guangdong Province, China. *Sci. Rep.* **2015**, *5*, 12507. [CrossRef] [PubMed]

16. Centers for Disease Control. Take Action to Prevent the Spread of flu Between Pigs and People. Available online: https://www.cdc.gov/flu/swineflu/prevention.htm (accessed on 3 April 2019).

17. Sikkema, R.; Freidl, G.; de Bruin, E.; Koopmans, M. Weighing serological evidence of human exposure to animal influenza viruses—a literature review. *Euro. Surveill.* **2016**, *21*, C30388. [CrossRef] [PubMed]

18. National Farm Biosecurity Manual for Pork Production. 2013. Available online: http://www.farmbiosecurity. com.au/wp-content/uploads/2013/08/National-Farm-Biosecurity-Manual-for-Pork-Production.pdf (accessed on 24 April 2019).

19. Animal Health Australia. AUSVETPLAN Response Policy Brief: Influenza A Viruses in Swine. Version 4.0 2018. Available online: //hdwa.health.wa.gov.au/users/home34/he08408/Downloads/FLU-SWINE-03-FINAL18May18-1.pdf (accessed on 24 April 2019).

17

A Single Dose of Modified Vaccinia Ankara Expressing Lassa Virus-like Particles Protects Mice from Lethal Intra-cerebral Virus Challenge

Maria S. Salvato [1,†], Arban Domi [2,†], Camila Guzmán-Cardozo [1], Sandra Medina-Moreno [1], Juan Carlos Zapata [1]●, Haoting Hsu [1], Nathanael McCurley [3], Rahul Basu [4], Mary Hauser [2], Michael Hellerstein [2] and Farshad Guirakhoo [2,*]●

[1]   Institute of Human Virology, University of Maryland, Baltimore, MD 21201, USA
[2]   GeoVax, Inc., Smyrna, GA 30080, USA
[3]   Office of Technology Licensing and Commercialization, Georgia State University, Atlanta, GA 30303, USA
[4]   Department of Biology, Georgia State University, Atlanta, GA 30302, USA
*   Correspondence: fguirakhoo@geovax.com
†   Contributed equally to this work.

Abstract: Lassa fever surpasses Ebola, Marburg, and all other hemorrhagic fevers except Dengue in its public health impact. Caused by Lassa virus (LASV), the disease is a scourge on populations in endemic areas of West Africa, where reported incidence is higher. Here, we report construction, characterization, and preclinical efficacy of a novel recombinant vaccine candidate GEO-LM01. Constructed in the Modified Vaccinia Ankara (MVA) vector, GEO-LM01 expresses the glycoprotein precursor (GPC) and zinc-binding matrix protein (Z) from the prototype Josiah strain lineage IV. When expressed together, GP and Z form Virus-Like Particles (VLPs) in cell culture. Immunogenicity and efficacy of GEO-LM01 was tested in a mouse challenge model. A single intramuscular dose of GEO-LM01 protected 100% of CBA/J mice challenged with a lethal dose of ML29, a Mopeia/Lassa reassortant virus, delivered directly into the brain. In contrast, all control animals died within one week. The vaccine induced low levels of antibodies but Lassa-specific CD4$^+$ and CD8$^+$ T cell responses. This is the first report showing that a single dose of a replication-deficient MVA vector can confer full protection against a lethal challenge with ML29 virus.

Keywords: Lassa vaccine; replication-deficient MVA vector; VLP formation; single-dose efficacy; cell-mediated immunity

1. Introduction

Lassa fever (LF), a zoonotic disease caused by Lassa virus (LASV), can lead to acute hemorrhagic fever with a case fatality rate (CFR) of up to 50% [1]. The estimated annual incidence of LF across West African countries including Ghana, Guinea, Mali, Benin, Liberia, Sierra Leone, Togo, and Nigeria has been reported as high as 300,000 infections and 5000–10,000 deaths, but these figures are most likely underestimates due to inadequate diagnosis and surveillance [2–5]. Based on prospective studies performed in Guinea, Sierra Leone, Liberia, and Nigeria, it was estimated that 59 million people are at risk of LASV infections, with as many as 67,000 deaths per year [6]. The 2018 outbreak in Nigeria resulted in 3498 suspected cases in 22 states and 171 deaths with a CFR of 27% based on confirmed cases [7]. The fact that a virus that was first discovered in 1969 in Lassa village in Nigeria is still capable of causing outbreaks in the same geographical regions indicates challenges in eradicating its animal reservoir.

The main animal reservoir of LASV is the multimammate rat (*Mastomys natalensis*), which is common in West Africa, but the potential transmission of LASV to new rodent hosts could have serious implications for its spread beyond West Africa [8]. LASV is mainly transmitted to humans by consumption of contaminated food, by contact with rodent urine and droppings, or by inhalation of virus particles from the excreta of infected animals; it can also be transmitted from human to human through nosocomial infections [9]. Most LASV infections are asymptomatic or cause only mild symptoms, but some infections lead to multi-organ failure, fever, and, on occasion, hemorrhage and death [10,11].

LASV is a member of the family *Arenaviridae* and genus *Mammarenavirus,* which includes Old World and New World arenaviruses [12,13]. Furthermore, LASV strains are classified into four lineages, I–IV (with a newly proposed fifth lineage from Cote d'Ivoire and Mali) based on their genetic variations [12,13]. The LASV genome is composed of two ambisense RNA segments. The large (L) segment of 7.2 kb in length encodes the viral RNA-dependent RNA polymerase protein and the zinc finger (Z) protein, a multifunctional matrix protein [14,15]. The small (S) segment of 3.4 kb in length encodes the nucleoprotein (NP) and glycoprotein precursor (GPC). GPC is cleaved post-translationally to form a trimer of hetero-trimers, each consisting of a receptor binding protein (GP1), a fusion protein (GP2) and a stable signal peptide (SSP) [16,17]. GPC sequences, shown previously to be required for full protection, have been used as the protective antigen in the construction of a large number of vaccine candidates delivered by various platforms. Some of these candidates have undergone preclinical evaluations in mice, guinea pigs, and non-human primates (NHP) [12], and a DNA vaccine has entered clinical trials [18].

Here, we describe the construction, characterization and efficacy of a Lassa vaccine candidate that generates virus-like particles (VLPs) by expression of Lassa GPC and Z proteins from our Modified Vaccinia Ankara (MVA) vector. It has been previously demonstrated that co-expression of Z and GP proteins leads to the formation of VLPs [19]. A murine model was chosen initially to establish dose and route of vaccination and whether our constructs could elicit any protective immunity. In this model, ML29, an attenuated Mopeia -Lassa (MOP/LAS) reassortant, is delivered into the brain and primarily infects brain capillary endothelial and glial cells that present LASV antigens, triggering an influx of lymphocytes 5–6 days later. The infiltrating cells contribute to encephalitis that is lethal unless the mice had been previously vaccinated against LASV (Djavani and Salvato, unpublished). The intra-cerebral (IC) delivery we used was not "natural", since it models brain infections that are rare in LF, but it allows a rapid and simple read-out for whether or not we elicited a protective immunity. Here, we show that a single dose of the vaccine conferred full protection against a lethal challenge dose of the ML29 virus delivered IC.

2. Results

2.1. Vaccine Characterization

The recombinant GEO-LM01 was constructed by inserting sequences from the well-characterized LASV prototype strain Josiah from lineage IV into MVA. The Josiah strain is extensively used for vaccine development, since it has shown protection against homologous and heterologous challenges [20]. The GPC protein of Josiah, the major protective antigen, has 93.1%, 93.5, and 94.5% homologies with lineage I, II, and III, respectively [12]. GEO-LM01 is designed to co-express GPC and the LASV matrix protein Z (Figure 1a,b). Expression of GPC and Z lead to the formation of VLPs in the cells of the inoculated host as well as promoting their release from GEO-LM01-infected cells. GEO-LM01 is replication-competent in avian cells (producing both infectious progeny and expressed antigens) but is replication-deficient in mammalian cells (producing antigens in the form of VLPs but not infectious progeny) (Figure 1c) due to six deletions in the MVA genome which together resulted in high attenuation and mammalian cell host restriction [21]. The assembly of VLPs from proteins expressed by GEO-LM01 was verified by electron microscopy, demonstrating active release of VLPs from DF1 cells, a chicken fibroblast cell line (Figure 2a). The entire population of GEO-LM01 virions retains both GPC and Z transgenes as demonstrated by immunostaining (Figure 2b). Similar plaque numbers at each dilution in the GPC and Z wells showed that both transgenes are equally retained. Expression of both transgenes and cleavage of GPC into GP1 and GP2 subunits was further demonstrated in western blots (WB) using cell lysates and supernatants (released VLPs) of GEO-LM01 infected DF1 cells (Figure 2c,d).

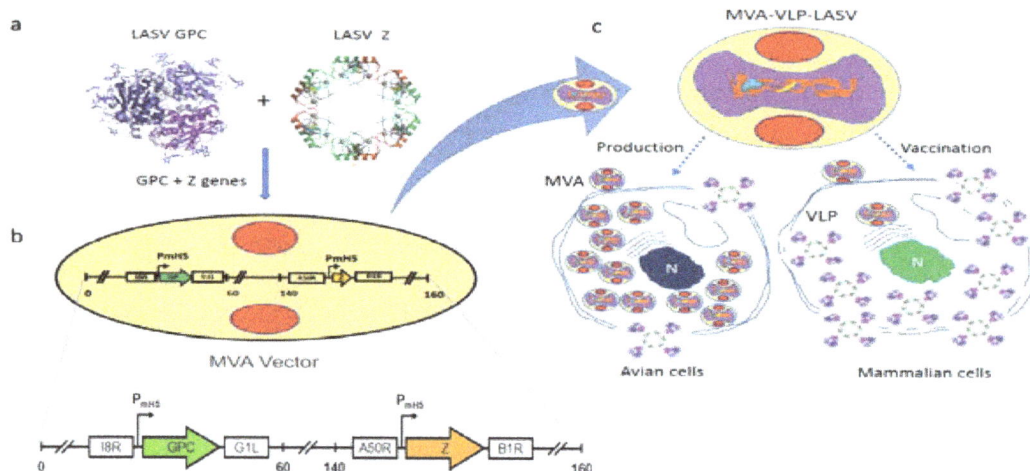

Figure 1. Construction of GEO-LM01 vaccine candidate. A Cartoon showing the vector design. (**a,b**) The Lassa virus (LASV) sequence for glycoprotein precursor (GPC) was inserted between the I8R and G1L genes and the Z sequence was inserted between the A50R and B1R genes. P$_{mH5}$, modified H5 promoter. Numbers are coordinates in the Modified Vaccinia Ankara (MVA) genome. (**c**) Similar to all MVA-derived vaccine viruses, GEO-LM01 is replication-competent in avian cells, used for propagation of the vaccine but replication-deficient in mammalian cells that are used for vaccination purposes. Image of the LASV GPC protein structure is courtesy of Dr. Erica O. Saphire, The Scripps Research Institute. The image of LASV Z structure is from RCSB PDB ID 5I72 [22].

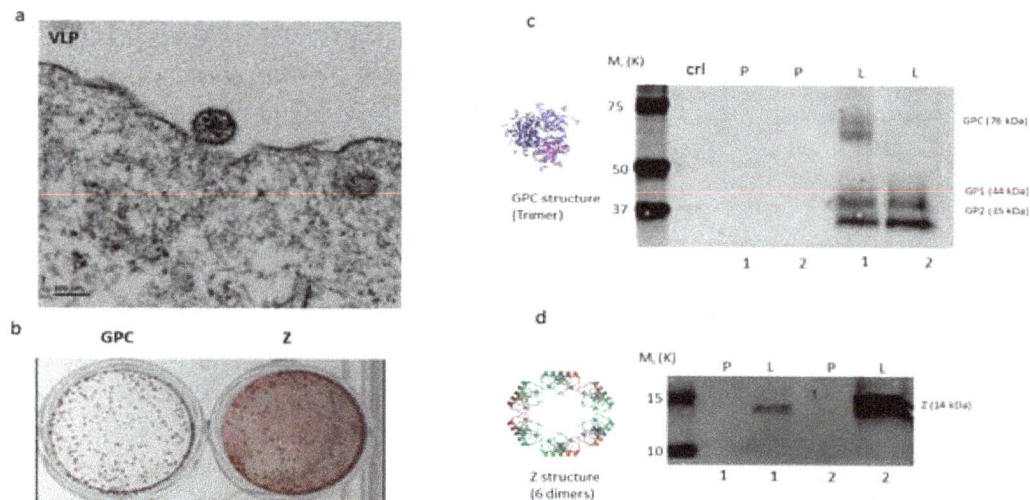

Figure 2.   Electron microscopy, Immunocytochemistry and Western blot of GEO-LM01 vaccine candidate. (**a**) Electron micrograph of virus-like particles (VLP) formed in cells infected with GEO-LM01. (**b**) Immunocytochemistry on infected duplicates of cell monolayers stained with GPC- (left) or Z- (right) specific antibodies. Western blots verified expression of LASV GP (**c**) and Z (**d**) proteins in cultured cells. DF1 cell lysates contained both the unprocessed GPC and the processed subunits GP1 and GP2, whereas the DF1 supernatants contained only the processed GP1 and GP2 subunits. P, Parental (empty) MVA; L, GEO-LM01; 1, cell lysate; 2, supernatant. A loading control lane (**crl lane c**) served as another negative control. The two GP bands correspond to LASV GP1 and GP2 with the molecular weights of 44kD and 35kD, respectively.

2.2. Vaccine Efficacy Testing in a ML29 Mouse Challenge Model

Immunogenicity and efficacy testing of GEO-LM01 was performed in a mouse model that uses ML29 virus for lethal challenge (Figure 3). In this model, young immune-competent CBA/J mice are vaccinated once and challenged 2 weeks later. Animals are monitored for weight loss, morbidity, and mortality. Blood and spleens from three mice were collected on day 11 prior to challenge for determination of vaccine-elicited antibody and T cell responses, respectively.

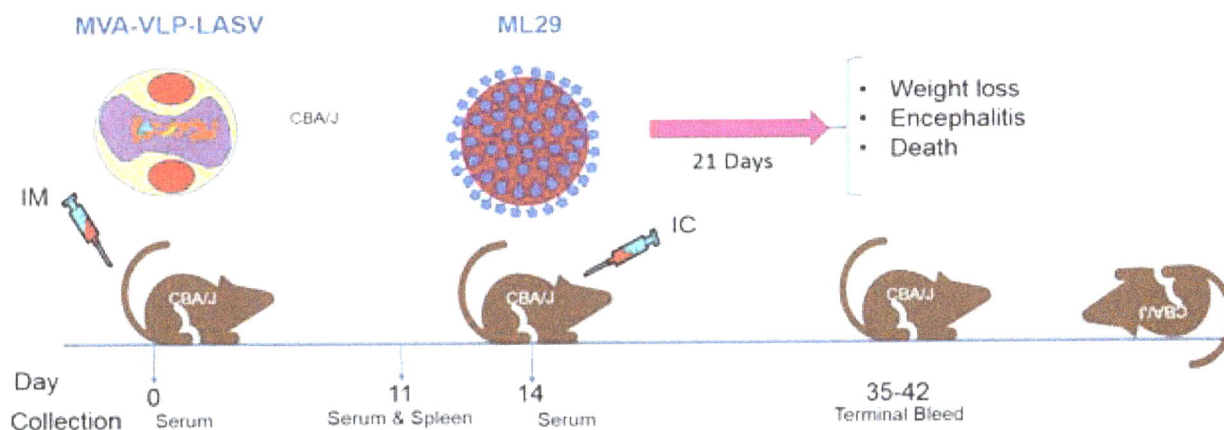

Figure 3. ML29 challenge model; schedule of vaccination, sample collections and intracerebral (IC) challenge. CBA/J mice are vaccinated with a single dose of GEO-LM01 (MVA-VLP-LASV) (1×10^7 $TCID_{50}$ in 100 μL volume) by the intramuscular (IM) route. Three mice are sacrificed on day 11, sera and spleens were collected for assessment of antibody and T cell responses. The remaining mice are challenged on day 14 by the IC route with 1000 plaque forming units (PFU) of ML29 virus. After challenge, mice are observed for weight loss, signs of encephalitis and death.

ML29 is a reassortant virus encoding the GPC and NP proteins of LASV (Josiah strain) and the L and Z proteins of MOPV virus [23]. The virus is uniformly lethal when administered by IC inoculation into immunocompetent CBA/J mice; however, when administered by intraperitoneal (IP) inoculation, ML29 elicits a strong immune response that protects CBA/J mice from death upon subsequent IC challenge [24]. To determine the best route of immunization, 4–6 week-old CBA/J mice were immunized with 10^7 $TCID_{50}$ of GEO-LM01 by IP, IM, or SC inoculation. Additionally, two groups of mice (n = 6) were injected IP with ML29 virus (1000 PFU) or saline, and served as positive and negative controls, respectively. On day 14, all mice were challenged by IC inoculation with ML29 virus and monitored for weight change, morbidity, and mortality. Mice immunized with ML29 virus (IP) (positive control) or with GEO-LM01 (IM) were 100% protected from lethal challenge and gained weight throughout the study (Figure 4a), whereas mice administered saline alone all died on day 7 or 8 after lethal challenge (Figure 4b). Some mice in the vaccinated groups exhibited minor weight loss after challenge, but they all regained weight and remained healthy (no ataxia or ruffled fur) until the end of the study. Mice immunized with GEO-LM01 by SC and IP administration showed less robust immunity to lethal challenge, as seen in the more appreciable weight loss in these groups as well as the death of one animal in each group (one animal in the SC group died early on day 2 post challenge, most likely due to problems with inoculation rather than virus growth; it was excluded from survival analysis). A second experiment to measure immunogenicity and efficacy was initiated in the same model system, in this instance examining only two conditions: Immunization with GEO-LM01 by IM inoculation (n = 10) and mock immunization with saline (n = 8) (Figure 4c). Spleens were harvested from immunized animals (n = 3) and saline-inoculated animals (n = 3) on day 11 after a single administration of the vaccine.

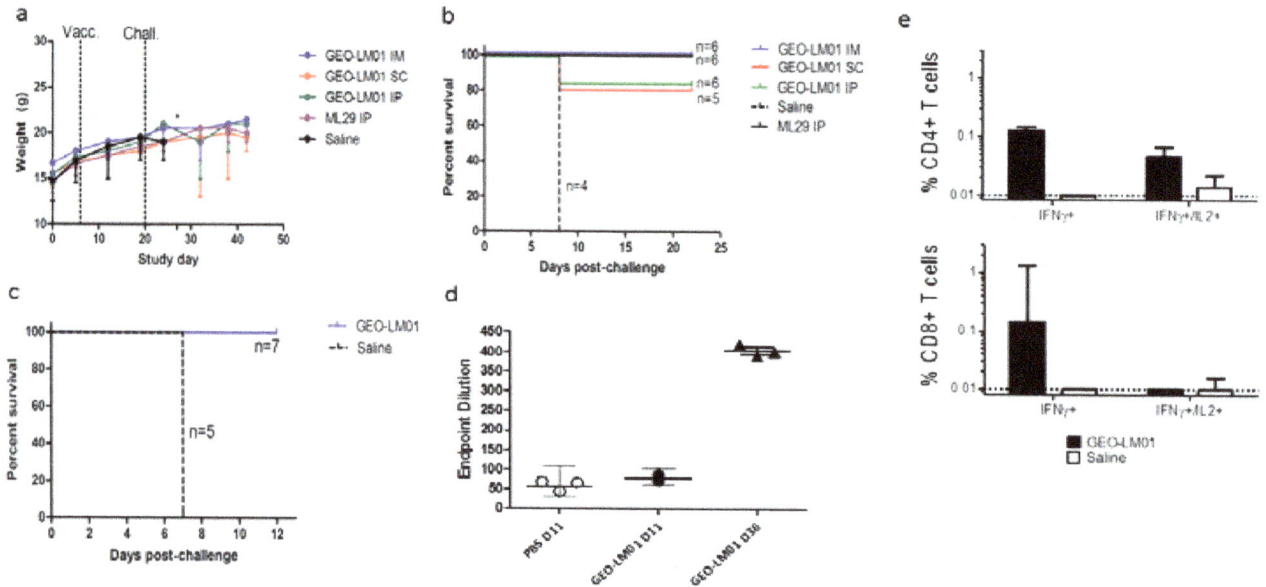

Figure 4. Efficacy and immunogenicity of GEO-LM01. Weight loss (**a**) and survival curves (**b**) following immunization by various routes then challenged with IC with ML29 virus 14 days later. * demonstrates death of control animals. (**c**) Survival curves of animals vaccinated by IM route only. (**d**) ML29-specific Ab titers from immunized on days 11 and 36 (22 days after challenge) and mock-immunized mice on day 11 as determined by ELISA. (**e**) Percentage of antigen-specific CD4+ and CD8+ T cells expressing IFNγ and IL2 in response to LASV GP peptides from GEO-LM01 or saline immunized animals were assessed by flow cytometry. These data demonstrate considerable differences between immunization groups but are not statistically significant.

Antigen-specific T cell responses were measured by Intracellular Cytokine Staining (ICS) for IFNγ and IL2 production by stimulating with peptides derived from immuno-dominant epitopes (IDE) present in GP1 and GP2 subunits [24–26]. IFNγ expression was evident in both CD4+ and CD8+ T cells of immunized but not mock immunized mice (Figure 4e). Some CD4+ T cells were also shown to be double positive for IFNγ and IL2, suggesting an expanding population. The remaining seven vaccinated and five control animals were challenged on day 14 as in the first experiment. All vaccinated animals survived the challenge, whereas all controls died by day 7 (Figure 4c) confirming the 100% single-dose efficacy of GEO-LM01 observed in the previous study. Four of the surviving GEO-LM01-vaccinated mice were housed for an additional year to see if they would be able to survive a second challenge long after the initial challenge. All four survived their second IC challenge (Table 1). A true test of durable immunity would not use mice surviving lethal challenge because the ML29 challenge itself may boost vaccine immunity; a better test would be to vaccinate mice and leave them unchallenged for a year to see whether or not the single vaccination could confer durable year-long protection.

Table 1. Surviving mice from Experiment 2 were re-challenged [1] one year later.

Experimental Mice	Number of Mice	Survivors after 2nd Challenge
Survivors of 1st challenge	4	4
Control mice (naïve adult CBA/J)	4	0

[1] All mice were challenged with a lethal dose of ML29 to see if the original vaccinated survivors could survive a second lethal challenge a year later. The naïve mice served as negative controls.

We additionally assayed for the presence of binding antibody (bAb) to GPC in the serum of the immunized mice. Despite the excellent protection from death afforded by GEO-LM01, we found no statistically significant level of bAb above background, we found low bAb at the early sampling days

11–14 post vaccination (Figure 4d). Similar results were observed previously with an ML29 vaccine that conferred protection from lethal challenge but yielded a minimal amount of bAb and neutralizing antibody (nAb) [24]. Substantial bAb were found in mice 36d after vaccination (Figure 4d) but these had been ML29 challenged, which could serve to boost the response to LASV antigens. We did not look for neutralizing antibodies.

3. Discussion

LF has a greater human impact than any other hemorrhagic fever, with the exception of Dengue fever [6]. Despite the severe impact of LF on populations in West Africa, no effective and practical medical countermeasure is available [18]. The one available treatment is the antiviral drug ribavirin, which is effective only if given within six days after infection [18]. A vaccine against LASV would be an ideal solution to the problem of LF, especially given the growing threat of outbreaks due to globalization and increased travel [27]. Several groups have developed vaccine candidates that have shown activity against LASV in animal models [20,23], but only one has progressed to the clinic [18]. Although a multi-dose immunization regiment is logistically feasible for medical providers and military personnel, a single dose vaccine is critical for epidemic response and is preferable and much more practical in under-resourced endemic areas. LF has been listed in the WHO R&D Blueprint among the 10 diseases and pathogens to prioritize for research and development in public health emergency contexts [28]. These diseases are identified as those that pose a public health risk because of their epidemic potential and for which there are insufficient countermeasures. For this reason, CEPI (Coalition for Epidemic Preparedness Innovations), founded to address the threat of epidemic diseases, has set aside a major portion of its $1 billion budget for the development of vaccines against LF [29].

GEO-LM01 provides a unique combination of advantages required for visitors or residents of LASV endemic countries. The potential for GEO-LM01 to protect after a single dose is favorable for travelers and military personnel who require a rapid onset of immunity (ideally ~<2 weeks post vaccination) as well as for epidemic/endemic vaccinations (due to the urgency of epidemic response and the complexity of locating vaccinated subjects in rural villages to administer a second dose for routine vaccination campaigns).

The GEO-LM01 reported here is designed to produce secreted as well as cell-associated LASV proteins in VLP (GPC+Z) formations in vaccinated subjects. This vaccine thereby provides two sources of viral antigens that mimic a natural viral infection promoting predominantly a balanced T cell response, which is critical for protection against LASV infection [30,31].

In our murine model, antibody responses occur too late to protect from an acute viral infection. We assessed binding antibodies in ML29-coated ELISA plates that are able to detect both the GP and Z components of VLP. Unfortunately, half of the Z protein is comprised of a RING structure that is common to many ligases and transcription factors in the normal cell, so it cross-reacts with many other proteins. In a recent publication [30], we posit that the value of the Z in VLP vectors is mostly to boost immunity by forming a 3-D structure with GP since conformational antigens are more immunogenic than linear antigens (boosting both CD4 and B cell responses).

As a vaccine candidate, GEO-LM01 has a unique combination of advantages that could potentially meet the preferred Target Product Profiles (TPP) of a LASV vaccine set by the WHO for both non-emergency (Preventive Use) and emergency settings (Reactive/Outbreak use) [28]. These include the immunological advantages of a live but safe (replication-deficient) vector that produces conformationally relevant VLPs; inclusion of multiple genes of LASV (GPC and Z) for induction of potentially broad immunity; the ability to immunize sequentially or concurrently with other MVA-vectored vaccines without generating any vector immunity [32] (potentially even combining GEO-LM01 with other hemorrhagic fever vaccines in a multivalent formulation); the likelihood of single-dose protection, as demonstrated with MVA-VLP-EBOV and MVA-Zika vaccines candidates [32,33] with the durability of the immune response attributed to MVA-vectored vaccines; and a temperature stable, simple, adjuvant-free presentation.

Considering the high prevalence of HIV in some LASV endemic areas of Sub-Saharan Africa (up to 68% in some populations) [34], an LASV vaccine must be safe and effective in immunocompromised populations [35]. Safety for the parental MVA vector was shown in more than 120,000 subjects in Europe, including immunocompromised individuals, during the initial development of MVA as a "safer smallpox vaccine" [36,37]. Furthermore, MVA has shown no reproductive toxicity in studies in pregnant rabbits or rats [38], and was used as a vector for malaria, influenza, and tuberculosis vaccines as well for cancer therapies in over 100 clinical trials since 1999 [32,33,39]. Our MVA-VLP HIV vaccine has demonstrated outstanding safety in clinical trials involving 500 humans [40,41], including immunocompromised individuals as well as HIV patients [40–42].

In this paper, we demonstrated that a single dose of GEO-LM01 confered full protection against the challenge virus ML29, which was directly inoculated into the brain. ML29 virus itself confers protection by the peripheral route, but its classification as a Risk group 3 (BSL3) agent creates major challenges for manufacturing in the US; in Europe it is considered Risk group 2 (BSL2). Similarly, commercial yellow fever (YF) vaccines (strains 17D and 17DD), approved more than half a century ago, are lethal for immunocompetent mice when inoculated by the IC route but can confer protection when administered by peripheral routes [43]. These strains are used as challenge viruses for the evaluation of new vaccines against YF virus. Our future work will continue in Hartley guinea pigs and NHP models (e.g., in cynomolgous macaques where signs of LASV infection mirror human disease) with live LASV under high laboratory containment, that is, Animal BSL4 (ABSL4) where the challenge virus is fully lethal by the parenteral route.

T cells are known to be a vital component of immune-mediated protection against LASV infection [44]. T cells also steer the B cell response and, therefore, a thorough investigation of the T cell response yields insight concerning the mechanisms of both cellular and humoral protection. Despite a strong T cell response, especially with CD4+ populations that are double positive for IFNγ and IL2 (an indication of expanding population), at day 11 after single-dose vaccination there was a low level of IgG antibodies produced at this timepoint. While administration of nAbs in the early stages of LASV infection by passive transfer has shown protection in animal models [45,46], the protection afforded by prior vaccination is thought to be strictly dependent on a T cell response [30,31,35,47,48]. Similarly, multiple vaccine vector platforms that showed high levels of protection in mice, guinea pigs, and NHP have not induced detectable levels of neutralizing Ab (reviewed in Ref 26).

In the 1980s, Clegg and Lloyd [49] expressed Lassa NP from a vaccinia vector and succeeded in protecting guinea pigs, but not primates, from lethal LF disease. Since then, researchers at Porton Down have used a safer vector, MVA, to express LASV NP and protect guinea pigs from LF disease progression [50]. Since they elicited both bAb and a robust cell-mediated immunity to NP in the guinea pig model, it is possible that the MVA-LAS NP could be a standalone vaccine.

GPC is the natural target for nAb responses since it contains epitopes involved in both entry and the endosomal fusion process. GPC, however, is highly glycosylated with 11 N-linked carbohydrate sites on each monomer comprising ~25% of the total mass of the protein, shielding critical residues from Ab access. nAb against GPC have been isolated from the sera of convalescent patients, but these are rare and appear very late in infection [51]. We have consistently elicited excellent functional antibody responses (e.g., bAb, nAb and antibody-dependent cell-mediated cytotoxicity, ADCC) with MVA vaccines that target other viruses such as HIV, Ebola, and Zika [32,33,40,41,50]. A recent publication elicits excellent bAb against an MVA vector expressing LASV NP that has no glycan shield [52]. The low natural bAb against LASV GPC speaks to the effectiveness of the immuno-evasive properties of the protein, including its glycan shield, explaining failures of nAb-based vaccines or therapies using convalescent sera [51]. The combination of the 33 glycans shield, leaving only a few regions vulnerable to antibody binding, and the metastability of the native protein further explain why bAb responses are altogether difficult to elicit by vaccination. Here, we saw robust bAb at d36 (Figure 4d), but that could be attributed to the boost from ML29 virus challenge. Neutralizing antibodies have been isolated from LF survivors as patients were recovering from illness during which the humoral response had time to mature [53]. Recently, by introducing a number of mutations in GPC, this protein could be "locked" in its prefusion state increasing its stability and enabling co-crystallization with human nAb 37.7 H [16]. We are currently exploring whether replacement of the locked GPC structure with native GPC or any other modifications thereof could result in a viable vaccine candidate, demasking the GPC from carbohydrate shields and exposing more epitopes for inducing binding and neutralizing antibodies in vaccinated hosts.

4. Materials and Methods

4.1. Vaccine Construction, Seed Stock Preparation, VLP Formation, and Protein Expression

A recombinant GEO-LM01 was constructed on GeoVax's MVA-VLP platform, utilizing the highly potent yet safe viral vector MVA [54,55]. The vaccine produces two LASV proteins, GPC and Z proteins from Josiah strain LASV lineage IV (GenBank JN650517.1 and JN650518.1). We used a parental MVA that had been harvested in 1974 before the appearance of Bovine Spongiform Encephalopathy /Transmissible Spongiform Encephalopathy (BSE/TSE) and sent in 2001 to Dr. Bernard Moss at NIAID, where it was plaque purified 3 times using certified reagents from sources free of BSE. The pLW76 shuttle vector (Wyatt and Moss, unpublished data) was used to insert the GPC sequences between two essential genes of MVA (I8R and G1L), and LASV Z gene into a restructured and modified deletion III between the A50R and B1R genes. These insertion sites have been identified as supporting high expression and insert stability. All inserted sequences were codon optimized for MVA. Silent mutations were introduced to interrupt homo-polymer sequences (>4G/C and >4A/T), which reduce RNA polymerase errors that possibly lead to frameshifts. The sequences were edited for vaccinia-specific terminators to remove motifs that could lead to premature termination [56]. All vaccine inserts were placed under the modified H5 early/late vaccinia promoter as described previously [57,58]. Vectors, Research Seed Virus (RSV), and Research Stocks (RS) were prepared in a dedicated room at GeoVax, with full traceability and complete documentation of all steps using BSE/TSE-free raw materials and therefore can be directly used for production of cGMP Master Seed Virus (MSV). For production of RSV for animal studies, specific pathogen-free CEF cells were acquired from Charles River Laboratories (cat#10100807), seeded into sterile tissue culture flasks, and infected with GEO-LM01 at MOIs of 0.01. Cells were recovered at 3 days post-infection, disrupted by sonication, and bulk harvest material clarified by low-speed centrifugation. The clarified viral harvest was purified using sucrose cushion ultracentrifugation. The purified viruses were titrated by limiting dilution in DF1 cells, diluted to 1×10^8 $TCID_{50}$/mL in sterile PBS + 7.5% sucrose, dispensed into sterile vials, and stored at $-80\,°C$. Generally, a minimum of 1×10^{10} $TCID_{50}$ of vaccines are produced per mL of harvest material. The VLP formation was evaluated by electron microscopy conducted on thin sections of 48 hour-infected DF-1 cell and was performed at the Emory University Apkarian Integrated Electron Microscopy Core, as previously described [59]. The expression of GPC and Z proteins by MVA was assessed by immunostaining of GEO-LM01 infected DF1 cells that had been fixed in 1:1 methanol:acetone and probed using LASV-specific GPC and Z antibodies (IBT 0307-001, rabbit anti-LASV GP pAb and IBT 0307-002, rabbit anti LASV Z pAb). Plaques were serially diluted (10-fold) from 1:100 to 1:100,000 and stained with anti-GPC or anti-Z monoclonal antibodies, respectively. Similar plaque numbers at each dilution in the GPC and Z wells show that both inserts are retained. The expression of full-length GP1 and GP2 (derived from cleavage of GPC) as well as Z protein, was confirmed by WB analysis conducted on supernatants and lysates of 293T cells 48 hours after infection using standard practices. A pool of human anti-GP1 and -GP2 antibodies (2.4F and 22.5D from Dr. James Robinson, Tulane University, New Orleans, LA) were used as the primary Abs for GP1 and GP2, and a polyclonal rabbit Ab as the primary Ab for Z (IBT Catalog# 0307-002).

4.2. Mouse Immunogenicity and Efficacy Studies

4.2.1. **Experiment 1**. Determination of Vaccine Efficacy by Different Routes

Vaccine challenge studies were performed in a mouse model as previously described [24]. Lethality of intracerebrally (IC)-administered ML29 virus was tested in several inbred mouse models and CBA/J mice were the most sensitive to challenge. ML29 is a reassortant virus with its large genome segment from MOPV and its small segment from LASV; subcutaneous administration protects guinea pigs and primates from lethal challenge with LASV [23], but in the absence of vaccination is lethal in this IC challenge model. According to the CDC, ML29 is classified as a BSL3 agent, but not as a Select Agent. In line with University of Maryland Biosafety protocols, all propagation and experiments with high-titer stocks of ML29 virus were performed under BSL3 containment. Day-to-day experiments performed with low-titer stocks were under BSL2 containment. According to biosafety and animal care and use protocols in place, animal studies with low-titer stocks of ML29 virus were performed under ABSL2 containment. The challenge dose was selected based on uniform lethality in unprotected mice as described previously [26]. Immunization doses were based on prior studies testing efficacy of MVA vectored vaccines [38,39].

To determine the best route of immunization, 4–6 week-old CBA/J mice (n = 6) were immunized with 10^7 TCID$_{50}$ of GEO-LM01 by intraperitoneal (IP), intramuscular (IM), or subcutaneous (SC) inoculations. Two groups of mice (n = 6 each) were injected IP with ML29 at 1000 plaque-forming units (PFU) or saline, and served as positive and negative controls, respectively. On day 14, all mice were challenged by IC inoculation with 1000 PFU of ML29 and monitored for weight change, morbidity, and mortality.ML29 titers in the brains of challenged mice were not high enough to be detected by plaque assay. However, ML29 was detectable in a sensitive co-culture assay described in ref [35]. Positive (+) detection was seen in the brains of dying mice, and negative (-) in the brains of surviving mice. Since successfully vaccinated mice survived whereas those given saline or empty vectors succumbed within a week of being challenged, the MVA-Lassa vaccine proved capable of controlling ML29 replication.

4.2.2. **Experiment 2**. Confirmation of Route and Immune Response

A second study to measure immunogenicity and efficacy was initiated in the same model system, in this instance examining only two conditions: immunization with GEO-LM01 by IM inoculation (n = 10) and mock immunization with saline (n = 8). Spleens were harvested from immunized animals (n = 3) and from saline-immunized animals on day 11 after a single administration of the vaccine, and antigen-specific T cell responses were measured by intracellular cytokine staining for IFNγ and IL-2 using LASV GPC immuno-dominant peptides for stimulation. The remaining animals from both groups were challenged on day 14 as in the first experiment. The serum obtained from the 3 animals sacrificed for T cell assays was additionally assayed for the presence of binding antibodies (bAb) against GPC, using ELISA.

4.3. Splenocyte Isolations and T Cell Assay

CBA/J mice immunized with saline or once with 10^7 TCID$_{50}$ GEO-LM01 vaccine were sacrificed on day 11 after immunization. Spleens were removed and homogenized through a cell strainer mounted on a 50 mL conical tube in DMEM-10 medium. Cells were centrifuged at 400× g for 5 minutes. Supernatants were aspirated and cells resuspended in 5mL 1× RBC lysis buffer. After 5 minutes at room temperature with occasional shaking, 25 mL HBSS were added to the tube, mixed by inversion, and cells centrifuged at 400× g for 5 minutes. Supernatants were discarded and pellets resuspended in 10mL DMEM-10. Isolated splenocytes were analyzed by ICS following standard protocols. In short, 10^6 splenocytes were stimulated with 0.1µg LASV GP1 (SLYKGVYEL; amino acids 60–68) or GP2 (YLISIFLHL; amino acids 441–480) immuno-dominant epitopes identified within the GPC protein sequence [24–26], or mock stimulated with saline. Incubation proceeded for 6 hours at 37 °C + 5% CO_2; GolgiPlug (BD Biosciences) was added at a concentration of 1.0 µL/mL for the last 4 hours of the incubation. The splenocytes were stained with Live/Dead Fixable Green Dead Cell Stain (ThermoFisher) at room temperature for 20 minutes. The samples were treated with Cytofix/Cytoperm (BD Biosciences) at 4 °C for 20 minutes and were stained with CD3-APC-CY7, CD4-PE-Cy7, CD8-PerCP, IL2-PE, and IFN-γ-Alexa647 (all flow cytometry antibodies from BD Biosciences). Samples were analyzed with a FACSCanto flow cytometer (BD Biosciences) utilizing FACSDiva software. Analysis was performed with FlowJo software. Responses to GP1 and GP2 stimulated cells were added together to represent the total GP stimulated response and then normalized to values from saline stimulated cells. Cytokine responses were scored as a percent of total $CD8^+$ or $CD4^+$ T cells.

4.4. ELISA

Whole blood samples were obtained by retro-orbital bleeding just prior to immunization on days 11–14 post vaccination, and at the termination of experiments. The terminal bleeds shown in Figure 4d were day 36 (22 days following challenge). Sera were obtained by centrifugation of the whole blood samples in serum separator tubes at 3500× g for 5 min. and used to measure bAb in ELISA as described previously [60]. Briefly, flat-bottom 96-well plates were coated overnight at 4 °C with sonication-inactivated ML29 virus, 10^5 PFU/mL in 100 mM bicarbonate buffer, pH 9.6. Plates were washed 4 times with phosphate buffered saline (PBS) + 0.05% Tween-20 (PBST). Next, the plates were blocked with StartingBlock Blocking Buffer (Thermo Fisher Scientific) for 5 minutes at room temperature. Serially-diluted heat-inactivated mouse serum samples were added to wells and incubated for 1 hour at 37 °C. After washing with PBST, goat anti-mouse IgG-HRP (ImmunoReagents) was added to each well and incubated for 1 hour at 37 °C. After a final washing, SureBlue TMB (3,3′, 5, 5′—Tetramethylbenzidine) 1-component substrate solution (KPL) was added to each well, incubated in the dark at room temperature for 10 minutes, and stopped with 1N hydrochloric acid (HCl). Optical density at 450 nm was determined using a Vmax Kinetic ELISA Absorbance Microplate Reader (Molecular Devices). Normalized absorbance values were determined by first subtracting optical density values of blank negative control wells. Endpoint titer was determined by the dilution at which the optical density equaled 0.03.

4.5. Statistical Analyses

Analysis of data was performed using GraphPad Prism (GraphPad Software). Comparisons between groups were performed using a Student's t-test. To test for pairwise differences between groups, an analysis of variance (ANOVA) and Tukey's test of multiple comparisons was performed. Correlations were performed by Spearman rank-correlation tests. A p-value less than 0.05 was considered statistically significant.

4.6. Regulatory Compliance

All methods were carried out in accordance with the relevant guidelines and regulations. All experimental protocols were approved by the University of Maryland School of Medicine Institutional Animal Care and Use Committee (IACUC Protocol # 0217017) and the Institutional Biosafety Committee (approval # IBC-00001495).

5. Conclusions

GEO-LM01 uses GeoVax's MVA-VLP vaccine platform that has been shown to be safe and to induce durable antibody and T cell responses in multiple human clinical trials for GeoVax's prophylactic HIV vaccine. In contrast to other LF vaccines in development that rely on a single glycoprotein antigen, GEO-LM01 includes an additional matrix protein that forms VLPs with the LASV glycoproteins. Upon infection of human cells, the MVA-driven expression of the two proteins leads to the formation of non-infectious VLPs that bear natively-folded glycoproteins on their surface, triggering an effective immune response that is predicted to be more broadly cross-protective than vaccines expressing only one viral antigen [30]. We previously demonstrated that our MVA-VLP-Ebola vaccine conferred full protection after a single dose in non-human primates. This vaccine induced near sterile immunity since no live virus could be detected in the blood of any vaccinated animal post challenge compared to controls ($>5\log_{10}$ $TCID_{50}$ per mL of blood). We are currently evaluating the efficacy of our LF vaccine in guinea pigs and non-human primate models. It remains to be seen whether this vaccine will also be a best-in class vaccine for LF, as shown for the MVA-VLP-Ebola vaccine [61].

Author Contributions: Conceptualization and data curation: M.S., F.G.; Investigation: A.D., C.G.-C., S.M.-M., J.C.Z., H.H., N.M. and R.J.B.; Methodology: M.S., F.G. and A.D.; Project administration: M.H.; Resources: J.C.Z.; Writing—original draft: M.S. and F.G. All authors contributed to reviewing and editing the manuscript.

Acknowledgments: We thank the Institute of Human Virology staff members Joseph Bryant, Harry Davis, Maurice White, and Sumiko Williams for their excellent contributions to animal husbandry and animal care needs throughout this study. We are indebted to Hong Yi and the Robert P. Apkarian Integrated Electron Microscopy Core of Emory University Medical School for thin section electron microscopy. We are thankful to Erica Saphire from Scripps Institute for providing the molecular structure of the GPC protein and James Robinson from Tulane University for providing antibodies to GP1 and GP2 polypeptides.

References

1. WHO. Epidemic Focus: Lassa fever Weekly Epidemiological Record. Available online: https://www.who.int/wer/2016/wer9121.pdf?ua=1 (accessed on 27 May 2016).

2. Shao, J.; Liang, Y.; Ly, H. Human Hemorrhagic Fever Causing Arenaviruses: Molecular Mechanisms Contributing to Virus Virulence and Disease Pathogenesis. *Pathogens* **2015**, *4*, 283–306. [CrossRef] [PubMed]

3. Leski, T.A.; Stockelman, M.G.; Moses, L.M.; Park, M.; Stenger, D.A.; Ansumana, R.; Bausch, D.G.; Lin, B. Sequence Variability and Geographic Distribution of Lassa Virus, Sierra Leone. *Emerg. Infect. Dis.* **2015**, *21*, 609–618. [CrossRef] [PubMed]

4. McCormick, J.B.; Webb, P.A.; Krebs, J.W.; Johnson, K.M.; Smith, E.S. A Prospective Study of the Epidemiology and Ecology of Lassa Fever. *J. Infect. Dis.* **1987**, *155*, 437–444. [CrossRef] [PubMed]

5. McCormick, J.B. *Lassa Fever, in Emergence and Control of Rodent-Borne Viral Diseases*; Saluzzo, J.F., Dodet, B., Eds.; Elsevier: Amsterdam, The Nertherlands, 1999; pp. 177–195.

6. Richmond, J.K.; Baglole, D.J. Lassa fever: Epidemiology, clinical features, and social consequences. *BMJ* **2003**, *327*, 1271–1275. [CrossRef] [PubMed]

7. Control, N.C.f.D. Disease Situation Reports. 2018. Available online: https://ncdc.gov.ng/diseases/sitreps (accessed on 2 September 2018).

8. Olayemi, A.; Cadar, D.; Magassouba, N.F.; Obadare, A.; Kourouma, F.; Oyeyiola, A.; Fasogbon, S.; Igbokwe, J.; Rieger, T.; Bockholt, S.; et al. New Hosts of The Lassa Virus. *Sci. Rep.* **2016**, *6*, 25280. [CrossRef] [PubMed]

9. Fisher-Hoch, S.P.; Tomori, O.; Nasidi, A.; I Perez-Oronoz, G.; Fakile, Y.; Hutwagner, L.; McCormick, J.B. Review of cases of nosocomial Lassa fever in Nigeria: The high price of poor medical practice. *BMJ* **1995**, *311*, 857–859. [CrossRef] [PubMed]

10. Mylne, A.Q.N.; Pigott, D.M.; Longbottom, J.; Shearer, F.; Duda, K.A.; Messina, J.P.; Weiss, D.J.; Moyes, C.L.; Golding, N.; Hay, S.I. Mapping the zoonotic niche of Lassa fever in Africa. *Trans. R. Soc. Trop. Med. Hyg.* **2015**, *109*, 483–492. [CrossRef] [PubMed]

11. Bowen, M.D.; Rollin, P.E.; Ksiazek, T.G.; Hustad, H.L.; Bausch, D.G.; Demby, A.H.; Bajani, M.D.; Peters, C.J.; Nichol, S.T. Genetic Diversity among Lassa Virus Strains. *J. Virol.* **2000**, *74*, 6992–7004. [CrossRef] [PubMed]

12. Hallam, H.J.; Hallam, S.; Rodriguez, S.E.; Barrett, A.D.T.; Beasley, D.W.C.; Chua, A.; Ksiazek, T.G.; Milligan, G.N.; Sathiyamoorthy, V.; Reece, L.M. Baseline mapping of Lassa fever virology, epidemiology and vaccine research and development. *NPJ Vaccines* **2018**, *3*, 11. [CrossRef]

13. Radoshitzky, S.R.; Bao, Y.; Buchmeier, M.J.; Charrel, R.N.; Clawson, A.N.; Clegg, C.S.; DeRisi, J.L.; Emonet, S.; Gonzalez, J.-P.; Kuhn, J.H.; et al. Past, present, and future of arenavirus taxonomy. *Arch. Virol.* **2015**, *160*, 1851–1874. [CrossRef] [PubMed]

14. Djavani, M.; Lukashevich, I.S.; Sanchez, A.; Nichol, S.T.; Salvato, M.S. Completion of the Lassa fever virus sequence and identification of a RING finger ORF at the L RNA 5′ end. *Virology* **1997**, *235*, 414–418. [CrossRef] [PubMed]

15. Lukashevich, I.S.; Nichol, S.T.; Shapiro, K.; Ravkov, E.; Sanchez, A.; Djavani, M.; Salvato, M.S. The Lassa fever virus L gene: Nucleotide sequence, comparison, and precipitation of a predicted 250 kDa protein with monospecific antiserum. *J. Gen. Virol.* **1997**, *78*, 547–551. [CrossRef] [PubMed]

16. Hastie, K.M.; Zandonatti, M.A.; Kleinfelter, L.M.; Heinrich, M.L.; Rowland, M.M.; Chandran, K.; Branco, L.M.; Robinson, J.E.; Garry, R.F.; Saphire, E.O. Structural basis for antibody-mediated neutralization of Lassa virus. *Science* **2017**, *356*, 923–928. [CrossRef] [PubMed]

17. Lenz, O.; Ter Meulen, J.; Klenk, H.-D.; Seidah, N.G.; Garten, W. The Lassa virus glycoprotein precursor GP-C is proteolytically processed by subtilase SKI-1/S1P. *Proc. Natl. Acad. Sci. USA* **2001**, *98*, 12701–12705. [CrossRef] [PubMed]

18. Ölschläger, S.; Flatz, L. Vaccination Strategies against Highly Pathogenic Arenaviruses: The Next Steps toward Clinical Trials. *PLoS Pathog.* **2013**, *9*, e1003212. [CrossRef] [PubMed]

19. Urata, S.; Yasuda, J. Cis- and cell-type-dependent trans-requirements for Lassa virus-like particle production. *J. Gen. Virol.* **2015**, *96 Pt 7*, 1626–1635. [CrossRef]

20. Safronetz, D.; Mire, C.; Rosenke, K.; Feldmann, F.; Haddock, E.; Geisbert, T.; Feldmann, H. A Recombinant Vesicular Stomatitis Virus-Based Lassa Fever Vaccine Protects Guinea Pigs and Macaques against Challenge with Geographically and Genetically Distinct Lassa Viruses. *PLoS Negl. Trop. Dis.* **2015**, *9*, e0003736. [CrossRef]

21. Verheust, C.; Goossens, M.; Pauwels, K.; Breyer, D. Biosafety aspects of modified vaccinia virus Ankara (MVA)-based vectors used for gene therapy or vaccination. *Vaccine* **2012**, *30*, 2623–2632. [CrossRef]

22. Hastie, K.M.; Zandonatti, M.; Liu, T.; Li, S.; Woods, V.L.; Saphire, E.O. Crystal Structure of the Oligomeric Form of Lassa Virus Matrix Protein Z. *J. Virol.* **2016**, *90*, 4556–4562. [CrossRef]

23. Lukashevich, I.S.; Patterson, J.; Carrion, R.; Moshkoff, D.; Ticer, A.; Zapata, J.; Brasky, K.; Geiger, R.; Hubbard, G.B.; Bryant, J.; et al. A Live Attenuated Vaccine for Lassa Fever Made by Reassortment of Lassa and Mopeia Viruses. *J. Virol.* **2005**, *79*, 13934–13942. [CrossRef]

24. Goicochea, M.A.; Zapata, J.C.; Bryant, J.; Davis, H.; Salvato, M.S.; Lukashevich, I.S. Evaluation of Lassa virus vaccine immunogenicity in a CBA/JML29 mouse model. *Vaccine* **2012**, *30*, 1445–1452. [CrossRef] [PubMed]

25. Botten, J.; Alexander, J.; Pasquetto, V.; Sidney, J.; Barrowman, P.; Ting, J.; Peters, B.; Southwood, S.; Stewart, B.; Rodriguez-Carreno, M.P.; et al. Identification of Protective Lassa Virus Epitopes That Are Restricted by HLA-A2. *J. Virol.* **2006**, *80*, 8351–8361. [CrossRef]

26. Boesen, A.; Sundar, K.; Coico, R. Lassa Fever Virus Peptides Predicted by Computational Analysis Induce Epitope-Specific Cytotoxic-T-Lymphocyte Responses in HLA-A2.1 Transgenic Mice. *Clin. Vaccine Immunol.* **2005**, *12*, 1223–1230. [CrossRef] [PubMed]

27. Kyei, N.N.; Abilba, M.M.; Kwawu, F.K.; Agbenohevi, P.G.; Bonney, J.H.; Agbemaple, T.K.; Nimo-Paintsil, S.C.; Ampofo, W.; Ohene, S.-A.; Nyarko, E.O. Imported Lassa fever: A report of 2 cases in Ghana. *BMC Infect. Dis.* **2015**, *15*, 217. [CrossRef] [PubMed]

28. Mehand, M.S.; Al Shorbaji, F.; Millett, P.; Murgue, B. The WHO R&D Blueprint: 2018 review of emerging infectious diseases requiring urgent research and development efforts. *Antivir. Res.* **2018**, *159*, 63–67. [PubMed]

29. CEPI. News. 2018. Available online: http://cepi.net/news (accessed on 2 September 2018).

30. Zapata, J.C.; Medina-Moreno, S.; Guzmán-Cardozo, C.; Salvato, M.S. Improving the Breadth of the Host's Immune Response to Lassa Virus. *Pathogens* **2018**, *7*, 84. [CrossRef] [PubMed]

31. Ter Meulen, V. Lassa fever: Implications of T-cell immunity for vaccine development. *J. Biotechnol.* **1999**, *73*, 207–212. [CrossRef]

32. Domi, A.; Feldmann, F.; Basu, R.; McCurley, N.; Shifflett, K.; Emanuel, J.; Hellerstein, M.S.; Guirakhoo, F.; Orlandi, C.; Flinko, R.; et al. A Single Dose of Modified Vaccinia Ankara expressing Ebola Virus Like Particles Protects Nonhuman Primates from Lethal Ebola Virus Challenge. *Sci. Rep.* **2018**, *8*, 864. [CrossRef]

33. Brault, A.C.; Domi, A.; McDonald, E.M.; Talmi-Frank, D.; McCurley, N.; Basu, R.; Robinson, H.L.; Hellerstein, M.; Duggal, N.K.; Bowen, R.A.; et al. A Zika Vaccine Targeting NS1 Protein Protects Immunocompetent Adult Mice in a Lethal Challenge Model. *Sci. Rep.* **2017**, *7*, 14769. [CrossRef]

34. Djomand, G.; Quaye, S.; Sullivan, P.S. HIV epidemic among key populations in west Africa. *Curr. Opin. HIV AIDS* **2014**, *9*, 506–513. [CrossRef]

35. Zapata, J.C.; Poonia, B.; Bryant, J.; Davis, H.; Ateh, E.; George, L.; Crasta, O.; Zhang, Y.; Slezak, T.; Jaing, C.; et al. An attenuated Lassa vaccine in SIV-infected rhesus macaques does not persist or cause arenavirus disease but does elicit Lassa virus-specific immunity. *Virol. J.* **2013**, *10*, 52. [CrossRef] [PubMed]

36. Sutter, G.; Moss, B. Nonreplicating vaccinia vector efficiently expresses recombinant genes. *Proc. Natl. Acad. Sci. USA* **1992**, *89*, 10847–10851. [CrossRef] [PubMed]

37. Overton, E.T.; Stapleton, J.; Frank, I.; Hassler, S.; Goepfert, P.A.; Barker, D.; Wagner, E.; Von Krempelhuber, A.; Virgin, G.; Weigl, J.; et al. Safety and Immunogenicity of Modified Vaccinia Ankara-Bavarian Nordic Smallpox Vaccine in Vaccinia-Naive and Experienced Human Immunodeficiency Virus-Infected Individuals: An Open-Label, Controlled Clinical Phase II Trial. *Open Forum Infect. Dis.* **2015**, *2*, ofv040. [CrossRef] [PubMed]

38. Committee for Medicinal Products for Human Use (CHMP). *Assessment Report, IMVANEX, Common Name: Modified Vaccinia Ankara Virus, Procedure No. EMEA/H/C/002596*; Committee for Medicinal Products for Human Use (CHMP), Ed.; European Medicines Agency: London, UK, 2013.

39. Bliss, C.M.; Bowyer, G.; Anagnostou, N.A.; Havelock, T.; Snudden, C.M.; Davies, H.; De Cassan, S.C.; Grobbelaar, A.; Lawrie, A.M.; Venkatraman, N.; et al. Assessment of novel vaccination regimens using viral vectored liver stage malaria vaccines encoding ME-TRAP. *Sci. Rep.* **2018**, *8*, 3390. [CrossRef] [PubMed]

40. Goepfert, P.A.; Elizaga, M.L.; Sato, A.; Qin, L.; Cardinali, M.; Hay, C.M.; Hural, J.; DeRosa, S.C.; Defawe, O.D.; Tomaras, G.D.; et al. Phase 1 Safety and Immunogenicity Testing of DNA and Recombinant Modified Vaccinia Ankara Vaccines Expressing HIV-1 Virus-like Particles. *J. Infect. Dis.* **2011**, *203*, 610–619. [CrossRef] [PubMed]

41. Goepfert, P.A.; Elizaga, M.L.; Seaton, K.; Tomaras, G.D.; Montefiori, D.C.; Sato, A.; Hural, J.; DeRosa, S.C.; Kalams, S.A.; McElrath, M.J.; et al. Specificity and 6-Month Durability of Immune Responses Induced by DNA and Recombinant Modified Vaccinia Ankara Vaccines Expressing HIV-1 Virus-Like Particles. *J. Infect. Dis.* **2014**, *210*, 99–110. [CrossRef] [PubMed]

42. Thompson, M.; Heath, S.L.; Sweeton, B.; Williams, K.; Cunningham, P.; Keele, B.F.; Sen, S.; Palmer, B.E.; Chomont, N.; Xu, Y.; et al. DNA/MVA Vaccination of HIV-1 Infected Participants with Viral Suppression on Antiretroviral Therapy, followed by Treatment Interruption: Elicitation of Immune Responses without Control of Re-Emergent Virus. *PLoS ONE* **2016**, *11*, 0163164. [CrossRef]

43. Maciel, M.M., Jr.; Cruz, F.D.S.P.; Cordeiro, M.T.; da Motta, M.A.; de Melo Cassemiro, K.M.S.; Maia, R.D.C.C.; de Figueiredo, R.C.B.Q.; Galler, R.; da Silva Freire, M.; August, J.T.; et al. A DNA Vaccine against Yellow Fever Virus: Development and Evaluation. *PLoS Negl. Trop. Dis.* **2015**, *9*, e0003693. [CrossRef]

44. Perdomo-Celis, F.; Salvato, M.S.; Medina-Moreno, S.; Zapata, J.C. T-Cell Response to Viral Hemorrhagic Fevers. *Vaccines* **2019**, *7*, 11. [CrossRef]

45. Cross, R.W.; Mire, C.E.; Branco, L.M.; Geisbert, J.B.; Rowland, M.M.; Heinrich, M.L.; Goba, A.; Momoh, M.; Grant, D.S.; Fullah, M.; et al. Treatment of Lassa virus infection in outbred guinea pigs with first-in-class human monoclonal antibodies. *Antivir. Res.* **2016**, *133*, 218–222. [CrossRef]

46. Mire, C.E.; Cross, R.W.; Geisbert, J.B.; Borisevich, V.; Agans, K.N.; Deer, D.J.; Heinrich, M.L.; Rowland, M.M.; Goba, A.; Momoh, M.; et al. Human-monoclonal-antibody therapy protects nonhuman primates against advanced Lassa fever. *Nat. Med.* **2017**, *23*, 1146–1149. [CrossRef] [PubMed]

47. Lukashevich, I.S.; Carrion, R.; Salvato, M.S.; Mansfield, K.; Brasky, K.; Zapata, J.; Cairo, C.; Goicochea, M.; Hoosien, G.E.; Ticer, A.; et al. Safety, immunogenicity, and efficacy of the ML29 reassortant vaccine for Lassa fever in small non-human primates. *Vaccine* **2008**, *26*, 5246–5254. [CrossRef] [PubMed]

48. Kiley, M. Protection of Rhesus Monkeys from Lassa Virus by Immunisation With Closely Related Arenavirus. *Lancet* **1979**, *314*, 738. [CrossRef]

49. Clegg, J.; Lloyd, G. Vaccinia Recombinant Expressing Lassa-Virus Internal Nucleocapsid Protein Protects Guinea pigs against Lassa Fever. *Lancet* **1987**, *330*, 186–188. [CrossRef]

50. McCurley, N.P.; Domi, A.; Basu, R.; Saunders, K.O.; Labranche, C.C.; Montefiori, D.C.; Haynes, B.F.; Robinson, H.L. HIV transmitted/founder vaccines elicit autologous tier 2 neutralizing antibodies for the CD4 binding site. *PLoS ONE* **2017**, *12*, e0177863. [CrossRef] [PubMed]

51. Sommerstein, R.; Flatz, L.; Remy, M.M.; Malinge, P.; Magistrelli, G.; Fischer, N.; Sahin, M.; Bergthaler, A.; Igonet, S.; Ter Meulen, J.; et al. Arenavirus Glycan Shield Promotes Neutralizing Antibody Evasion and Protracted Infection. *PLoS Pathog.* **2015**, *11*, e1005276. [CrossRef] [PubMed]

52. Kennedy, E.; Dowall, S.; Salguero, F.; Yeates, P.; Aram, M.; Hewson, R. A vaccine based on recombinant modified Vaccinia Ankara containing the nucleoprotein from Lassa virus protects against disease progression in a guinea pig model. *Vaccine* **2019**, *37*, 5404–5413. [CrossRef] [PubMed]

53. Robinson, J.E.; Hastie, K.M.; Cross, R.W.; Yenni, R.E.; Elliott, D.H.; Rouelle, J.A.; Kannadka, C.B.; Smira, A.A.; Garry, C.E.; Bradley, B.T.; et al. Most neutralizing human monoclonal antibodies target novel epitopes requiring both Lassa virus glycoprotein subunits. *Nat. Commun.* **2016**, *7*, 11544. [CrossRef]

54. Altenburg, A.F.; Kreijtz, J.H.C.M.; De Vries, R.D.; Song, F.; Fux, R.; Rimmelzwaan, G.F.; Sutter, G.; Volz, A. Modified Vaccinia Virus Ankara (MVA) as Production Platform for Vaccines against Influenza and Other Viral Respiratory Diseases. *Viruses* **2014**, *6*, 2735–2761. [CrossRef]

55. Moss, B.; Carroll, M.W.; Wyatt, L.S.; Bennink, J.R.; Hirsch, V.M.; Goldstein, S.; Elkins, W.R.; Fuerst, T.R.; Lifson, J.D.; Piatak, M.; et al. Host Range Restricted, Non-Replicating Vaccinia Virus Vectors as Vaccine Candidates. *Results Probl. Cell Differ.* **1996**, *397*, 7–13.

56. Wyatt, L.S.; Earl, P.L.; Vogt, J.; Eller, L.A.; Chandran, D.; Liu, J.; Robinson, H.L.; Moss, B. Correlation of immunogenicities and in vitro expression levels of recombinant modified vaccinia virus Ankara HIV vaccines. *Vaccine* **2008**, *26*, 486–493. [CrossRef] [PubMed]

57. Wyatt, L.S.; Earl, P.L.; Xiao, W.; Americo, J.L.; Cotter, C.A.; Vogt, J.; Moss, B. Elucidating and Minimizing the Loss by Recombinant Vaccinia Virus of Human Immunodeficiency Virus Gene Expression Resulting from Spontaneous Mutations and Positive Selection. *J. Virol.* **2009**, *83*, 7176–7184. [CrossRef] [PubMed]

58. Earl, P.L.; Cotter, C.; Moss, B.; VanCott, T.; Currier, J.; Eller, L.A.; McCutchan, F.; Birx, D.L.; Michael, N.L.; Marovich, M.A.; et al. Design and evaluation of multi-gene, multi-clade HIV-1 MVA vaccines. *Vaccine* **2009**, *27*, 5885–5895. [CrossRef] [PubMed]

59. Hellerstein, M.; Xu, Y.; Marino, T.; Lu, S.; Yi, H.; Wright, E.R.; Robinson, H.L. Co-expression of HIV-1 virus-like particles and granulocyte-macrophage colony stimulating factor by GEO-D03 DNA vaccine. *Hum. Vaccines Immunother.* **2012**, *8*, 1654–1658. [CrossRef] [PubMed]

60. Salvato, M.S.; Lukashevich, I.S.; Medina-Moreno, S.; Zapata, J.C. *Diagnostics for Lassa Fever: Detecting Host Antibody Responses, in Hemorrhagic Fever Viruses: Methods and Protocols*; Humana Press: New York, NY, USA, 2018.

61. Lázaro-Frías, A.; Gomez-Medina, S.; Sánchez-Sampedro, L.; Ljungberg, K.; Ustav, M.; Liljeström, P.; Muñoz-Fontela, C.; Esteban, M.; García-Arriaza, J. Distinct Immunogenicity and Efficacy of Poxvirus-Based Vaccine Candidates against Ebola Virus Expressing GP and VP40 Proteins. *J. Virol.* **2018**, *92*, e00363–e00418. [CrossRef]

18

Clostridium difficile in Asia: Opportunities for One Health Management

Deirdre A. Collins [1] and **Thomas V. Riley** [1,2,3,*]

[1]   School of Medical & Health Sciences, Edith Cowan University, Joondalup 6027, Australia;
       deirdre.collins@ecu.edu.au
[2]   Department of Microbiology, PathWest Laboratory Medicine, Nedlands 6009, Australia
[3]   School of Veterinary & Life Sciences, Murdoch University, Murdoch 6150, Australia
*   Correspondence: thomas.riley@uwa.edu.au.

Abstract: *Clostridium difficile* is a ubiquitous spore-forming bacterium which causes toxin-mediated diarrhoea and colitis in people whose gut microflora has been depleted by antimicrobial use, so it is a predominantly healthcare-associated disease. However, there are many One Health implications to *C. difficile*, given high colonisation rates in food production animals, contamination of outdoor environments by use of contaminated animal manure, increasing incidence of community-associated *C. difficile* infection (CDI), and demonstration of clonal groups of *C. difficile* shared between human clinical cases and food animals. In Asia, the epidemiology of CDI is not well understood given poor testing practices in many countries. The growing middle-class populations of Asia are presenting increasing demands for meat, thus production farming, particularly of pigs, chicken and cattle, is rapidly expanding in Asian countries. Few reports on *C. difficile* colonisation among production animals in Asia exist, but those that do show high prevalence rates, and possible importation of European strains of *C. difficile* like ribotype 078. This review summarises our current understanding of the One Health aspects of the epidemiology of CDI in Asia.

Keywords: *Clostridium difficile*; Asia; epidemiology; One Health

1. Introduction

Clostridium difficile is a ubiquitous spore-forming anaerobic bacterium which colonises the infant mammalian and avian gastrointestinal tract before the gut microflora has been established [1]. This "virgin" gut environment is replicated in mammals of all ages during and after antimicrobial exposure, or because of other circumstances that deplete or change the gut microflora. While human infants may not yet express the receptor for *C. difficile* toxins [2], older children and adults who become infected with toxigenic *C. difficile* can experience toxin-mediated disease ranging from self-limiting diarrhoea to life-threatening pseudomembranous colitis (PMC) and/or toxic megacolon.

C. difficile infection (CDI) has been predominantly a healthcare-associated illness, with the majority of cases being of advanced age, with comorbidities and a history of recent hospitalisation or treatment for illness. Increasing reported incidence rates in many regions [3] can partly be explained by the adoption of highly sensitive PCR testing [4] over the past decade, however, rates of community-associated (CA)-CDI are also rising [5,6]. While *C. difficile* spores can survive for long periods of time in healthcare environments due to their resistance to many disinfectants, recent advances in whole genome sequencing (WGS) studies have shown that up to 50% of CDI cases may be acquired from sources outside of healthcare facilities [7], implying environmental exposure accounts for a considerable proportion of CDI cases. High rates of *C. difficile* colonisation among food production livestock in which antimicrobials are frequently overused [8] have increased the risk of zoonotic transmission of *C. difficile* to humans [1]. Studies show high prevalence of *C. difficile* contamination of outdoor environments [9,10] and root vegetables [11] due to the use of contaminated animal manure as fertiliser. WGS has identified clonal groups of *C. difficile* isolated from both humans and animals [12], further supporting the possibility of zoonotic transmission of *C. difficile* from production animals to humans.

Intercontinental epidemics of CDI demonstrate the potential for international spread of *C. difficile*. Examples include the severe outbreaks in North America and Europe caused by clonal strains of ribotype (RT) 027 *C. difficile* originating in North America [13], and outbreaks of clindamycin-resistant strains of RT 017 across Asia, Europe and North America [14–17]. CDI epidemiology has been well documented in North America, Europe and, to a lesser extent, in Australia [5,6,18,19]. Different molecular types of *C. difficile* circulate in these respective regions, primarily ribotype (RT) 027 in North America and, until recently, Europe [20,21], and RT 014/020 in Australia [22]. To date, CDI has been largely under-diagnosed, under-reported and under-investigated in Asia, despite being home to 60% of the world's population, due to poor awareness among physicians and often inappropriate testing [23].

Over recent decades, growing economies and expanding populations across Asia have led to a rising middle class and ageing population with increasing demands for medical and aged care facilities. This wealth increase has also led to a greater appetite for meat and meat products, which has triggered a massive increase in meat consumption [24] and huge population expansion among meat production livestock, most notably pigs, chicken and cattle. This large-scale production farming, growing populations accessing healthcare facilities and widespread overuse of antimicrobials [25] make Asia an environment which is highly conducive to transmission of *C. difficile*, among both humans and animals.

The One Health paradigm approaches public health from a collaborative, multi-sectorial point of view, aiming to integrate policies, legislation and research to achieve better public health outcomes. It is particularly relevant to biosecurity, encompassing zoonotic infection, the rise of antimicrobial resistance and food safety. Given widespread colonisation of production animals and environmental contamination with *C. difficile* spores, management and control of CDI should use a One Health-based approach. This review examines our current knowledge of *C. difficile* in Asia from a One Health perspective.

2. Epidemiology of CDI in Asia

2.1. Diagnostic Practices in Asia

The prevalence and incidence rates of CDI can vary widely according to the testing method used. Diagnostic assays range from enzyme immunoassays (EIAs) detecting glutamate dehydrogenase (GDH) and/or toxin (A, B or both) to PCR for the *tcdA* or *tcdB* genes, to traditional culture and cell culture cytotoxicity assay (CCCA). No diagnostic test besides CCCA is suitable as a stand-alone test since toxin EIAs have low sensitivity, and PCR, GDH EIA and culture cannot rule out cases of transient colonisation [26]. CCCA is laborious and time-consuming so it is not routinely employed in diagnostic settings. Reports from Asia have indicated inappropriate testing in the past, particularly use of toxin A EIAs, which will underdiagnose CDI in Asia due to the high prevalence of toxin A-negative/toxin B-positive (A-B+) RT 017 and RT 369 strains [23]. According to a systematic review of studies in Asia, the most commonly performed tests were culture (71%) followed by EIA (52%) and PCR (51%) [27].

2.2. Estimated Prevalence and Incidence of CDI in Asia

Culture and PCR identify toxigenic *C. difficile* at high prevalence ranging from 9%–11% [28–30] in South-East Asia, while toxin EIA was positive in only 3%–5% of the same study specimens [28,29]. A systematic review of studies of CDI from Asia found a mean overall prevalence of 14.8% among hospital inpatients and outpatients, varying significantly from 2.0% to 61.4% across studies, and

16.4% among hospitalised patients with diarrhoea. The pooled incidence rate of CDI in Asia was calculated by meta-analysis at 5.3/10,000 patient days (95% CI 4.0–6.7) [27]. The random effects pooled CDI-related death rate was estimated at 8.9% (95% CI 5.4%–12.3%) by meta-analysis of existing studies [27], while a 13-country descriptive study with 600 recruited CDI cases found a lower mortality rate of 5.2% [31].

Studies in Singapore have demonstrated how changing testing practices have affected incidence rates. The incidence of CDI in Singapore was reported as increasing during the early 2000s, and from 2001 to 2006 the number of samples tested each year increased from 906 to 3508, with the percentage of positive samples increasing from 7% to 11% over the same period [32]. Subsequently, the incidence rate appeared to reduce, which was due to continuing increases in the number of samples being tested (4348 in 2006 to 6738 in 2008 between two hospitals) [33]. This suggests that increasing awareness and vigilance among physicians for possible cases of CDI led to more extensive testing among patients with diarrhoeal disease. Limited resources in some settings have resulted in still inadequate or no testing for CDI. For example, in a study in the Philippines, patients with CDI were frequently misdiagnosed with amoebiasis according to endoscopic detection of colitis [34].

2.3. Burden of CDI in Asia

Despite a high prevalence of C. difficile in Asia [27,28,30,35], reports of severe outcomes of CDI are rare. Few reports of PMC and toxic megacolon exist from Asian countries [36–43], suggesting they may be less commonly seen than in other regions. Where reports do appear, they are frequently associated with infection with A-B+ strains [36,40]. Recurrence rates are also lower at 9%–13% [31,44–46] than those reported from North America (15%–20%) [6] and Europe (16%–22%) [19,47], however definitions of recurrence can vary from 8 weeks to 90 days for reappearance of symptoms after resolution of disease. The apparent rarity of severe outcomes of CDI in the region, such as PMC or toxic megacolon, is likely influenced by the poor awareness of CDI among physicians. As demonstrated in the study in the Philippines, CDI is misdiagnosed as amoebiasis and treated with metronidazole which is often sufficient for resolution of milder cases of CDI, resulting in missed cases [34].

2.4. Molecular Epidemiology of CDI in Asia

2.4.1. A-B+ C. difficile Strains

The most commonly used molecular typing methods for C. difficile are PCR ribotyping and multi-locus sequence typing (MLST). Phylogenetic analyses based on MLST describe at least five major population clades of C. difficile [48]. As mentioned before, RT 017/ST37, a clade 4 strain [49], is A-B+ [48] and the predominant strain identified in Asia [23,27,28,35,50]. In China, Korea, Indonesia and Malaysia, RT 017 is generally the most common C. difficile strain in circulation, and it is also prevalent in Japan (referred to in older papers as ribotype "fr"), Taiwan, Hong Kong, Thailand and Singapore [28–30,51–56]. Exposure to antineoplastic agents, use of nasal feeding tubes and care in one particular hospital ward were associated with infection with RT 017 strains in a hospital in Japan [57]. C. difficile RT 017 has also caused major outbreaks of CDI outside of Asia, in Canada [58] and Europe [15,16], and is frequently reported as having enhanced fluoroquinolone and clindamycin resistance [15,16], a feature that has most likely contributed to its success as an epidemic strain.

The emergence of C. difficile RT 369/ST81, another clade 4 A-B+ strain, is also of interest and warrants close monitoring [31,59,60]. This strain apparently emerged first in Japan, where historically it was referred to in the literature using local nomenclature as "trf" [60,61]. It appears that RT 369 caused outbreaks of CDI in hospitals in 2000 and 2001, when ribotyping was not performed [57,60,62]. The first report of RT 369 was in a study conducted on isolates collected from outbreak and non-outbreak situations from 2009–2013 in Japan. This study detected RT 369 in an outbreak setting in a hospital in 2009 [60], and it is now one of the most common strains in circulation there [31,59]. RT 369 has since been reported in studies from China as the cause of a nosocomial outbreak among hospital patients in

Shanghai in 2014 and 2015 where it was the most common strain in circulation. RT 369/ST81 strains are also reported to have higher rates of resistance to clindamycin, ciprofloxacin and moxifloxacin compared with other strains, and a higher sporulation rate than RT 017/ST37 strains [63,64].

2.4.2. Binary Toxin-Positive *C. difficile* Strains

Many but not all binary toxin-positive (CDT+) *C. difficile* strains tend to group in phylogenetic clades 2 and 5, and have been associated with epidemics of CDI in North America (RT 027/ST1, clade 2) [13,65], Europe (RT 078/ST11, clade 5, and RT 027/ST1) [19,21] and Australia (RT 244/ST41, clade 2) [66] in recent times. In contrast, CDT+ strains have been only sporadically reported from Asia and major epidemics like those seen elsewhere have not occurred [67]. Most cases of RT 027 infection to date have been reported from China, where 11 cases were reported from one hospital over 3 years [68]. RT 027 also caused CDI among seven patients across four hospitals in Seoul and Gyenngi province in Korea [69], and may be increasing in prevalence in Taiwan, where it was never reported prior to 2015 [70,71]. Most Asian RT 027 *C. difficile* strains investigated to date have not been related to either of the two main epidemic RT 027 lineages referred to as FQR1 and FQR2 [13], and many have been reported as fluoroquinolone-susceptible, unlike the epidemic lineages.

C. difficile RT 078 (CDT+) was reported among eight cases of CDI across three hospitals in China, where it was also isolated from environmental surfaces suggesting nosocomial transmission [72]. RT 078-related strains RT 126 and 127 (both ST11) are more common in Taiwan, where they were the most common CDT+ strains reported from Southern Taiwan between 2011 and 2013 [73]. A subsequent nationwide study from 2015–2016 identified RTs 078, 126 and 127 at significant prevalence among 842 toxigenic isolates (1.5%, 3.1% and 2.9%, respectively), mainly confined to two hospitals [70].

2.4.3. A+B+ *C. difficile* Strains

C. difficile clade 1 strains that are mainly A+B+ are also frequently reported from Asia. RT 018/ST17 is the predominant clade 1 strain found in the region with the earliest reports coming from Japan (referred to as ribotype "smz") [23]. A closely related strain, "smz'"/QX 239/ST17 is now also circulating at high prevalence in Japan [59,60]. RT 018 is now the most common *C. difficile* strain reported from Korea, where it has largely replaced RT 017 [23,74]. RT 012/ST54 and RT 046/ST35 localise to China in particular [75–79], RT 014/020/ST2/14 is widespread across the continent [31], and RT 002/ST8 is most frequently reported from Taiwan and Hong Kong [31,80].

2.4.4. Non-Toxigenic *C. difficile* Strains

A notable aspect of the molecular epidemiology of *C. difficile* in Asia is the high prevalence of non-toxigenic strains, particularly in South-East Asia. In recent studies in Thailand, Indonesia and Malaysia [28,30,35], non-toxigenic strains of *C. difficile*, most commonly RTs 009 and 010, QX 083, QX 002 and QX 083, were isolated at a prevalence of 50% among all study isolates. Further north in Asia, non-toxigenic strains are reported less frequently (24%, Taiwan [70] 8%–11%, China [76,79,81]), however, this may be a reflection of the use of diagnostic methods other than culture, which would not detect non-toxigenic strains. These strains are incapable of causing CDI but can colonise the gut when the normal flora are disrupted due to antimicrobial use. Many group in the predominantly non-toxigenic MLST clade 4 [49]. The high prevalence of RT 017 and non-toxigenic strains [28,30,35] suggests that clade 4 may have evolved in the Asian region, but further studies on non-toxigenic strains both in Asia and elsewhere are required to determine whether this is the case.

The unique molecular epidemiology of *C. difficile* in Asia (described in more detail in Collins et al. [23]), particularly the high prevalence of non-toxigenic strains, likely plays a role in the overall apparently less severe manifestations of disease seen in the region. Therapeutic administration of non-toxigenic *C. difficile* can protect against recurrent CDI [82], which occurs more rarely among Asian patients (9.1% of cases) than elsewhere [31]. Thus, it is highly plausible that the high prevalence of non-toxigenic strains is protective against recurrence and possibly reduces risk of exposure to virulent strains in Asia. However, many non-toxigenic Asian *C. difficile* strains are resistant to multiple antimicrobials, possibly due to inappropriate antimicrobial use in the region, and they may pose a risk in terms of transmission of antimicrobial resistance (AMR) genes. There have been concerning, albeit rare, reports of metronidazole-resistant non-toxigenic strains [79,83], which should be closely monitored in the region.

3. Prevalence and Molecular Epidemiology of *C. difficile* among Production Animals in Asia

3.1. Prevalence of C. difficile Colonisation and Strain Types in Asian Production Animals

While there are few reports on *C. difficile* in animals in Asia, the prevalence appears to be high among production swine across the continent. A study of 120 neonatal piglets in Japan found a prevalence of *C. difficile* of 57.5%; 61.0% of strains were toxigenic [84]. A high prevalence of 19.3% among 910 pigs of all ages across 47 farms has been reported in Korea, with peak prevalence in diarrheic suckling piglets (53.6%) followed by diarrheic sows (40.0%); again, the majority of isolates (86.9%) was toxigenic [85]. In Taiwan, the prevalence of *C. difficile* among 204 pigs on 13 commercial farms was 49% [86]. The only report to date of *C. difficile* among production animals in South-East Asia comes from Thailand, where the prevalence of *C. difficile* was 35% among piglets (*n* = 165), with all 58 isolates reported as non-toxigenic [87]. RT 078 and closely-related strains including RTs 126 and 127 are the most commonly reported toxigenic strains in pigs in Korea (RT 078 86.5%, RT 126 13.5% of toxigenic strains) [85], Taiwan (RT 078 18%, RT 126 28%, RT 127 43% of toxigenic strains) [86] and Japan (RT 078 third most common strain; 19.7% of toxigenic strains) [84], countries where demand for pork and pork products has surged in recent decades.

3.2. Possible International Sources of C. difficile among Asian Production Animals

To date, *C. difficile* RT 078 and related strains RT 126 and 127 have rarely infected humans in Asia apart from in Taiwan [70,73,88] and, given the apparent endemicity of RT 078 among production animals and human infections in mainland Europe and North America, it is plausible that the strain was introduced into northern Asia via live animal imports. Supporting evidence has been reported from Japan; multi-locus variable number tandem repeat analysis (MLVA) found that Japanese piglet isolates clustered with European human and pig RT 078 strains, giving a strong likelihood that they were imported into Japan from Europe via live breeding pig imports [84]. Live breeding pigs and cattle are imported from Europe, Australia and North America to many Asian countries including Japan [89], China, Taiwan, Vietnam, Cambodia, Malaysia and Thailand (ahdb.org.uk). RTs 078 and 127 are common among cattle and pigs in Europe [90] and RTs 126 and 127 are frequently reported in cattle in Australia [91].

C. difficile RT 078 has also been reported in thoroughbred racehorses, which are frequently traded internationally, in Japan. Five cases of postoperative colitis were documented from the same facility, indicating contamination with a single clone [92]. Further analysis using WGS of RT 078 strains from Japanese racehorses identified a sub-lineage associated with a nosocomial outbreak. RT 027 and RT 017 were also reported, with high relatedness to several reported European strains including clinical isolates from Ireland [93], a prolific producer of racehorses.

4. Discussion

4.1. Systematic Testing Is Required to Identify True CDI Cases in Asia

Introduction of systematic, comprehensive testing for CDI across Asia could provide a better understanding of the epidemiology of CDI in the region, particularly accurate measurement of incidence and prevalence, and deepen our understanding of the burden of CDI. While there is still considerable international debate about optimal testing practices for CDI, colonisation rates with both toxigenic and non-toxigenic *C. difficile* among hospital inpatients are particularly high in

South-East Asia. Many Asian countries are popular destinations for "medical tourism" and there is a risk of transmission of strains via medical tourists returning to their own countries after their treatment. Due to the high prevalence of colonization, it is important to use a diagnostic test which will discriminate true cases of CDI from cases of colonization. GDH and toxin EIA can be performed at relatively low cost and will identify most cases of true infection, despite its lower sensitivity, so it may be the best choice currently for Asian laboratories in developing countries.

Given the apparently uniquely high prevalence of non-toxigenic *C. difficile* strains in Asia, particularly in South-East Asia, it is important to monitor colonization as well. The high prevalence suggests that hospital environments may be heavily contaminated due to poor cleaning or hand hygiene, which puts vulnerable patients at higher risk of CDI. Monitoring of *C. difficile* colonization would also allow further investigation of whether non-toxigenic *C. difficile* colonization is protecting Asian patients from developing CDI and reducing their risk of recurrent disease.

4.2. One Health Implications of CDI in Asia

4.2.1. C. difficile in Asian Production Animals Warrants Close Observation

While there are still relatively few reports of *C. difficile* among Asian production animals, and no reports yet of environmental contamination, the prevalence of *C. difficile* among pigs across Asia is markedly high. Given the significantly increasing demands for pork and pork products, particularly in China and Taiwan, biosecurity measures to ensure these meat products do not pose a threat to humans should include monitoring for *C. difficile* contamination. A spatial epidemiology study in the USA identified increased risk of CA-CDI among people living close to livestock farms [94]. China currently holds half the world's pig population in addition to being the most populated country in the world, so there is a significant risk of infection of a substantial population. In Taiwan, the presence of "hypervirulent" RT 078 and related strains among pigs and increasing prevalence of these strains among clinical cases of CDI suggests transmission of strains between pigs and humans has already occurred. This could be confirmed using WGS studies, as described in an Australian study showing clonal relationships between *C. difficile* isolates from human clinical cases and pigs located thousands of kilometres apart [12].

4.2.2. Live Animal Imports and Exports: Plausible International Routes of Transmission of C. difficile

Genotypic studies of pig and racehorse *C. difficile* isolates from Japan are showing a possibly significant international transmission route of *C. difficile* via live animal imports and exports. The international live animal trade market is a growing sector. From a One Health perspective, it is most important to monitor animals traded with the intention of farming for meat production, as these are kept in close quarters and are thus frequently prophylactically treated with antimicrobials to reduce risk of infection and loss of stock.

5. Conclusions

A One Health approach will be important in management and control of CDI in Asia. It is most important to establish comprehensive testing policies, to identify the true incidence of CDI in Asia before being able to implement effective control measures.

References

1.   Moono, P.; Foster, N.F.; Hampson, D.J.; Knight, D.R.; Bloomfield, L.E.; Riley, T.V. *Clostridium difficile* infection in production animals and avian species: A review. *Foodborne Pathog. Dis.* **2016**, *13*, 647–655. [CrossRef]

2. Eglow, R.; Pothoulakis, C.; Itzkowitz, S.; Israel, E.J.; O'Keane, C.J.; Gong, D.; Gao, N.; Xu, Y.L.; Walker, W.A.; LaMont, J.T. Diminished *Clostridium difficile* toxin A sensitivity in newborn rabbit ileum is associated with decreased toxin A receptor. *J. Clin. Investig.* **1992**, *90*, 822–829. [CrossRef] [PubMed]

3. Martin, J.S.; Monaghan, T.M.; Wilcox, M.H. *Clostridium difficile* infection: Epidemiology, diagnosis and understanding transmission. *Nat. Rev. Gastroenterol. Hepatol.* **2016**, *13*, 206–216. [CrossRef] [PubMed]

4. Polage, C.R.; Gyorke, C.E.; Kennedy, M.A.; Leslie, J.L.; Chin, D.L.; Wang, S.; Nguyen, H.H.; Huang, B.; Tang, Y.W.; Lee, L.W.; et al. Overdiagnosis of *Clostridium difficile* infection in the molecular test era. *JAMA Intern. Med.* **2015**, *175*, 1792–1801. [CrossRef] [PubMed]

5. Slimings, C.; Armstrong, P.; Beckingham, W.D.; Bull, A.L.; Hall, L.; Kennedy, K.J.; Marquess, J.; McCann, R.; Menzies, A.; Mitchell, B.G.; et al. Increasing incidence of *Clostridium difficile* infection, Australia, 2011–2012. *Med. J. Aust.* **2014**, *200*, 272–276. [CrossRef] [PubMed]

6. Lessa, F.C.; Mu, Y.; Bamberg, W.M.; Beldavs, Z.G.; Dumyati, G.K.; Dunn, J.R.; Farley, M.M.; Holzbauer, S.M.; Meek, J.I.; Phipps, E.C.; et al. Burden of *Clostridium difficile* infection in the United States. *N. Engl. J. Med.* **2015**, *372*, 825–834. [CrossRef] [PubMed]

7. Eyre, D.W.; Cule, M.L.; Wilson, D.J.; Griffiths, D.; Vaughan, A.; O'Connor, L.; Ip, C.L.; Golubchik, T.; Batty, E.M.; Finney, J.M.; et al. Diverse sources of *C. difficile* infection identified on whole-genome sequencing. *N. Engl. J. Med.* **2013**, *369*, 1195–1205. [CrossRef]

8. Van Boeckel, T.P.; Brower, C.; Gilbert, M.; Grenfell, B.T.; Levin, S.A.; Robinson, T.P.; Teillant, A.; Laxminarayan, R. Global trends in antimicrobial use in food animals. *Proc. Natl. Acad. Sci. USA* **2015**, *112*, 5649–5654. [CrossRef]

9. Moono, P.; Lim, S.C.; Riley, T.V. High prevalence of toxigenic *Clostridium difficile* in public space lawns in Western Australia. *Sci. Rep.* **2017**, *7*, 41196. [CrossRef]

10. Lim, S.C.; Androga, G.O.; Knight, D.R.; Moono, P.; Foster, N.F.; Riley, T.V. Antimicrobial susceptibility of *Clostridium difficile* isolated from food and environmental sources in Western Australia. *Int. J. Antimicrob. Agents* **2018**, *52*, 411–415. [CrossRef]

11. Lim, S.C.; Foster, N.F.; Elliott, B.; Riley, T.V. High prevalence of *Clostridium difficile* on retail root vegetables, Western Australia. *J. Appl. Microbiol.* **2018**, *124*, 585–590. [CrossRef] [PubMed]

12. Knight, D.R.; Squire, M.M.; Collins, D.A.; Riley, T.V. Genome analysis of *Clostridium difficile* PCR ribotype 014 lineage in Australian pigs and humans reveals a diverse genetic repertoire and signatures of long-range interspecies transmission. *Front. Microbiol.* **2017**, *7*, 2138. [CrossRef] [PubMed]

13. He, M.; Miyajima, F.; Roberts, P.; Ellison, L.; Pickard, D.J.; Martin, M.J.; Connor, T.R.; Harris, S.R.; Fairley, D.; Bamford, K.B.; et al. Emergence and global spread of epidemic healthcare-associated *Clostridium difficile*. *Nat. Genet.* **2013**, *45*, 109–113. [CrossRef] [PubMed]

14. al-Barrak, A.; Embil, J.; Dyck, B.; Olekson, K.; Nicoll, D.; Alfa, M.; Kabani, A. An outbreak of toxin A negative, toxin B positive *Clostridium difficile*-associated diarrhea in a Canadian tertiary-care hospital. *Can. Commun. Dis. Rep.* **1999**, *25*, 65–69. [PubMed]

15. Kuijper, E.J.; de Weerdt, J.; Kato, H.; Kato, N.; van Dam, A.P.; van der Vorm, E.R.; Weel, J.; van Rheenen, C.; Dankert, J. Nosocomial outbreak of *Clostridium difficile*-associated diarrhoea due to a clindamycin-resistant enterotoxin A-negative strain. *Eur. J. Clin. Microbiol. Infect. Dis.* **2001**, *20*, 528–534. [CrossRef] [PubMed]

16. Drudy, D.; Harnedy, N.; Fanning, S.; Hannan, M.; Kyne, L. Emergence and control of fluoroquinolone-resistant, toxin A-negative, toxin B-positive *Clostridium difficile*. *Infect. Control. Hosp. Epidemiol.* **2007**, *28*, 932–940. [CrossRef]

17. Cairns, M.D.; Preston, M.D.; Hall, C.L.; Gerding, D.N.; Hawkey, P.M.; Kato, H.; Kim, H.; Kuijper, E.J.; Lawley, T.D.; Pituch, H.; et al. Comparative genome analysis and global phylogeny of the toxin variant *Clostridium difficile* PCR ribotype 017 reveals the evolution of two independent sublineages. *J. Clin. Microbiol.* **2017**, *55*, 865–876. [CrossRef]

18. Centers for Disease Control and Prevention (CDC). *Antibiotic Resistance Threats in the United States, 2013*; CDC: Atlanta, GA, USA, 2013.

19. Bauer, M.P.; Notermans, D.W.; van Benthem, B.H.; Brazier, J.S.; Wilcox, M.H.; Rupnik, M.; Monnet, D.L.; van Dissel, J.T.; Kuijper, E.J.; ECDIS Study Group. *Clostridium difficile* infection in Europe: A hospital-based survey. *Lancet* **2011**, *377*, 63–73. [CrossRef]

20. Tickler, I.A.; Goering, R.V.; Whitmore, J.D.; Lynn, A.N.; Persing, D.H.; Tenover, F.C.; Healthcare Associated Infection Consortium. Strain types and antimicrobial resistance patterns of *Clostridium difficile* isolates from the United States, 2011 to 2013. *Antimicrob. Agents Chemother.* **2014**, *58*, 4214–4218. [CrossRef]

21. Freeman, J.; Vernon, J.; Morris, K.; Nicholson, S.; Todhunter, S.; Longshaw, C.; Wilcox, M.H.; Pan-European Longitudinal Surveillance of Antibiotic Resistance among Prevalent *Clostridium difficile* Ribotypes' Study Group. Pan-European longitudinal surveillance of antibiotic resistance among prevalent *Clostridium difficile* ribotypes. *Clin. Microbiol. Infect.* **2015**, *21*, 248.e9–248.e16. [CrossRef]

22. Collins, D.A.; Putsathit, P.; Elliott, B.; Riley, T.V. Laboratory-based surveillance of *Clostridium difficile* strains circulating in the Australian healthcare setting in 2012. *Pathology* **2017**, *49*, 309–313. [CrossRef] [PubMed]

23. Collins, D.A.; Hawkey, P.M.; Riley, T.V. Epidemiology of *Clostridium difficile* infection in Asia. *Antimicrob. Resist. Infect. Control* **2013**, *2*, 21. [CrossRef] [PubMed]

24. Larsen, J. China's Growing Hunger for Meat Shown by Move to Buy Smithfield, World's Leading Pork Producer. In *Data Highlights*; Earth Policy Institute: Washington, DC, USA, 2013.

25. Van Boeckel, T.P.; Gandra, S.; Ashok, A.; Caudron, Q.; Grenfell, B.T.; Levin, S.A.; Laxminarayan, R. Global antibiotic consumption 2000 to 2010: An analysis of national pharmaceutical sales data. *Lancet Infect. Dis.* **2014**, *14*, 742–750. [CrossRef]

26. McDonald, L.C.; Gerding, D.N.; Johnson, S.; Bakken, J.S.; Carroll, K.C.; Coffin, S.E.; Dubberke, E.R.; Garey, K.W.; Gould, C.V.; Kelly, C.; et al. Clinical practice guidelines for *Clostridium difficile* infection in adults and children: 2017 update by the Infectious Diseases Society of America (IDSA) and Society for Healthcare Epidemiology of America (SHEA). *Clin. Infect. Dis.* **2018**, *66*, e1–e48. [CrossRef] [PubMed]

27. Borren, N.Z.; Ghadermarzi, S.; Hutfless, S.; Ananthakrishnan, A.N. The emergence of *Clostridium difficile* infection in Asia: A systematic review and meta-analysis of incidence and impact. *PLoS ONE* **2017**, *12*, e0176797. [CrossRef] [PubMed]

28. Collins, D.A.; Gasem, M.H.; Habibie, T.H.; Arinton, I.G.; Hendriyanto, P.; Hartana, A.P.; Riley, T.V. Prevalence and molecular epidemiology of *Clostridium difficile* infection in Indonesia. *New Microbe New Infect.* **2017**, *18*, 34–37. [CrossRef] [PubMed]

29. Riley, T.V.; Collins, D.A.; Karunakaran, R.; Kahar, M.A.; Adnan, A.; Hassan, S.A.; Zainul, N.H.; Rustam, F.R.M.; Wahab, Z.A.; Ramli, R.; et al. High prevalence of toxigenic and nontoxigenic *Clostridium difficile* strains in Malaysia. *J. Clin. Microbiol.* **2018**, *56*. [CrossRef]

30. Putsathit, P.; Maneerattanaporn, M.; Piewngam, P.; Kiratisin, P.; Riley, T.V. Prevalence and molecular epidemiology of *Clostridium difficile* infection in Thailand. *New Microbe New Infect.* **2017**, *15*, 27–32. [CrossRef]

31. Collins, D.A.; Sohn, K.M.; Wu, Y.; Ouchi, K.; Ishii, Y.; Elliott, B.; Riley, T.V.; Tateda, K.; for the Clostridium difficile Asia Pacific (CDAP) Study Group. Clostridium difficile infection in the Asia-Pacific region. In Proceedings of the 27th European Congress of Clinical Microbiology and Infectious Diseases, Vienna, Austria, 22–25 April 2017.

32. Lim, P.L.; Barkham, T.M.; Ling, L.M.; Dimatatac, F.; Alfred, T.; Ang, B. Increasing incidence of *Clostridium difficile*-associated disease, Singapore. *Emerg. Infect. Dis.* **2008**, *14*, 1487–1489. [CrossRef]

33. Hsu, L.Y.; Tan, T.Y.; Koh, T.H.; Kwa, A.L.; Krishnan, P.; Tee, N.W.; Jureen, R. Decline in *Clostridium difficile*-associated disease rates in Singapore public hospitals, 2006 to 2008. *BMC Res. Notes* **2011**, *4*, 77. [CrossRef]

34. Warren, C.A.; Labio, E.; Destura, R.; Sevilleja, J.E.; Jamias, J.D.; Daez, M.L. *Clostridium difficile* and *Entamoeba histolytica* infections in patients with colitis in the Philippines. *Trans. R. Soc. Trop. Med. Hyg.* **2012**, *106*, 424–428. [CrossRef] [PubMed]

35. Zainul, N.H.; Ma, Z.F.; Besari, A.; Siti Asma, H.; Rahman, R.A.; Collins, D.A.; Hamid, N.; Riley, T.V.; Lee, Y.Y. Prevalence of *Clostridium difficile* infection and colonization in a tertiary hospital and elderly community of North-Eastern Peninsular Malaysia. *Epidemiol. Infect.* **2017**, *145*, 3012–3019. [CrossRef] [PubMed]

36. Shin, B.M.; Kuak, E.Y.; Yoo, S.J.; Shin, W.C.; Yoo, H.M. Emerging toxin A-B+ variant strain of *Clostridium difficile* responsible for pseudomembranous colitis at a tertiary care hospital in Korea. *Diagn. Microbiol. Infect. Dis.* **2008**, *60*, 333–337. [CrossRef] [PubMed]

37. Shin, J.Y.; Ko, E.J.; Lee, S.H.; Shin, J.B.; Kim, S.I.; Kwon, K.S.; Kim, H.G.; Shin, Y.W.; Bang, B.W. Refractory pseudomembranous colitis that was treated successfully with colonoscopic fecal microbial transplantation. *Intest. Res.* **2016**, *14*, 83–88. [CrossRef] [PubMed]

38. Nishimura, S.; Kou, T.; Kato, H.; Watanabe, M.; Uno, S.; Senoh, M.; Fukuda, T.; Hata, A.; Yazumi, S. Fulminant pseudomembranous colitis caused by *Clostridium difficile* PCR ribotype 027 in a healthy young woman in Japan. *J. Infect. Chemother.* **2014**, *20*, 729–731. [CrossRef] [PubMed]

39. Wang, J.; Xiao, Y.; Lin, K.; Song, F.; Ge, T.; Zhang, T. Pediatric severe pseudomembranous enteritis treated with fecal microbiota transplantation in a 13-month-old infant. *Biomed. Rep.* **2015**, *3*, 173–175. [CrossRef] [PubMed]

40. Toyokawa, M.; Ueda, A.; Tsukamoto, H.; Nishi, I.; Horikawa, M.; Sunada, A.; Asari, S. Pseudomembranous colitis caused by toxin A-negative/toxin B-positive variant strain of *Clostridium difficile*. *J. Infect. Chemother.* **2003**, *9*, 351–354. [CrossRef]

41. Chen, T.C.; Lu, P.L.; Lin, W.R.; Lin, C.Y.; Wu, J.Y.; Chen, Y.H. Rifampin-associated pseudomembranous colitis. *Am. J. Med. Sci.* **2009**, *338*, 156–158. [CrossRef]

42. Huang, S.C.; Yang, Y.J.; Lee, C.T. Rectal prolapse in a child: An unusual presentation of *Clostridium difficile*-associated pseudomembranous colitis. *Pediatr. Neonatol.* **2011**, *52*, 110–112. [CrossRef]

43. Shen, B.J.; Lin, S.C.; Shueng, P.W.; Chou, Y.H.; Tseng, L.M.; Hsieh, C.H. Pseudomembranous colitis within radiotherapy field following concurrent chemoradiation therapy: A case report. *Onco Targets Ther.* **2013**, *6*, 25–28. [CrossRef]

44. Ryu, H.S.; Kim, Y.S.; Seo, G.S.; Lee, Y.M.; Choi, S.C. Risk factors for recurrent *Clostridium difficile* infection. *Intest. Res.* **2012**, *10*, 176–182. [CrossRef]

45. Choi, H.K.; Kim, K.H.; Lee, S.H.; Lee, S.J. Risk factors for recurrence of *Clostridium difficile* infection: Effect of vancomycin-resistant Enterococci colonization. *J. Korean Med. Sci.* **2011**, *26*, 859–864. [CrossRef] [PubMed]

46. Ho, J.; Dai, R.Z.W.; Kwong, T.N.Y.; Wang, X.; Zhang, L.; Ip, M.; Chan, R.; Hawkey, P.M.K.; Lam, K.L.Y.; Wong, M.C.S.; et al. Disease burden of *Clostridium difficile* infections in adults, Hong Kong, China, 2006–2014. *Emerg. Infect. Dis.* **2017**, *23*, 1671–1679. [CrossRef] [PubMed]

47. Eyre, D.W.; Walker, A.S.; Wyllie, D.; Dingle, K.E.; Griffiths, D.; Finney, J.; O'Connor, L.; Vaughan, A.; Crook, D.W.; Wilcox, M.H.; et al. Predictors of first recurrence of *Clostridium difficile* infection: Implications for initial management. *Clin. Infect. Dis.* **2012**, *55*, S77–S87. [CrossRef] [PubMed]

48. Dingle, K.E.; Elliott, B.; Robinson, E.; Griffiths, D.; Eyre, D.W.; Stoesser, N.; Vaughan, A.; Golubchik, T.; Fawley, W.N.; Wilcox, M.H.; et al. Evolutionary history of the *Clostridium difficile* pathogenicity locus. *Genome Biol. Evol.* **2014**, *6*, 36–52. [CrossRef] [PubMed]

49. Stabler, R.A.; Dawson, L.F.; Valiente, E.; Cairns, M.D.; Martin, M.J.; Donahue, E.H.; Riley, T.V.; Songer, J.G.; Kuijper, E.J.; Dingle, K.E.; et al. Macro and micro diversity of *Clostridium difficile* isolates from diverse sources and geographical locations. *PLoS ONE* **2012**, *7*, e31559. [CrossRef] [PubMed]

50. Putsathit, P.; Kiratisin, P.; Ngamwongsatit, P.; Riley, T.V. *Clostridium difficile* infection in Thailand. *Int. J. Antimicrob. Agents* **2015**, *45*, 1–7. [CrossRef]

51. Huang, H.; Weintraub, A.; Fang, H.; Wu, S.; Zhang, Y.; Nord, C.E. Antimicrobial susceptibility and heteroresistance in Chinese *Clostridium difficile* strains. *Anaerobe* **2010**, *16*, 633–635. [CrossRef]

52. Kim, H.; Jeong, S.H.; Roh, K.H.; Hong, S.G.; Kim, J.W.; Shin, M.G.; Kim, M.N.; Shin, H.B.; Uh, Y.; Lee, H.; et al. Investigation of toxin gene diversity, molecular epidemiology, and antimicrobial resistance of *Clostridium difficile* isolated from 12 hospitals in South Korea. *Korean J. Lab. Med.* **2010**, *30*, 491–497. [CrossRef]

53. Kim, S.J.; Kim, H.; Seo, Y.; Yong, D.; Jeong, S.H.; Chong, Y.; Lee, K. Molecular characterization of toxin A-negative, toxin B-positive variant strains of *Clostridium difficile* isolated in Korea. *Diagn Microbiol. Infect. Dis.* **2010**, *67*, 198–201. [CrossRef] [PubMed]

54. Huang, H.; Wu, S.; Wang, M.; Zhang, Y.; Fang, H.; Palmgren, A.C.; Weintraub, A.; Nord, C.E. Molecular and clinical characteristics of *Clostridium difficile* infection in a University Hospital in Shanghai, China. *Clin. Infect. Dis.* **2008**, *47*, 1606–1608. [CrossRef] [PubMed]

55. Tan, X.Q.; Verrall, A.J.; Jureen, R.; Riley, T.V.; Collins, D.A.; Lin, R.T.; Balm, M.N.; Chan, D.; Tambyah, P.A. The emergence of community-onset *Clostridium difficile* infection in a tertiary hospital in Singapore: A cause for concern. *Int. J. Antimicrob. Agents* **2014**, *43*, 47–51. [CrossRef] [PubMed]

56. Ngamskulrungroj, P.; Sanmee, S.; Putsathit, P.; Piewngam, P.; Elliott, B.; Riley, T.V.; Kiratisin, P. Molecular epidemiology of *Clostridium difficile* infection in a large teaching hospital in Thailand. *PLoS ONE* **2015**, *10*, e0127026. [CrossRef]

57. Komatsu, M.; Kato, H.; Aihara, M.; Shimakawa, K.; Iwasaki, M.; Nagasaka, Y.; Fukuda, S.; Matsuo, S.; Arakawa, Y.; Watanabe, M.; et al. High frequency of antibiotic-associated diarrhea due to toxin A-negative, toxin B-positive *Clostridium difficile* in a hospital in Japan and risk factors for infection. *Eur. J. Clin. Microbiol. Infect. Dis.* **2003**, *22*, 525–529. [CrossRef] [PubMed]

58. Alfa, M.J.; Kabani, A.; Lyerly, D.; Moncrief, S.; Neville, L.M.; Al-Barrak, A.; Harding, G.K.; Dyck, B.; Olekson, K.; Embil, J.M. Characterization of a toxin A-negative, toxin B-positive strain of *Clostridium difficile* responsible for a nosocomial outbreak of *Clostridium difficile*-associated diarrhea. *J. Clin. Microbiol.* **2000**, *38*, 2706–2714. [PubMed]

59. Mori, N.; Yoshizawa, S.; Saga, T.; Ishii, Y.; Murakami, H.; Iwata, M.; Collins, D.A.; Riley, T.V.; Tateda, K. Incorrect diagnosis of *Clostridium difficile* infection in a university hospital in Japan. *J. Infect. Chemother.* **2015**, *21*, 718–722. [CrossRef] [PubMed]

60. Senoh, M.; Kato, H.; Fukuda, T.; Niikawa, A.; Hori, Y.; Hagiya, H.; Ito, Y.; Miki, H.; Abe, Y.; Furuta, K.; et al. Predominance of PCR-ribotypes, 018 (smz) and 369 (trf) of *Clostridium difficile* in Japan: A potential relationship with other global circulating strains? *J. Med. Microbiol.* **2015**, *64*, 1226–1236. [CrossRef]

61. Iwashima, Y.; Nakamura, A.; Kato, H.; Kato, H.; Wakimoto, Y.; Wakiyama, N.; Kaji, C.; Ueda, R. A retrospective study of the epidemiology of *Clostridium difficile* infection at a university hospital in Japan: Genotypic features of the isolates and clinical characteristics of the patients. *J. Infect. Chemother.* **2010**, *16*, 329–333. [CrossRef]

62. Sato, H.; Kato, H.; Koiwai, K.; Sakai, C. [A nosocomial outbreak of diarrhea caused by toxin A-negative, toxin B-positive *Clostridium difficile* in a cancer center hospital]. *Kansenshogaku Zasshi* **2004**, *78*, 312–319. [CrossRef]

63. Wang, B.; Peng, W.; Zhang, P.; Su, J. The characteristics of *Clostridium difficile* ST81, a new PCR ribotype of toxin A- B+ strain with high-level fluoroquinolones resistance and higher sporulation ability than ST37/PCR ribotype 017. *FEMS Microbiol. Lett.* **2018**, *365*. [CrossRef]

64. Qin, J.; Dai, Y.; Ma, X.; Wang, Y.; Gao, Q.; Lu, H.; Li, T.; Meng, H.; Liu, Q.; Li, M. Nosocomial transmission of *Clostridium difficile* genotype ST81 in a general teaching hospital in China traced by whole genome sequencing. *Sci. Rep.* **2017**, *7*, 9627. [CrossRef] [PubMed]

65. Loo, V.G.; Poirier, L.; Miller, M.A.; Oughton, M.; Libman, M.D.; Michaud, S.; Bourgault, A.M.; Nguyen, T.; Frenette, C.; Kelly, M.; et al. A predominantly clonal multi-institutional outbreak of *Clostridium difficile*-associated diarrhea with high morbidity and mortality. *N. Engl. J. Med.* **2005**, *353*, 2442–2449. [CrossRef]

66. Eyre, D.W.; Tracey, L.; Elliott, B.; Slimings, C.; Huntington, P.G.; Stuart, R.L.; Korman, T.M.; Kotsiou, G.; McCann, R.; Griffiths, D.; et al. Emergence and spread of predominantly community-onset *Clostridium difficile* PCR ribotype 244 infection in Australia, 2010 to 2012. *Euro Surveill.* **2015**, *20*, 21059. [CrossRef] [PubMed]

67. Collins, D.A.; Riley, T.V. *Clostridium difficile* guidelines. *Clin. Infect. Dis.* **2018**, *67*, 1639. [CrossRef]

68. Jia, H.; Du, P.; Yang, H.; Zhang, Y.; Wang, J.; Zhang, W.; Han, G.; Han, N.; Yao, Z.; Wang, H.; et al. Nosocomial transmission of *Clostridium difficile* ribotype 027 in a Chinese hospital, 2012–2014, traced by whole genome sequencing. *BMC Genom.* **2016**, *17*, 405. [CrossRef] [PubMed]

69. Kim, H.; Lee, Y.; Moon, H.W.; Lim, C.S.; Lee, K.; Chong, Y. Emergence of *Clostridium difficile* ribotype 027 in Korea. *Korean J. Lab. Med.* **2011**, *31*, 191–196. [CrossRef] [PubMed]

70. Hung, Y.P.; Tsai, P.J.; Lee, Y.T.; Tang, H.J.; Lin, H.J.; Liu, H.C.; Lee, J.C.; Tsai, B.Y.; Hsueh, P.R.; Ko, W.C. Nationwide surveillance of ribotypes and antimicrobial susceptibilities of toxigenic *Clostridium difficile* isolates with an emphasis on reduced doxycycline and tigecycline susceptibilities among ribotype 078 lineage isolates in Taiwan. *Infect. Drug Resist.* **2018**, *11*, 1197–1203. [CrossRef]

71. Hung, Y.P.; Cia, C.T.; Tsai, B.Y.; Chen, P.C.; Lin, H.J.; Liu, H.C.; Lee, J.C.; Wu, Y.H.; Tsai, P.J.; Ko, W.C. The first case of severe *Clostridium difficile* ribotype 027 infection in Taiwan. *J. Infect.* **2015**, *70*, 98–101. [CrossRef]

72. Jin, H.; Ni, K.; Wei, L.; Shen, L.; Xu, H.; Kong, Q.; Ni, X. Identification of *Clostridium difficile* RT078 from patients and environmental surfaces in Zhejiang Province, China. *Infect. Control Hosp. Epidemiol.* **2016**, *37*, 745–746. [CrossRef]

73. Hung, Y.P.; Huang, I.H.; Lin, H.J.; Tsai, B.Y.; Liu, H.C.; Liu, H.C.; Lee, J.C.; Wu, Y.H.; Tsai, P.J.; Ko, W.C. Predominance of *Clostridium difficile* ribotypes 017 and 078 among toxigenic clinical isolates in southern Taiwan. *PLoS ONE* **2016**, *11*, e0166159. [CrossRef]

74. Seo, M.R.; Kim, J.; Lee, Y.; Lim, D.G.; Pai, H. Prevalence, genetic relatedness and antibiotic resistance of hospital-acquired *Clostridium difficile* PCR ribotype 018 strains. *Int. J. Antimicrob. Agents* **2018**, *51*, 762–767. [CrossRef] [PubMed]

75. Cheng, J.-W.; Xiao, M.; Kudinha, T.; Kong, F.; Xu, Z.-P.; Sun, L.-Y.; Zhang, L.; Fan, X.; Xie, X.-L.; Xu, Y.-C. Molecular epidemiology and antimicrobial susceptibility of *Clostridium difficile* isolates from a university teaching hospital in China. *Front. Microbiol.* **2016**, *7*, 1621. [CrossRef] [PubMed]

76. Chen, Y.B.; Gu, S.L.; Wei, Z.Q.; Shen, P.; Kong, H.S.; Yang, Q.; Li, L.J. Molecular epidemiology of *Clostridium difficile* in a tertiary hospital of China. *J. Med. Microbiol.* **2014**, *63*, 562–569. [CrossRef] [PubMed]

77. Wang, B.; Lv, Z.; Zhang, P.; Su, J. Molecular epidemiology and antimicrobial susceptibility of human *Clostridium difficile* isolates from a single institution in Northern China. *Medicine* **2018**, *97*, e11219. [CrossRef] [PubMed]

78. Tian, T.T.; Zhao, J.H.; Yang, J.; Qiang, C.X.; Li, Z.R.; Chen, J.; Xu, K.Y.; Ciu, Q.Q.; Li, R.X. Molecular characterization of *Clostridium difficile* isolates from human subjects and the environment. *PLoS ONE* **2016**, *11*, e0151964. [CrossRef] [PubMed]

79. Jin, D.; Luo, Y.; Huang, C.; Cai, J.; Ye, J.; Zheng, Y.; Wang, L.; Zhao, P.; Liu, A.; Fang, W.; et al. Molecular epidemiology of *Clostridium difficile* infection in hospitalized patients in Eastern China. *J. Clin. Microbiol.* **2017**, *55*, 801–810. [CrossRef] [PubMed]

80. Cheng, V.C.; Yam, W.C.; Lam, O.T.; Tsang, J.L.; Tse, E.Y.; Siu, G.K.; Chan, J.F.; Tse, H.; To, K.K.; Tai, J.W.; et al. *Clostridium difficile* isolates with increased sporulation: Emergence of PCR ribotype 002 in Hong Kong. *Eur. J. Clin. Microbiol. Infect. Dis.* **2011**, *30*, 1371–1381. [CrossRef]

81. Gao, Q.; Wu, S.; Huang, H.; Ni, Y.; Chen, Y.; Hu, Y.; Yu, Y. Toxin profiles, PCR ribotypes and resistance patterns of *Clostridium difficile*: A multicentre study in China, 2012–2013. *Int. J. Antimicrob. Agents* **2016**, *48*, 736–739. [CrossRef]

82. Gerding, D.N.; Meyer, T.; Lee, C.; Cohen, S.H.; Murthy, U.K.; Poirier, A.; Van Schooneveld, T.C.; Pardi, D.S.; Ramos, A.; Barron, M.A.; et al. Administration of spores of nontoxigenic *Clostridium difficile* strain M3 for prevention of recurrent *C. difficile* infection: A randomized clinical trial. *JAMA* **2015**, *313*, 1719–1727. [CrossRef]

83. Moura, I.; Spigaglia, P.; Barbanti, F.; Mastrantonio, P. Analysis of metronidazole susceptibility in different *Clostridium difficile* PCR ribotypes. *J. Antimicrob. Chemother.* **2013**, *68*, 362–365. [CrossRef]

84. Usui, M.; Nanbu, Y.; Oka, K.; Takahashi, M.; Inamatsu, T.; Asai, T.; Kamiya, S.; Tamura, Y. Genetic relatedness between Japanese and European isolates of *Clostridium difficile* originating from piglets and their risk associated with human health. *Front. Microbiol.* **2014**, *5*, 513. [CrossRef] [PubMed]

85. Kim, H.Y.; Cho, A.; Kim, J.W.; Kim, H.; Kim, B. High prevalence of *Clostridium difficile* PCR ribotype 078 in pigs in Korea. *Anaerobe* **2018**, *51*, 42–46. [CrossRef]

86. Wu, Y.C.; Lee, J.J.; Tsai, B.Y.; Liu, Y.F.; Chen, C.M.; Tien, N.; Tsai, P.J.; Chen, T.H. Potentially hypervirulent *Clostridium difficile* PCR ribotype 078 lineage isolates in pigs and possible implications for humans in Taiwan. *Int. J. Med. Microbiol.* **2016**, *306*, 115–122. [CrossRef] [PubMed]

87. Putsathit, P.; Ngamwongsatit, B.; Riley, T.V. Epidemiology and antimicrobial susceptibility of Clostridium difficile in piglets in Thailand. In Proceedings of the 6th International Clostridium difficile Symposium, Bled, Slovenia, 12–14 September 2018.

88. Hung, Y.P.; Lin, H.J.; Tsai, B.Y.; Liu, H.C.; Liu, H.C.; Lee, J.C.; Wu, Y.H.; Wilcox, M.H.; Fawley, W.N.; Hsueh, P.R.; et al. *Clostridium difficile* ribotype 126 in southern Taiwan: A cluster of three symptomatic cases. *Anaerobe* **2014**, *30*, 188–192. [CrossRef] [PubMed]

89. Baba, K.; Ishihara, K.; Ozawa, M.; Tamura, Y.; Asai, T. Isolation of meticillin-resistant *Staphylococcus aureus* (MRSA) from swine in Japan. *Int. J. Antimicrob. Agents* **2010**, *36*, 352–354. [CrossRef] [PubMed]

90. Spigaglia, P.; Drigo, I.; Barbanti, F.; Mastrantonio, P.; Bano, L.; Bacchin, C.; Puiatti, C.; Tonon, E.; Berto, G.; Agnoletti, F. Antibiotic resistance patterns and PCR-ribotyping of *Clostridium difficile* strains isolated from swine and dogs in Italy. *Anaerobe* **2015**, *31*, 42–46. [CrossRef]

91. Knight, D.R.; Putsathit, P.; Elliott, B.; Riley, T.V. Contamination of Australian newborn calf carcasses at slaughter with *Clostridium difficile*. *Clin. Microbiol. Infect.* **2016**, *22*, 266.e1–266.e7. [CrossRef]

92. Niwa, H.; Kato, H.; Hobo, S.; Kinoshita, Y.; Ueno, T.; Katayama, Y.; Hariu, K.; Oku, K.; Senoh, M.; Kuroda, T.; et al. Postoperative *Clostridium difficile* infection with PCR ribotype 078 strain identified at necropsy in five Thoroughbred racehorses. *Vet. Rec.* **2013**, *173*, 607. [CrossRef]

93. Niwa, H.; Sekizuka, T.; Kuroda, M.; Uchida, E.; Kinoshita, Y.; Katayama, Y.; Senoh, M.; Kato, H. Whole-genome analysis of Clostridioides difficile strains isolated from horses in Japan. In Proceedings of the 6th International Clostridium difficile Symposium, Bled, Slovenia, 12–14 September 2018.

94. Anderson, D.J.; Rojas, L.F.; Watson, S.; Knelson, L.P.; Pruitt, S.; Lewis, S.S.; Moehring, R.W.; Sickbert Bennett, E.E.; Weber, D.J.; Chen, L.F.; et al. Identification of novel risk factors for community-acquired *Clostridium difficile* infection using spatial statistics and geographic information system analyses. *PLoS ONE* **2017**, *12*, e0176285. [CrossRef]

Permissions

List of Contributors

Andrea Reiss, Keren Cox-Witton and Tiggy Grillo
Wildlife Health Australia, Mosman, NSW 2088, Australia

Rupert Woods
Wildlife Health Australia, Mosman, NSW 2088, Australia
World Organisation for Animal Health Working
Group on Wildlife, 75017 Paris, France

Andrew Peters
School of Animal and Veterinary Sciences, E. H.
Graham Centre for Agricultural Innovation, Charles
Sturt University, Boorooma St, Wagga Wagga, New
South Wales 2678, Australia

**Katherine A. Willard, Jacob T. Alston and Marissa
Acciani**
Department of Infectious Diseases, College of Veterinary
Medicine, University of Georgia, Athens, GA 30602, USA

Melinda A. Brindley
Department of Infectious Diseases, Department
of Population Health, Center for Vaccines and
Immunology, College of Veterinary Medicine,
University of Georgia, Athens, GA 30602, USA

**Andrew F. van den Hurk, Alyssa T. Pyke and Sonja
Hall-Mendelin**
Public Health Virology, Forensic and Scientific Services,
Department of Health, Queensland Government,
Archerfield, QLD 4108, Australia

John S. Mackenzie
Faculty of Medical Sciences, Curtin University, and
Division of Microbiology and Infectious Diseases,
PathWest, Locked Bag 2009, Nedlands, WA 6909,
Australia

Scott A. Ritchie
College of Public Health, Medical and Veterinary
Sciences, and Australian Institute of Tropical Health
and Medicine, James Cook University, Cairns, QLD
4870, Australia

Kavita M. Berger and Margaret Rush
Gryphon Scientific, LLC, 6930 Carroll Avenue, Suite
810, Takoma Park, MD 20912, USA

James L. N. Wood
Disease Dynamics Unit, Department of Veterinary
Medicine, University of Cambridge, Madingley Road,
Cambridge CB3 0ES, UK

Bonnie Jenkins
Brookings Institution, 1775 Massachusetts Avenue
NW, Washington, DC 20036, USA

Women of Color Advancing Peace, Security and
Conflict Transformation, 3695 Ketchum Court,
Woodbridge, VA 22193, USA

Jennifer Olsen
Rosalynn Carter Institute for Caregiving, Georgia
Southwestern State University, 800 GSW State
University Drive, Americus, GA 31709, USA

Stephen S. Morse
Department of Epidemiology, Mailman School of
Public Health, Columbia University, 722 West 168th
St, New York, NY 10032, USA

Louise Gresham
Ending Pandemics and San Diego State University,
San Diego, CA 92182, USA

J. Jeffrey Root
U.S. Department of Agriculture, National Wildlife
Research Center, Fort Collins, CO 80521, USA

David Pigott
Institute for Health Metrics and Evaluation, Department
of Health Metrics Sciences, University of Washington,
2301 Fifth Avenue, Suite 600, Seattle, WA 98121, USA
Wellcome Centre for Human Genetics, Nuffield
Department of Medicine, University of Oxford,
Roosevelt Drive, Oxford OX3 7BN, UK

Taylor Winkleman
Next Generation Global Health Security Network,
Washington, DC 20001, USA

Melinda Moore
RAND Corporation, 1200 South Hayes St., Arlington,
VA 22202, USA

James N. Mills
Population Biology, Ecology, and Evolution Program,
Emory University, Atlanta, GA 30322, USA

Thomas R. Gillespie
Population Biology, Ecology, and Evolution Program,
Emory University, Atlanta, GA 30322, USA
Department of Environmental Health, Rollins School
of Public Health, 1518 Clifton Road, Atlanta, GA
30322, USA

Jennifer B. Nuzzo
Center for Health Security, Johns Hopkins University
School of Public Health, Pratt Street, Baltimore, MD
21202, USA

Barbara A. Han
Cary Institute of Ecosystem Studies, Box AB Millbrook, NY 12545, USA

Patricia Olinger
Environmental, Health and Safety Office (EHSO), Emory University, 1762 Clifton Rd., Suite 1200, Atlanta, GA 30322, USA

William B. Karesh
EcoHealth Alliance, 460 West 34th Street, New York, NY 10001, USA

Joseph F. Annelli
Practical One Health Solutions, LLC, New Market, MD 21774, USA

Jamie Barnabei
Plum Island Animal Disease Center, Department of Homeland Security, Greenport, NY 11944, USA

Daniel Lucey
Department of Medicine Infectious Disease, Georgetown University, 600 New Jersey Avenue, NW Washington, DC 20001, USA

David T. S. Hayman
EpiLab, Infectious Disease Research Centre, School of Veterinary Science, Massey University, Private Bag, 11 222, Palmerston North 4442, New Zealand

María Eugenia Loureiro, Alejandra D'Antuono and Nora López
Centro de Virología Animal (CEVAN), CONICET-SENASA, Av Sir Alexander Fleming 1653, Martínez, Provincia de Buenos Aires B1640CSI, Argentina

Aminul Islam, John Stenos and Gemma Vincent
Australian Rickettsial Reference Laboratory, University Hospital Geelong, Geelong, VIC 3220, Australia

Stephen Graves
Australian Rickettsial Reference Laboratory, University Hospital Geelong, Geelong, VIC 3220, Australia
New South Wales Health Pathology, Nepean Hospital, Penrith, NSW 2751, Australia

Anna George
Centre on Global Health Security, Chatham House, London SW1Y 4LE, UK
Public Policy and International Affairs, Murdoch University, Murdoch, WA 6150, Australia

Christopher M. Ziegler, Philip Eisenhauer and Emily A. Bruce
Department of Medicine, Division of Immunobiology, University of Vermont, Burlington, VT 05405, USA

Inessa Manuelyan
Department of Medicine, Division of Immunobiology, University of Vermont, Burlington, VT 05405, USA
Cellular, Molecular and Biomedical Sciences Graduate Program, University of Vermont, Burlington, VT 05405, USA

Marion E. Weir and Bryan A. Ballif
Department of Biology, University of Vermont, Burlington, VT 05405, USA

Jason Botten
Department of Medicine, Division of Immunobiology, University of Vermont, Burlington, VT 05405, USA
Department of Microbiology and Molecular Genetics, University of Vermont, Burlington, VT 05405, USA

Peter Jolly, Nelly Marquetoux and Joanna McKenzie
School of Veterinary Science, Massey University, Palmerston North 4442, New Zealand

Kezang Dorji
School of Veterinary Science, Massey University, Palmerston North 4442, New Zealand
Samdrup Jongkhar Hospital, Ministry of Health, Samdrup Jongkhar 41001, Bhutan

Yoenten Phuentshok
School of Veterinary Science, Massey University, Palmerston North 4442, New Zealand
National Centre for Animal Health, Department of Livestock, Ministry of Agriculture and Forests, Serbithang, Thimphu 11001, Bhutan

Tandin Zangpo
School of Veterinary Science, Massey University, Palmerston North 4442, New Zealand
Dechencholing BHU-I, Ministry of Health, Thimphu 11001, Bhutan

Sithar Dorjee and Chencho Dorjee
Faculty of Nursing and Public Health, Khesar Gyalpo University of Medical Sciences of Bhutan, Thimphu 11001, Bhutan

Roger Morris
Morvet Ltd., Consultancy Services in Health Risk Management and Food Safety Policy and Programs, Masterton 5885, New Zealand

Diana Prada, Bethany Jackson and Mark O'Dea
School of Veterinary Medicine, Murdoch University, Perth, WA 6150, Australia

Victoria Boyd and Michelle Baker
Australian Animal Health Laboratory, CSIRO, Geelong, VIC 3220, Australia

Rachel A. Sattler, Slobodan Paessler and Cheng Huang
Department of Pathology, University of Texas Medical Branch, 301 University Blvd., Galveston, TX 77555-0609, USA

Hinh Ly
Department of Veterinary Biomedical Sciences, University of Minnesota, Twin Cities, 1988 Fitch Ave., 295H Animal Science Veterinary Medicine Bldg., Saint Paul, MN 55108, USA

Peter J. Collignon
Infectious Diseases and Microbiology, Canberra Hospital, Garran, ACT 2605, Australia
Medical School, Australian National University, Acton ACT 2601, Australia

Scott A. McEwen
Department of Population Medicine, University of Guelph, Guelph N1G 2W1, Canada

Dylan M. Johnson
Department of Microbiology and Immunology, University of Louisville Health Sciences Center, Louisville, KY 40292, USA

Jenny D. Jokinen and Igor S. Lukashevich
Department of Pharmacology and Toxicology, University of Louisville Health Sciences Center, Louisville, KY 40292, USA
Center for Predictive Medicine for Biodefense and Emerging Infectious Diseases, NIH Regional Biocontainment Laboratory, Louisville, KY 40222, USA

Delia Grace
Department of Biosciences, International Livestock Research Institute, Nairobi 00100, Kenya

Johanna F. Lindahl
Department of Biosciences, International Livestock Research Institute, Nairobi 00100, Kenya
Department of Clinical Sciences, Swedish University of Agricultural Sciences, SE-750 07 Uppsala, Sweden
Zoonosis Science Centre, Department of Medical Biochemistry and Microbiology, Uppsala University, SE-751 23 Uppsala, Sweden

Jatinder Paul Singh Gill and Jasbir S. Bedi
Guru Angad Dev Veterinary and Animal Sciences University, Ludhiana 141004, Punjab, India

Razibuddin Ahmed Hazarika
Department of Veterinary Public Health, Assam Agricultural University, Khanapara Campus

Nadeem Mohamed Fairoze
Department of LPT, Veterinary College, Karnataka Veterinary Animal & Fisheries Sciences University Bangalore, Bangalore 560024, India

Ian Dohoo
Atlantic Veterinary College, University of Prince Edward Island, Charlottetown, C1A 4P3, Canada

Manish Kakkar
Public Health Foundation India, Gurgaon 122002, India

Abhimanyu Singh Chauhan
Public Health Foundation India, Gurgaon 122002, India
Department of Public Health Sciences, Faculty of Medicine, University of Liège, 4000 Liege, Belgium

Juan Carlos Zapata, Sandra Medina-Moreno, Camila Guzmán-Cardozo and Maria S. Salvato
Institute of Human Virology, School of Medicine, University of Maryland, Baltimore, MD 21201, USA

Avram Levy
Department of Microbiology, PathWest Laboratory Medicine WA, Nedlands, WA 6009, Australia

David W. Smith
Department of Microbiology, PathWest Laboratory Medicine WA, Nedlands, WA 6009, Australia
Faculty of Health and Medical Sciences, University of Western Australia, Nedlands, WA 6009, Australia

Paul V. Effler
Faculty of Health and Medical Sciences, University of Western Australia, Nedlands, WA 6009, Australia
Communicable Disease Control Directorate, Department of Health Western Australia, Perth WA 6004, Australia

Ian G. Barr
World Health Organization (WHO) Collaborating Centre for Reference and Research on Influenza, at The Peter Doherty Institute for Infection and Immunity, Melbourne, VIC 3000, Australia
Department of Microbiology and Immunology, University of Melbourne, at the Peter Doherty Institute for Infection and Immunity, Melbourne, VIC 3000, Australia

Richmond Loh
Sustainability and Biosecurity, Department of Primary Industries and Regional Development, Perth, WA 6151, Australia

Simone Tempone
Communicable Disease Control Directorate, Department of Health Western Australia, Perth, WA 6004, Australia

Mark O'Dea
School of Veterinary Medicine, Murdoch University, Perth, WA 6150, Australia

James Watson and Frank Y. K. Wong
CSIRO Australian Animal Health Laboratory, Geelong, VIC 3219, Australia

Maria S. Salvato Camila Guzmán-Cardozo, Sandra Medina-Moreno, Juan Carlos Zapata and Haoting Hsu
Institute of Human Virology, University of Maryland, Baltimore, MD 21201, USA

Arban Domi, Mary Hauser, Michael Hellerstein and Farshad Guirakhoo
GeoVax, Inc, Smyrna, GA 30080, USA

Nathanael McCurley
Office of Technology Licensing and Commercialization, Georgia State University, Atlanta, GA 30303, USA

Rahul Basu
Department of Biology, Georgia State University, Atlanta, GA 30302, USA

Deirdre A. Collins
School of Medical & Health Sciences, Edith Cowan University, Joondalup 6027, Australia

Thomas V. Riley
School of Medical & Health Sciences, Edith Cowan University, Joondalup 6027, Australia
Department of Microbiology, PathWest Laboratory Medicine, Nedlands 6009, Australia
School of Veterinary & Life Sciences, Murdoch University, Murdoch 6150, Australia

Index